MW01713864

Nutrition and Healthy Eating

CHOICES, PRACTICES, AND PATTERNS

Authors

Cindy Ghartey
Applewood Heights Secondary School
Peel District School Board

Denise Nembhard
Dr. Charles Best Secondary School
School District 43 Coquitlam

Recipe Tester

Diane O'Shea
Oakridge Secondary School
Thames Valley District School Board

Mc Graw Hill Education | McGraw-Hill Ryerson

McGraw-Hill Ryerson

Nutrition and Healthy Eating

CHOICES, PRACTICES, AND PATTERNS

COPIES OF THIS BOOK MAY BE OBTAINED BY CONTACTING:
McGraw-Hill Ryerson Ltd.

Web Site:
www.mcgrawhill.ca

E-MAIL:
orders@mcgrawhill.ca

TOLL-FREE FAX:
1-800-463-5885

TOLL-FREE, CALL:
1-800-565-5758

OR BY MAILING YOUR ORDER TO:
McGraw-Hill Ryerson
Order Department
300 Water Street
Whitby, ON L1N 9B6

Please quote the ISBN and title when placing your order.

Copyright © 2013, McGraw-Hill Ryerson Limited, a Subsidiary of The McGraw-Hill Companies. All rights reserved. No part of this publication may be reproduced or transmitted in any form or by any means, or stored in a data base or retrieval system, without the prior written permission of McGraw-Hill Ryerson Limited, or, in the case of photocopying or other reprographic copying, a license from the Canadian Copyright Licensing Agency (Access Copyright). For an Access Copyright licence, visit *www.accesscopyright.ca* or call toll free to 1-800-893-5777.

Any request for photocopying, recording, or taping of this publication shall be directed in writing to Access Copyright.

ISBN-10: 1-25-903086-5

ISBN-13: 978-1-25-903086-4

www.mcgrawhill.ca

1 2 3 4 5 6 7 8 9 10 TCP 1 9 8 7 6 5 4 3

Printed and bound in Canada.

Care has been taken to trace ownership of copyright material contained in this text. The publishers will gladly accept any information that will enable them to rectify any reference or credit in subsequent printings.

PUBLISHER: Ian Nussbaum

PROGRAM MANAGER: Marilyn Wilson

DEVELOPMENTAL EDITORS: First Folio Resource Group Inc.:
Julie Kretchman, Loretta Johnson

MANAGER, EDITORIAL SERVICES: Crystal Shortt

SUPERVISING EDITOR: Jennifer Keay, Shannon Martin

COPY EDITOR: Sheila Harris, Linda Jenkins

PHOTO RESEARCH AND PERMISSIONS: Monika Schurmann

REVIEW COORDINATOR: Melanie Berthier

EDITORIAL ASSISTANT: Michelle Malda

MANAGER, PRODUCTION SERVICES: Yolanda Pigden

PRODUCTION COORDINATOR: Lena Keating, Tammy Mavroudi

COVER DESIGN: Liz Harasymczuk

INTERIOR DESIGN: First Image

ELECTRONIC PAGE MAKE-UP: First Image

COVER IMAGE: **Main** © barbaradudzinska /Shutterstock, **tr** Ingram Publishing/ SuperStock, **bl** © Brenda Carson /Shutterstock

Table of Contents

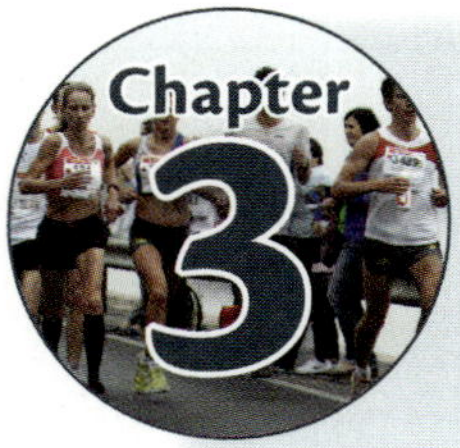
Chapter
3

Chapter
4

Chapter
5

Chapter
6

Advisors

Paula Aquino
G. W. Graham Middle-Secondary School
School District 33
British Columbia

Laura Benati
Family Studies/Religion Teacher
Christ the King Catholic Secondary School
Halton Catholic District School Board
Ontario

Jenell DeFehr Wiebe
Curriculum Advisor
Windsor Park Collegiate
Louis Riel School Division
Manitoba

Laura Featherstone
Instructional Leader
Social Science and Humanities, Family Studies
Toronto District School Board
Ontario

Valerie Hodowanski
Social Science and Humanities Department Head
Pine Ridge Secondary School
Durham District School Board
Ontario

Lou Anne Massey
Assistant Curriculum Leader
Social Sciences and Humanities, Family Studies
Lester B. Pearson Collegiate Institute
Toronto District School Board
Ontario

Mary E. Nowlan, B.Ed., M. Sc.
Blessed Cardinal Newman Catholic High School
Toronto Catholic District School Board
Ontario

Diane O'Shea
Family Studies and Social Sciences Department Head
Medway High School
Thames Valley District School Board
Ontario

Diane Parr
Curriculum Advisor
Central Memorial High School
Calgary Board of Education
Alberta

Frances Samouilhan
Department Head, Home Economics
Thomas Haney Secondary School
School District 42
British Columbia

Mary Gale Smith, Ph.D.
Home Economics Education, Department of Curriculum and Pedagogy
Faculty of Education, University of British Columbia

Lori Stryker, OCT
Subject Head, Social Sciences
Alexander Mackenzie High School
York Region District School Board
Ontario

Deanna Tan Francoeur
Registered Dietitian
New Westminster
British Columbia

Patricia Warecki
Sacred Heart Catholic High School
York Catholic District School Board
Ontario

Jim Wiese
Teacher Education Program
University of the Fraser Valley
British Columbia

Marlene Yellow Horn, B.Mgt., B.Ed., M.Ed.
Likiinayookaa | Gentle Sleeper
Learning Leader
First Nations Curriculum Advisor
Calgary Board of Education
Alberta

Mary Leah de Zwart, Ph.D.
Home Economics Education, Department of Curriculum and Pedagogy
Faculty of Education, University of British Columbia

Elements: Food Studies Reviewers

Connie Cameron
Fredericton High School
School District 18
British Columbia

Susan Cawker
Heritage Woods Secondary School
Coquitlam School District 43
British Columbia

Sally Cogswell
Grand Manan Community School
Anglophone South West School District
New Brunswick

Jolene Conti
Holy Name of Mary Catholic Secondary School
Dufferin-Peel Catholic District School Board
Ontario

Lorraine Dulder
Darwin School
Louis Riel School Division
Manitoba

Erin Ewen
Wynyard Composite High School
Horizon School Division
Saskatchewan

Michelle Hardy
Bethlehem Catholic High School
Greater Saskatoon Catholic Schools
Saskatchewan

Kristen Lee
Tisdale Middle and Secondary School
North East School Division
Saskatchewan

Denice Marr
South Kamloops Secondary School
School District 73
British Columbia

Kathryn Marrie
St. Mary's District Collegiate and Vocational Institute
Avon Maitland District School Board
Ontario

Marybeth Morrow
Calgary Board of Education
Alberta

Anna Niessen
Mount Royal Collegiate
Saskatoon Public School Division
Saskatchewan

Catherine Rose
St. Peter Secondary School
Peterborough Victoria Northumberland and Clarington Catholic District School Board
Ontario

Kevin Senra
Holy Name of Mary Catholic Secondary School
Dufferin-Peel Catholic District School Board
Ontario

Lisa Sidorkewicz
Sir Alan MacNab Secondary School
Hamilton-Wentworth District School Board
Ontario

Irene Sifrer
Forest Lawn High School
Calgary Board of Education
Alberta

Janice Skene
Retired
Evergreen School Division
Manitoba

Elaine Wilkie
Halifax West High School
Halifax Regional School Board District 4
Nova Scotia

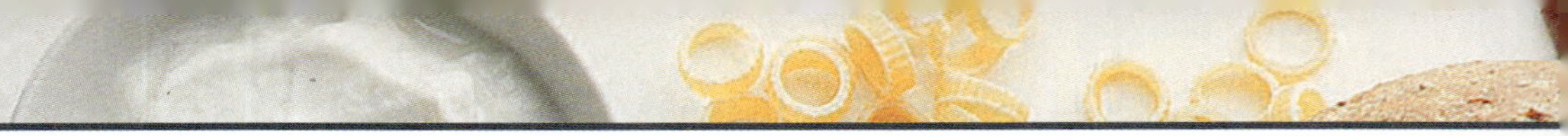

Unit 1 Healthy Eating

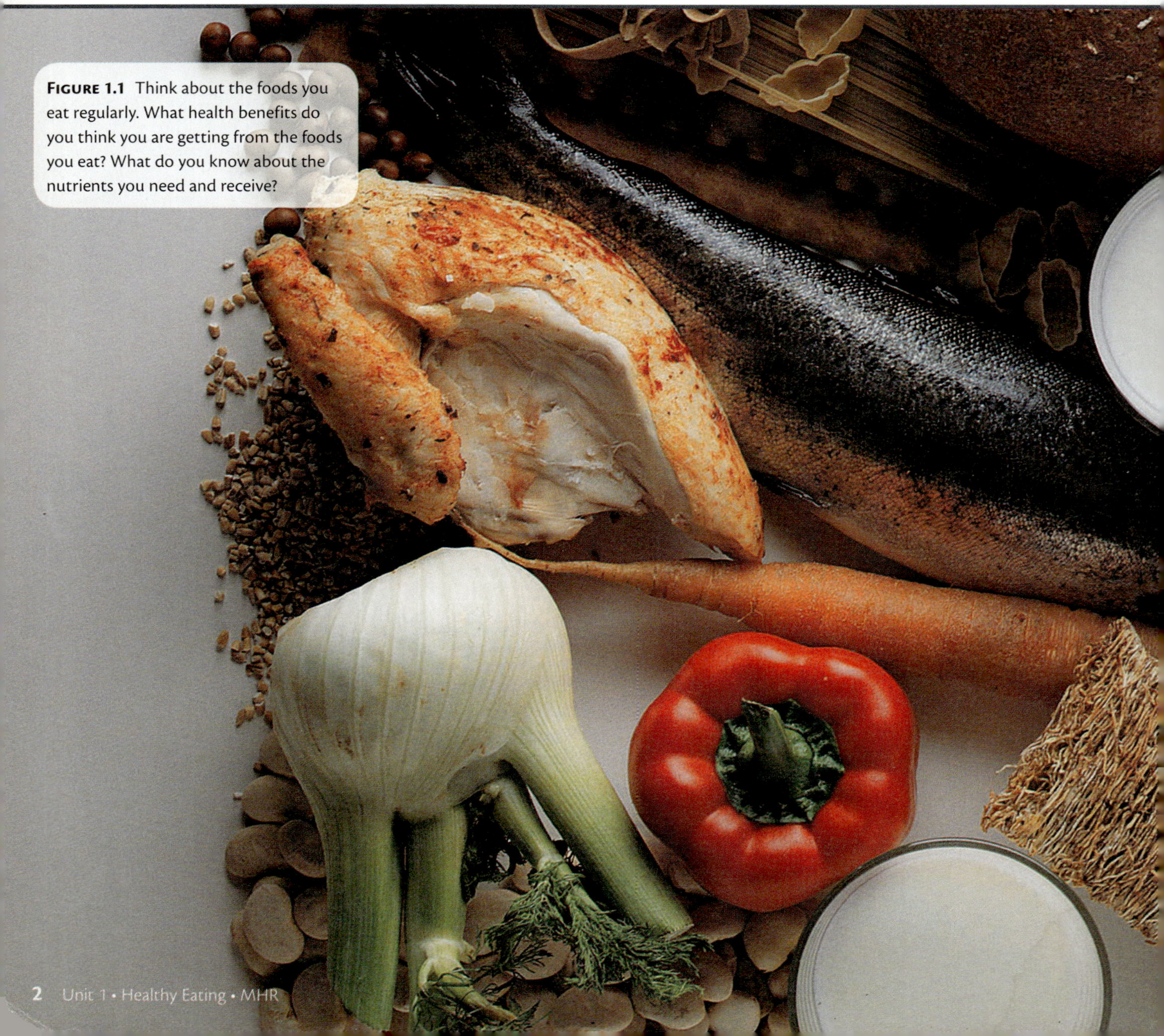

FIGURE 1.1 Think about the foods you eat regularly. What health benefits do you think you are getting from the foods you eat? What do you know about the nutrients you need and receive?

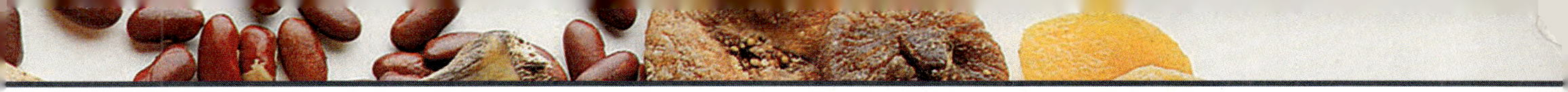

the BIG idea

What is healthy eating? What strategies can you use to ensure you obtain the nutrients your body needs?

- What are nutrients?
- Can different diets be healthier for different people?
- Is one diet healthier than others?
- How can you ensure you obtain the nutrients you need from your food?

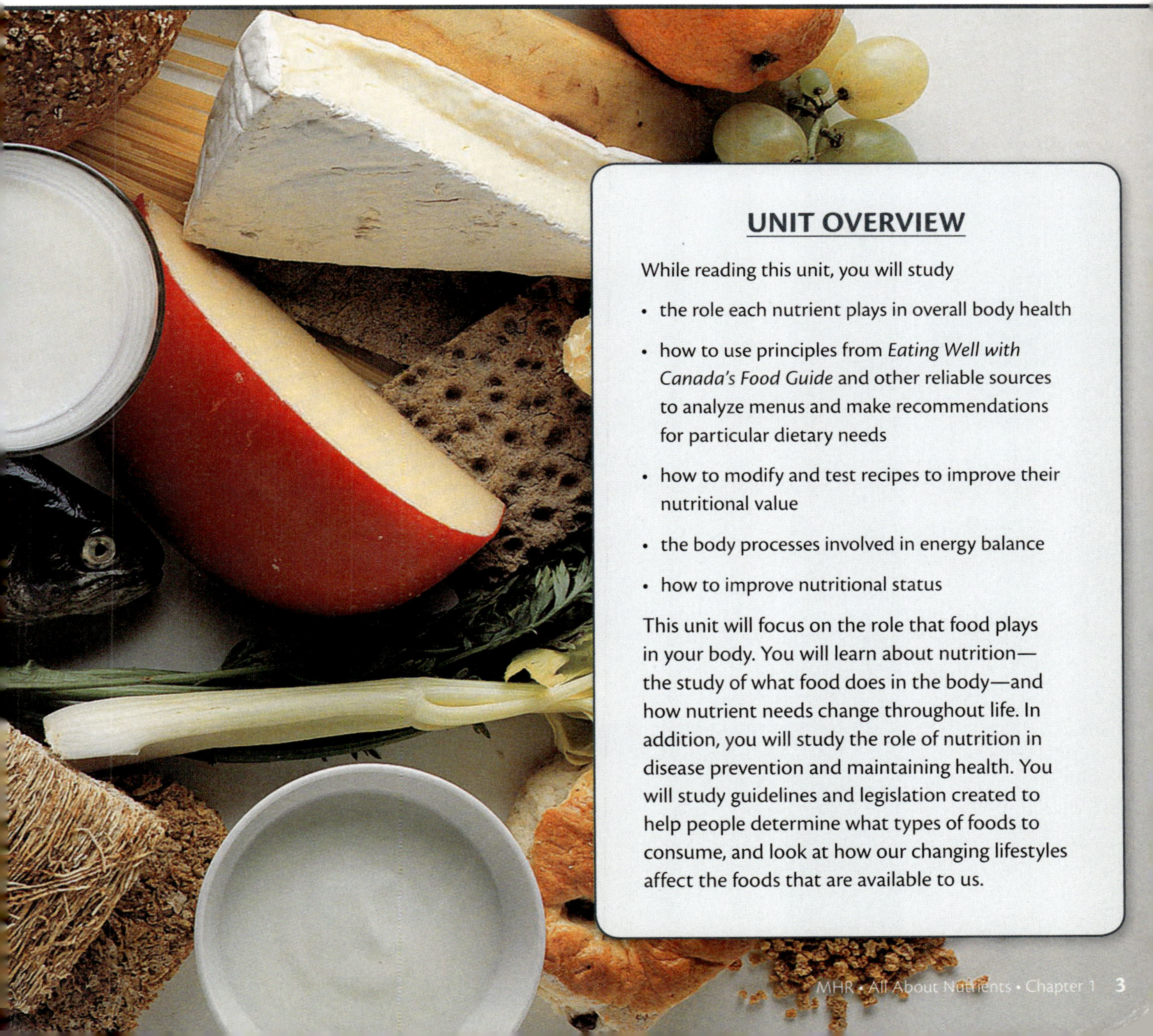

UNIT OVERVIEW

While reading this unit, you will study

- the role each nutrient plays in overall body health
- how to use principles from *Eating Well with Canada's Food Guide* and other reliable sources to analyze menus and make recommendations for particular dietary needs
- how to modify and test recipes to improve their nutritional value
- the body processes involved in energy balance
- how to improve nutritional status

This unit will focus on the role that food plays in your body. You will learn about nutrition—the study of what food does in the body—and how nutrient needs change throughout life. In addition, you will study the role of nutrition in disease prevention and maintaining health. You will study guidelines and legislation created to help people determine what types of foods to consume, and look at how our changing lifestyles affect the foods that are available to us.

Chapter

1

All About Nutrients

Key Terms

adipose tissue
anemia
bioavailability
coenzyme
empty Calorie
free radical
hemorrhoids
kilocalorie
malnutrition
nutrient deficiency
nutrient dense
oxidation

Research and Inquiry Skills

- Collect primary data
- Evaluate online information

Chapter Introduction

While reading this chapter, you will study

- **the components, sources, and functions of each nutrient group**
- **how to use nutrition information on food labels to determine nutrients found in foods**
- **nutrient deficiencies and toxicities**
- **how interests, skills, previous experience, and education requirements relate to a specific career opportunity in the food industry**

The foods you eat provide many nutrients that interact within your body to help maintain good health and prevent disease. It can be a challenge to decide what foods to consume to maintain and improve your health given the many choices available. In this chapter, you will learn the nutritional merits of various foods, the effects of food consumption on nutritional status and the effects of preparation techniques on nutrient values. This information will help you to evaluate the healthfulness of your diet.

The nutrients in the foods you eat have many effects on your health. They can act alone and in combination. Consuming too little or too much of a nutrient can have adverse effects. Think about what you already know about the nutrients in the foods you eat. Where did you learn what you know? How confident are you that your information is correct?

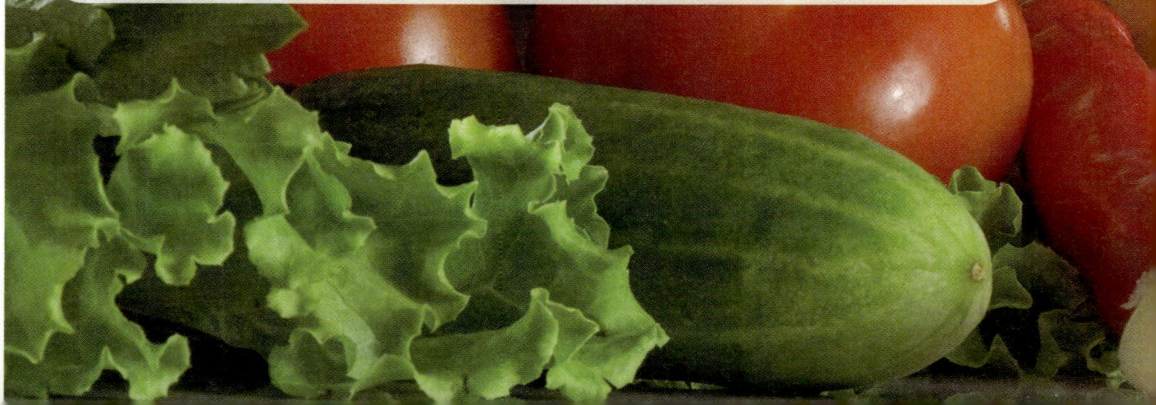

Figure 1.2 Each of these foods is rich in nutrients and part of a healthy diet. Which of these foods do you eat regularly?

Spotlight On...

Test Your Nutrient IQ

At this point in your life, you most likely know basic facts about healthy eating: Eat protein with every meal, eat plenty of vegetables and fruits, and reduce consumption of saturated fat. But do you know which foods contain fibre, vitamins, or minerals? What is your nutrient IQ? To find out, complete the following nutrient IQ quiz, based on one developed by Canadian Registered Dietitian Leslie Beck.

Decide whether each statement, 1 through 15, is true or false.

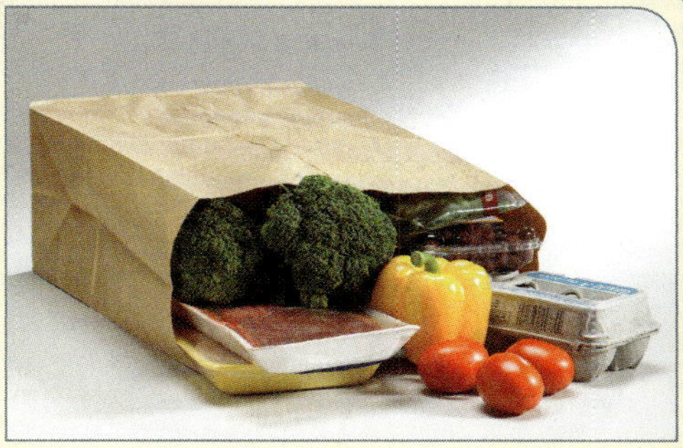

FIGURE 1.3 How knowledgable are you about different types of foods and the nutrients they contain?

Questions:

1. A healthier food will always contain fewer grams of total fat.
2. Honey is more nutritious than white sugar.
3. One large baked potato with the skin on has more fibre than two slices of whole-wheat bread.
4. Sunflower oil contains more vitamin E than olive oil.
5. The best source of magnesium is meat.
6. Coffee does not count toward your daily total water intake.
7. A restaurant side dish serving of garlic mashed potatoes usually contains more sodium than a serving of French fries.
8. Nutrition Facts tables on processed foods tell you what amount of sugar is in the package.
9. One celery stalk contains fewer nutrients than one tablespoon of white sugar.
10. While vitamins are essential nutrients, some vitamins are toxic in large amounts.
11. Soybeans are a good substitute for milk for people who are lactose intolerant.
12. Iron is available in foods from both animal and vegetable sources. The iron in foods from animal sources is easier for our bodies to use.
13. Dairy products and fortified foods are the only significant sources of calcium in our diets.
14. Apples are a significant source of vitamin C.
15. I know some steps I could take to improve my diet.

Check the answers (with explanations) on page 30. Which questions did you answer correctly? What do you need to learn more about?

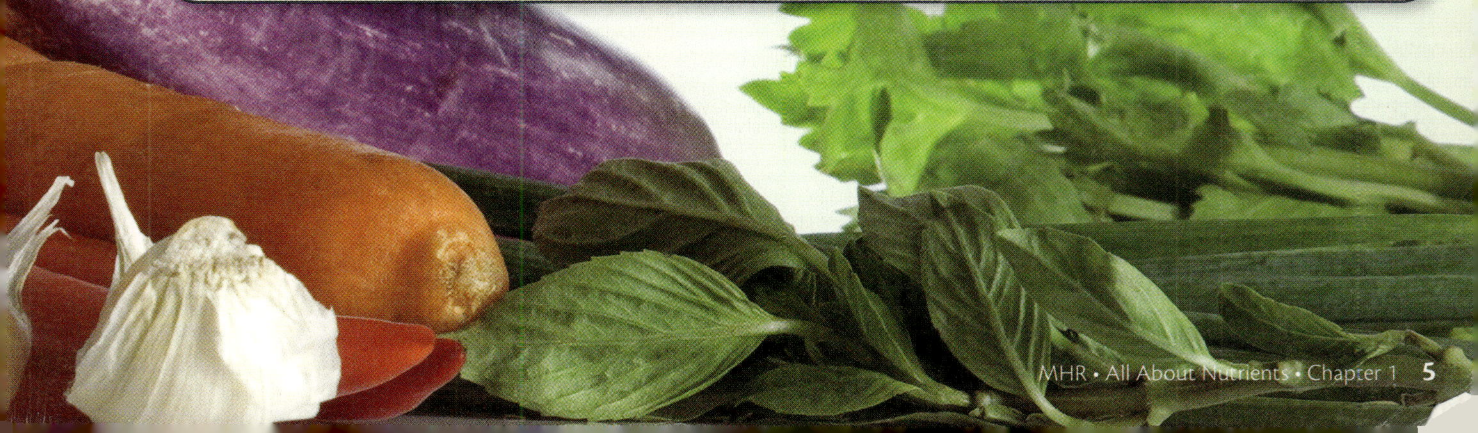

Research and Inquiry Skills

Collecting Primary Nutrition Data

Researchers collect data about nutrition from many sources. Data that others have already analyzed and written about, for example reports in books and articles in journals, is called *secondary data*. Data collected directly from a source is called *primary data*. There are many ways to collect primary research data.

Questionnaires

Questionnaires such as the quiz in *Spotlight On...* are one method of collecting primary data. In the case of the nutrition quiz, the data collected was about people's knowledge of nutrients. The most common way nutrition researchers obtain primary data is asking people what they eat. They then make inferences from the information they collect. Questionnaires can be administered by interview or by asking the participant to complete a form. Researchers learn to write questions that will provide answers they can easily compare, categorize, or tabulate. For example, providing answers to choose from, or providing a scale for responses that are opinions can ensure answers are useful.

Food Records

Asking what people eat may be done retrospectively, such as asking people to list everything they have eaten in the past 24 hours, or prospectively, such as asking people to record everything they eat as they eat it. The quality of retrospective data collected depends on people's memory. The quality of prospective data collected depends on the quality of instructions given and the motivation to write down everything that is eaten. Both methods only give information about food intake at one particular time. A questionnaire about eating habits can obtain more long-term information from a large number of people, but long-term memory can be unreliable.

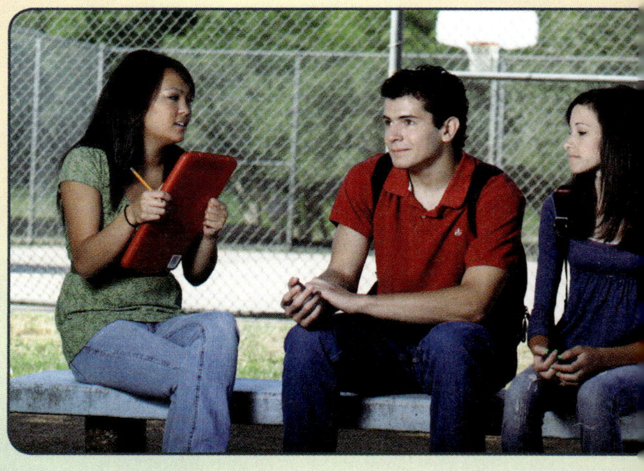

FIGURE 1.4 A trained interviewer can obtain valuable information on what people are eating in order to give advice on diets and establish dietary guidelines. How would data be affected if a researcher followed an individual all day to observe his or her food intake?

Retail and Distribution Surveys

To supplement information about nutrition, Statistics Canada gathers information about the food that is purchased in Canada. For example, they may collect data about the quantity of skim, 1%, 2% and homogenized milk sold, or the quantity of white bread sold in different provinces. This information can be used to estimate the nutritional qualities of diets of specific population groups. The major limitation of this method is that the data does not provide information about how the food is being used or who is consuming it.

Experiments

Nutrition researchers conduct experiments to gather information about people's behaviours. For example, they may provide packaged snacks and record how many people look at the Nutrition Facts table on the package before eating the snack. Researchers also conduct experiments to gather data about the nutrients found in foods. For example, researchers may combust (burn) a food to determine the amount of energy it contains.

Questions:

1. Write a question about people's nutrition knowledge or habits that you would like to have answered.
2. Develop a short questionnaire that you can use to gather data to answer your question. Include five questions. Work with one or more classmates to evaluate your questionnaire and make sure it is fair, unbiased, and clear, and that it will provide data that will help you answer your question.
3. Ask 20 students in your school to complete your questionnaire. Then ask five of them to evaluate the questionnaire for clarity, fairness, and usefulness. What did you learn?

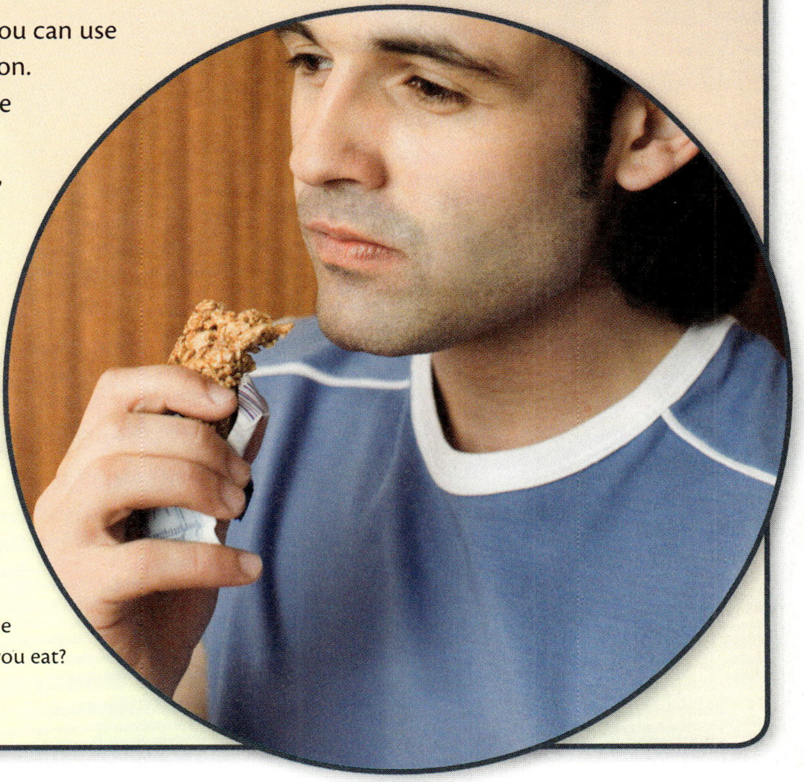

FIGURE 1.5 Do you read the Nutrition Facts for snacks you eat?

Nutrients

NUTRITION LITERACY

"Like" Nutrition
Enhance your nutrition knowledge by using nutrition-related hashtags and following or "liking" credible sources on social-media platforms. The Center for Science in the Public Interest (CSPI) and Dietitians of Canada are good places to start.

The ultimate purpose of food is to provide nourishment for healthy growth and development. The components of food that do this are known as *nutrients*. Some nutrients are required in large amounts to provide energy for all of the body's functions. Fat, carbohydrate, and protein make up these essential macronutrients. Vitamins, minerals, and water do not provide the body with energy but play an important role in keeping the body healthy. Vitamins minerals, and phytochemicals are needed in small quantities in the body and are categorized as micronutrients.

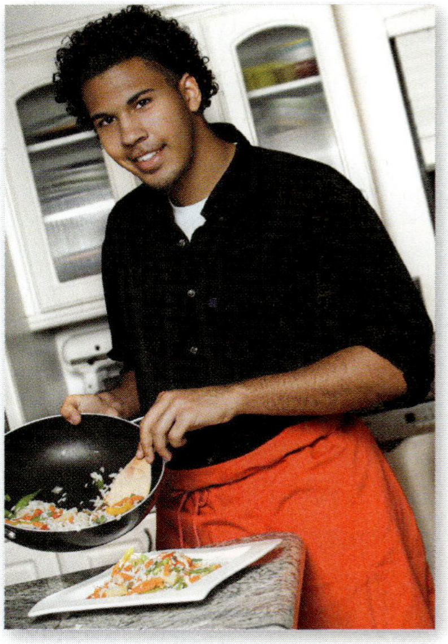

FIGURE 1.6 *Eating Well with Canada's Food Guide* helps individuals and families plan and prepare meals that provide all the nutrients required for good health, in appropriate serving sizes.

To help make the best food choices, health professionals study the actions of these nutrients in the body and create plans and suggestions for healthy eating. Like any science, nutrition is an ever-changing discipline: new discoveries are constantly being made, and recommendations change to incorporate new information.

malnutrition: a condition in which a person's diet is inadequate to meet minimum daily requirements for nutrients

Eating too little food, eating foods with insufficient amounts of particular nutrients, or not absorbing nutrients well can lead to **malnutrition**. Eating too much food, especially high-energy food like fats and sugars, can lead to obesity. The best way to ensure that you are obtaining the most from your diet is to eat a variety of foods and follow the guidelines in *Eating Well with Canada's Food Guide*.

kilocalorie: the amount of heat energy required to raise one kilogram of water one degree Celsius

The amount of energy obtained from macronutrients in food is measured in **kilocalories** (often referred to as Calories—with a capital C—to differentiate it from the smaller unit: calorie). An important aspect of healthy eating is consuming the appropriate amount of food to obtain the optimal amount of energy.

nutrient dense: describes foods that are relatively low in Calories, while high in a variety of nutrients

empty Calorie: describes foods that are high in Calories and low in other nutrients, also known as nutrient-poor foods

High-quality nutrition is necessary for optimal health and resistance to disease. The nutrients provided by food should be considered and compared to the energy the food contains, measured in Calories. **Nutrient dense** foods such as whole grains and fish should be consumed more often than **empty Calorie** foods such as pop and chips.

Pause and Think
Think of the food you ate most recently. Would you categorize it as nutrient dense or empty Calorie? Why?

Dietary Reference Intake

Specific amounts of each nutrient are required to prevent **nutrient deficiencies**. Health Canada has established Dietary Reference Intakes (DRIs) as a set of nutrient reference values for healthy individuals. These values are based on the most current Canadian and American scientific knowledge.

nutrient deficiency: inadequate amounts in the diet of nutrients necessary for good health and the prevention of disease

Estimated Average Requirement (EAR): the amount of a nutrient that is estimated to meet the requirement of half of all healthy individuals in a defined group.

Recommended Dietary Allowance (RDA): the average daily dietary intake level that is sufficient to meet the nutrient requirement of nearly all (97 to 98 percent) healthy individuals in a particular life stage and gender group.

Adequate Intake (AI): only established when an EAR and RDA cannot be determined.

Tolerable Upper Intake Level (UL): the maximum daily intake of a nutrient that is likely to pose no health risks for almost all individuals.

NUTRITION LITERACY

Summarize the differences between the dietary reference intakes. When might a health professional choose to use each one?

CAREER CONNECTION

Dietary Food Service Worker

Dietary food service workers are employed as dietary aides and food servers in hospitals, long-term care facilities, group homes, and other health care settings. They work as part of a nutritional care team to provide patients with safe, nutritious, customized diets in a commercial kitchen setting. While a solid understanding of nutrition is crucial, communication skills are also important, since dietary food service workers are often the main point of contact with patients at mealtimes. Several community colleges offer diplomas in this field.

Dietary food service workers may perform the following tasks, depending on where they work:

- interview patients to discuss food preferences
- help develop menus and nutrition care plans for patients
- ensure food is safely and correctly prepared and attractively presented
- help to train staff to prepare and serve meals for patients with particular diets

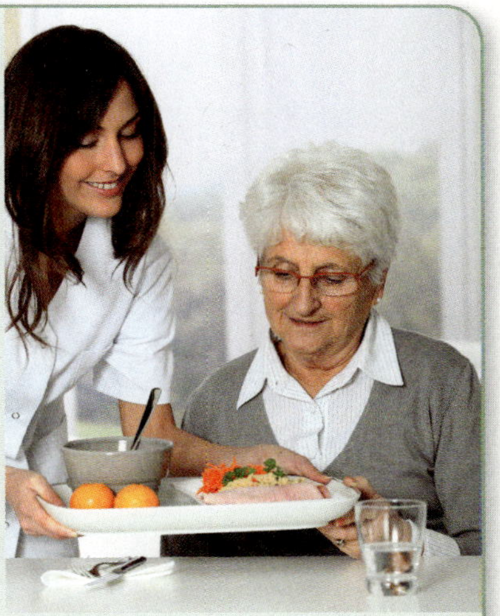

FIGURE 1.7 Dietary food service workers handle food and interact with people in health care settings.

Questions:

1. What relevant work and/or volunteer experience could provide skills transferable to this career?
2. What sources of information could provide reliable and useful nutrition information for a dietary food service worker?

Macronutrients

"A diet based on quantity rather than quality has ushered a new creature onto the world stage: the human being who manages to be both overfed and undernourished, two characteristics seldom found in the same body in the long natural history of our species."
– Michael Pollan

Macronutrients provide your body with the energy it needs to function. Carbohydrates, proteins, and fats are macronutrients; they are consumed in large amounts to provide energy and maintain health. You can use the Acceptable Macronutrient Distribution Range (AMDR) to estimate the percent of your daily energy that you should obtain from protein, fat, and carbohydrate in order to provide adequate intakes of essential nutrients and minimize the risk of chronic disease.

Acceptable Macronutrient Distribution Ranges (AMDR)

Males & Females	Total Carbohydrate	Total Protein	Total Fat
	Percent of Energy	*Percent of Energy*	*Percent of Energy*
1–3 years	45–65%	5–20%	30–40%
4–18 years	45–65%	10–30%	25–35%
19 years and over	45–65%	10–35%	20–35%
Note: These are reference values for normal, apparently healthy individuals (including pregnant women) eating a typical mixed North American diet. An individual may have physiological, health, or lifestyle characteristics that may require tailoring of specific nutrient values.			

Source: Health Canada (2005).

FIGURE 1.8 Find the AMDR that applies to you. How does your AMDR compare to another age group?

OPEN FOR DEBATE

Should the term *malnutrition* be used to describe being undernourished as well as being overnourished?

To understand how a particular meal or total meals throughout the day compares to the recommended balance of macronutrients, you need to determine the energy available from the foods you eat. You can calculate the percent of Calories from each macronutrient in the foods you eat by using the nutrition facts provided on labels, as well as the following formulas.

Food Energy Availability Formulas

Macronutrient	Energy (kcal/g)	Formula to calculate percent (%) of Calories from macronutrient
Protein	4	(grams of protein × 4 kcal/g) ÷ total energy (kcal) × 100
Fat	9	(total fat in grams × 9 kcal/g) ÷ total energy (kcal) × 100
Carbohydrate	4	(grams of carbohydrate – fibre/2) × 4 kcal/g, ÷ total energy (kcal) × 100

FIGURE 1.9 A large egg contains approximately 6 g of protein, 5 g of fat, and 1 g of carbohydrates. What percent of the energy in an egg does each macronutrient provide?

TIP for Healthy Living

Many health professionals do not recommend counting Calories to regulate the amount of energy you consume because everyone has different energy needs and Calories are only one aspect of healthy eating

ACTIVE LEARNING

Determine the macronutrient composition of this tofu berry smoothie, using the formulas in **Figure 1.9** table and the Calorie, fat, protein, carbohydrate, and fibre information in the recipe.

Tofu Berry Smoothie

Yield: 2 servings

This creamy milk-free shake is a great way to use up ripe bananas that have been frozen. When bananas start to get brown, pop them in the freezer and take out as needed.

Ingredients

250 mL (1 c) pineapple juice

1 ripe banana

125 mL (½ c) fresh or frozen strawberries

125 mL (½ c) silken tofu

15–30 mL (1–2 tbsp) honey

2.5 mL (½ tsp) vanilla

Method

Combine all the ingredients in a blender until smooth. Pour into glasses and enjoy.

Nutrients per Serving	
Calories	170.8 kcal
fat	2.2 g
saturated fat	0.3 g
sodium	7.3 mg
protein	4.4 g
carbohydrate	35.6 g
fibre	1.9 g

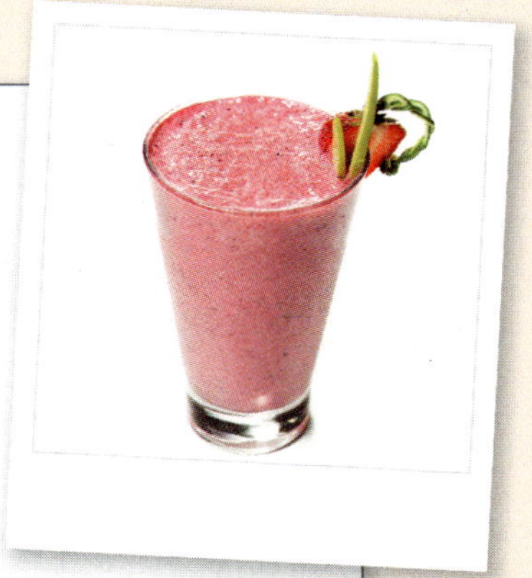

FIGURE 1.10 Describe four substitutions you could make to this recipe and why you might make each one.

Questions:

1. How does the macronutrient composition of this smoothie compare to the AMDR for your age group?
2. Can foods with compositions outside the AMDR be part of a healthy diet? Explain.
3. Why do you think the total percent of calories from protein, fat, and carbohydrates does not equal 100 percent?

THINK CRITICALLY

1. How does understanding the role of macronutrients help make you food literate?
2. If carbohydrates, proteins, and fats are all good sources of energy, why do you think dietitians recommend obtaining more of our energy from carbohydrates, and less from protein and fat?

Carbohydrates

Nutrition Literacy

You can often use prefixes and suffixes to identify components of foods. For example, different types of sugar all have the suffix *ose*.

Carbohydrates are naturally occurring compounds composed of carbon, hydrogen, and oxygen, and the most important source of energy for your body. Besides providing energy, carbohydrates are necessary for many other functions such as

- protein sparing—preventing your body from using protein tissue (muscles) as a source of energy
- regulating the amount of sugar circulating in your blood so that all your cells get the energy that they need
- providing nutrients for the bacteria in your intestinal tract that help you digest food
- assisting in your body's absorption of calcium (Gebo, 2011)

Sugars, starches, glycogen, and dietary fibre are carbohydrates. Because they play so many important roles, carbohydrates should form a large part of your diet.

Carbohydrates are chains of sugar molecules. Before long chains can be used, our bodies convert them to single sugar molecules—glucose. Glucose supplies energy for most processes in the body. Even our brain requires glucose in order to work properly.

Monosaccharides

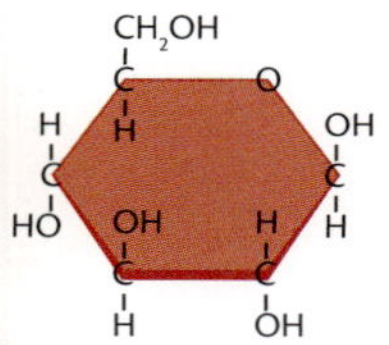

Figure 1.11 The monosaccharide glucose.

Monosaccharides are simple sugars and consist of a single unit. The three most common sugars in this group are glucose, found in fruits and vegetables; fructose, found in honey and in many fruits and vegetables; and galactose, derived from the more complex milk sugar *lactose*. These carbohydrates pass directly through the small intestine into the blood. Your body then converts fructose and galactose to glucose, making these simple sugars a quick source of energy (Novak, 2012).

Disaccharides

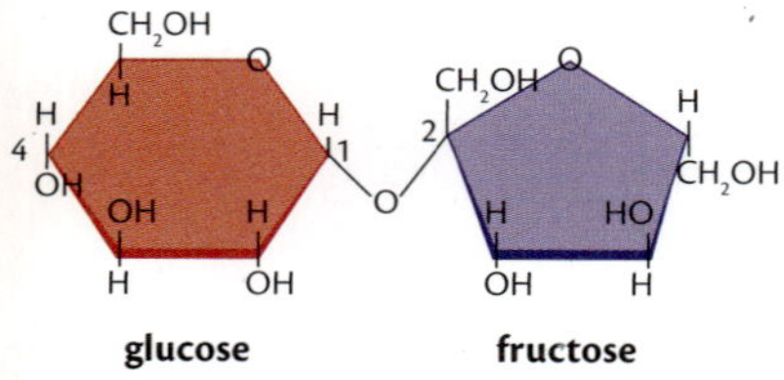

Figure 1.12 Sucrose is made up of one glucose molecule and one fructose molecule.

Disaccharides consist of molecules of two simple sugars linked together. The body digests disaccharides to form monosaccharides. The three most nutritionally important disaccharides are sucrose (table sugar from plants such as sugar cane or sugar beets), maltose (found in grains), and lactose (found in milk).

Polysaccharides

Polysaccharides are complex chains of three to several thousand simple sugars. As a result, digesting polysaccharides releases glucose into your bloodstream more slowly and evenly than monosaccharides or disaccharides (King, 2003). Polysaccharides include starch (found in foods such as cereal grains, beans, potatoes, and other plants), glycogen (the form in which the body stores glucose), and fibre.

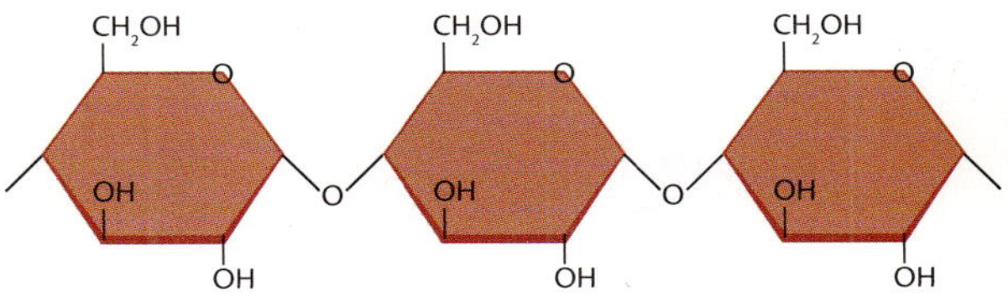

FIGURE 1.13 Amylose is a chain of many monosaccharides.

Fibre

Fibre is found in the cell walls of plants, in the outer layer of whole grains, and in the skin of fruits and vegetables. Fibre is made up of carbohydrates that humans are not able to digest, so it does not provide you with energy. Although fibre cannot be digested, it is an essential nutrient for good health. Insoluble fibre such as cellulose helps keep your bowel movements regular and helps prevent constipation and **hemorrhoids** (King, 2003). It does not dissolve in water but instead absorbs water in your digestive tract much like a sponge and helps you feel full. Research shows that fibre may also help you maintain a healthy body weight and lower your risk of heart disease and some cancers, such as colon cancer (Dietitians of Canada, 2012). Many fruits and vegetables, and the bran of whole grains are good sources of insoluble fibre.

hemorrhoids: a condition in which the veins in the rectum become enlarged and may be painful

Soluble fibre such as that found in apples, oranges, carrots, okra, eggplant, oats, barley, psyllium, pecans, walnuts, almonds, peanuts, beans and lentils (Royston, 2011) ferment in the intestinal tract, forming a gel and regulating the absorption of several substances. This, in turn, helps lower cholesterol and control blood glucose.

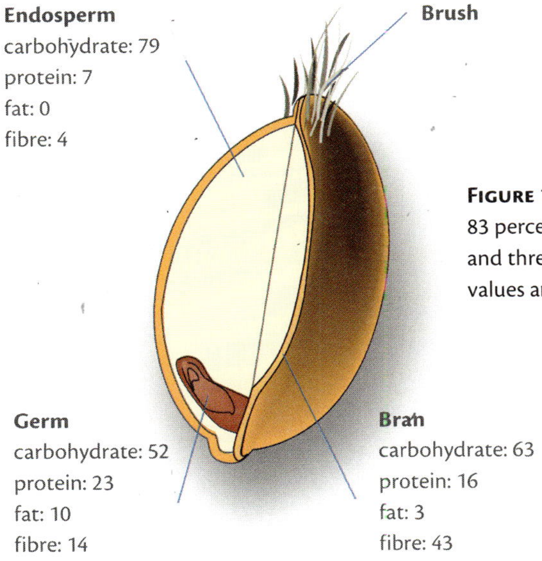

FIGURE 1.14 A wheat kernel consists of 83 percent endosperm, 14 percent bran, and three percent germ. Nutritional values are shown in grams per 100 g.

"Eat food. Not too much. Mostly plants."
– Michael Pollan

TRENDS AND CHANGE

The Glycemic Index

You may have noticed that if you eat a handful of nuts or a piece of cheese you don't feel hungry for a while, but if you eat a chocolate bar you feel hungry more quickly. This is because the body digests some foods much more slowly than others. Researchers have determined several factors that determine the rate at which foods are digested and their energy is released. In general, simple sugars and refined carbohydrates are digested quickly and can lead to a rapid rise in blood sugar levels for a short time, followed by a rapid decline. Complex carbohydrates, protein, and foods with large amounts of fibre are digested more slowly and tend to result in more consistent blood sugar levels. The glycemic index (GI) is a scale that was developed to show the effects of different carbohydrates on the body's blood sugar levels. The glycemic index uses glucose as the standard and assigns it a value of 100. Foods with a score of 70 or higher are said to have a high glycemic index. Foods with a score of 55 to 69 have a medium glycemic index. Foods with a score of 54 or below have a low glycemic index. Generally, a lower score indicates a healthier food.

GI Index	Examples	Resulting Blood Sugar Level
High GI (70 and above)	white potatoes, refined grains, dried dates, watermelon 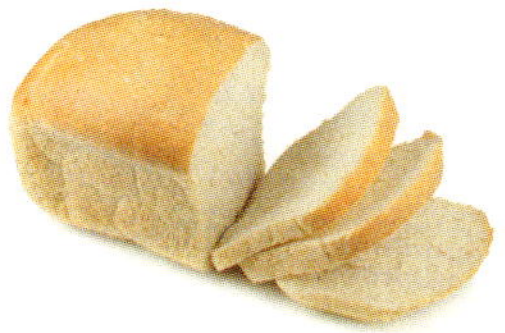	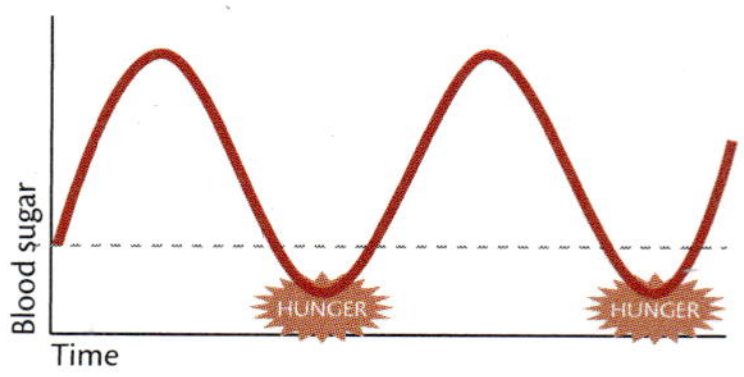
Medium GI (55 to 69)	unrefined grains, bananas, raisins, popcorn 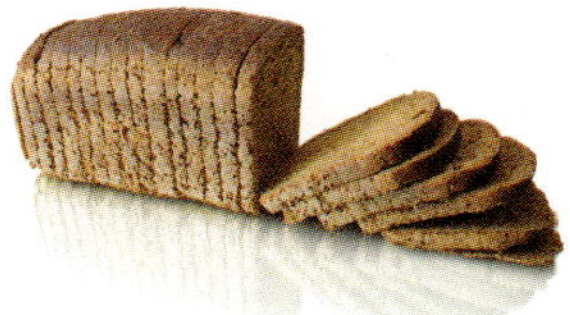	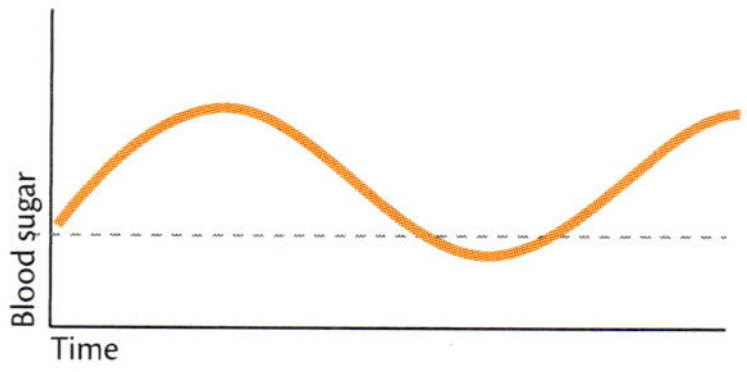
Low GI (54 and below)	legumes, sweet potatoes, apples, milk 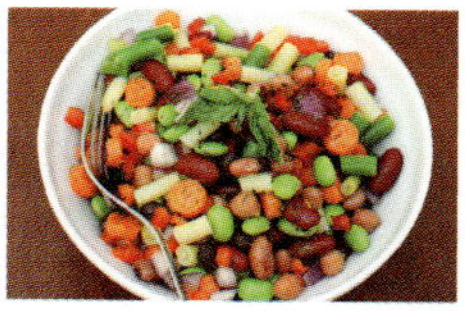	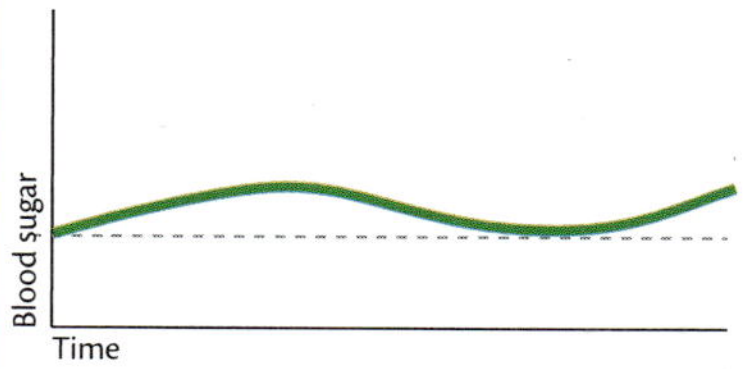

FIGURE 1.15 The GI values of some common foods. Where would a food you ate recently fall on the glycemic index?

Questions:

1. Why might watermelon have a high GI value, but apples have a low GI value?
2. What might be some consequences of rapid rises and drops in blood sugar?

Daily Fibre Requirement

Recommended amount per day

Age Group	Boys	Girls
9–13 years old	31 g	26 g
14–18 years old	38 g	26 g

Source: Dietitians of Canada (2011).

FIGURE 1.16 Most Canadians only consume half of their daily fibre requirement. Excellent sources of fibre include 250 mL (1 cup) of kidney beans (16 g of fibre) and 250 mL (1 cup) of raspberries (8 g of fibre).

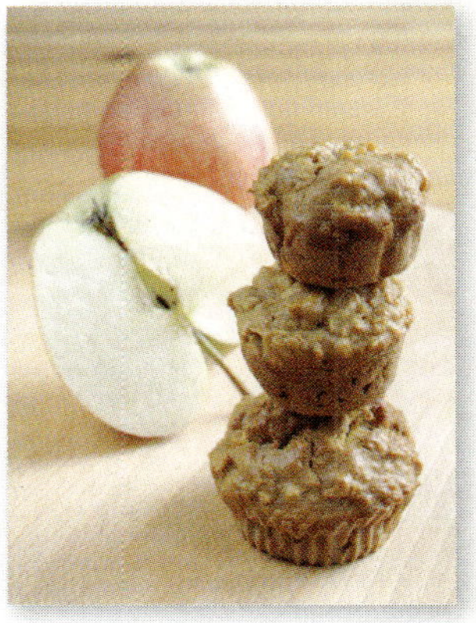

FIGURE 1.17 These foods are good sources of carbohydrates and fibre. Which food item provides more energy? Which food item provides more fibre?

Carbohydrate Toxicity and Deficiency

Your body stores excess glucose as glycogen in muscle and liver cells. If these are full, it stores the excess glycogen as fat in **adipose tissue**. If your diet includes more energy than you require, this could lead to weight gain, which in turn can increase the risk of cardiovascular disease and type 2 diabetes.

adipose tissue: body tissue that contains stored fat cells

If your diet provides too little energy as carbohydrates, your body breaks down stored glycogen to use as energy. If glycogen stores are insufficient, the body breaks down fatty tissue instead. Finally, the body begins to break down its own protein tissue (muscle) for energy. When this occurs, the body will eventually run out of energy, possibly leading to death. Carbohydrate deficiency can result from a carbohydrate-restricted diet or a medical condition that prevents you from using the carbohydrates you consume.

If your diet provides too little fibre, your digestive system will work slowly and sluggishly. This may lead to constipation and hemorrhoids and increase the risk of developing colon cancer (Royston, 2011).

On the other hand, if your diet provides too much fibre, you may experience indigestion, diarrhea and excessive gas. If you do not consume enough liquids to soften the fibre that you eat, then too much fibre in your diet can obstruct your intestines and cause constipation. Chronic constipation can lead to several other intestinal disorders including diverticulosis.

THINK CRITICALLY

1. Why is fibre an essential nutrient if it does not provide us with energy?
2. Refined grains such as white rice and white flour have had the bran and germ removed. What are the advantages of refined grains? What are the disadvantages?

OPEN FOR DEBATE

Pop contains large amounts of glucose but few other nutrients. Since pop does not contribute to a healthy diet, should it be priced higher than other beverages to discourage consumption?

Lipids

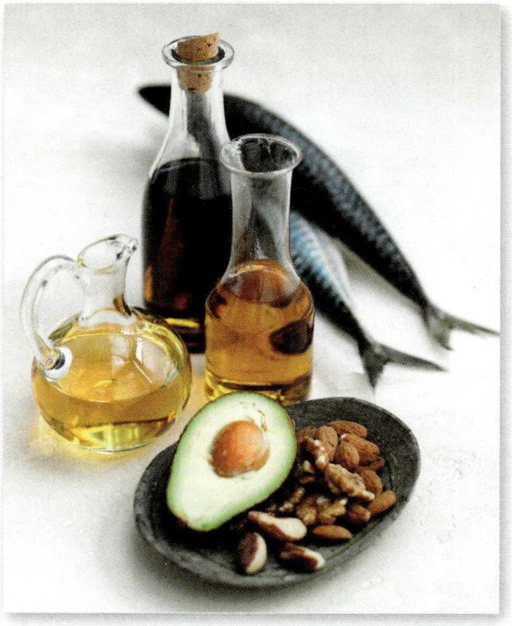

FIGURE 1.18 Lipids, such as those found in olive oil, cold-water fish, nuts, and avocado, are nutritious and help maintain health.

Fats, oils, and related compounds such as cholesterol are known as lipids. With the exception of cholesterol, lipids are energy-rich compounds. Fats and oils provide a concentrated source of energy. One gram of fat provides more than twice the amount of energy to your body than one gram of carbohydrate or protein does. Besides providing energy, lipids are necessary for many other functions in your body such as

- helping with ingestion and absorption of the fat-soluble vitamins A, D, E and K. These vitamins are only available in foods that contain lipids.
- giving shape to your body, promoting healthy skin and helping to insulate the body against extreme temperatures. The thin layer of fat under your skin helps perform all three functions.
- transmitting nerve signals efficiently. Nerve cells are surrounded by a thin layer of fat, which helps control and speed up signalling. Your brain is about 60 percent fat.
- cushioning and protecting organs such as your liver.
- helping the body fight off bacteria and repairing damaged tissue.
- forming parts of hormones and other biochemicals.

(Powell, 2003)

TIP for Healthy Living

Dietary cholesterol has little impact on the blood cholesterol level in most people. Consumption of saturated and trans fats has a greater impact on your blood cholesterol level.

Cholesterol

Cholesterol is part of every cell in the body. It helps you make vitamin D, bile, estrogen and testosterone. Your body makes all the cholesterol it needs, called *blood cholesterol*. Dietary cholesterol is found in some foods from animal sources, such as shrimp and eggs. The cholesterol in the food you eat is used primarily for energy and energy storage.

Cholesterol is a waxy lipid that does not dissolve in blood. Cholesterol forms part of lipoproteins, which are carried throughout your bloodstream. There are two types of lipoproteins: low-density lipoprotein (LDL) and high-density lipoprotein (HDL).

- LDL cholesterol that is not used in your body eventually settles in your arteries, hardens, and becomes plaque. The plaque can restrict blood flow and make the arteries less flexible.
- HDL cholesterol gathers up all the excess cholesterol in your arteries and transports it to the liver to be broken down. It works like a sponge to clean out your blood vessels.

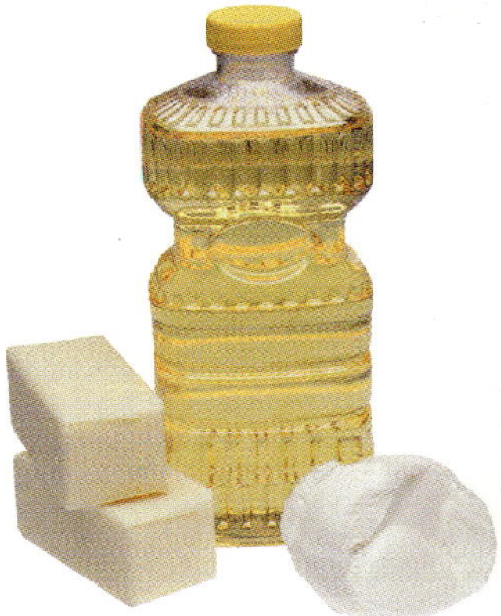

FIGURE 1.19 Oils are lipids that are liquid at room temperature. Fats are lipids that are solid at room temperature.

Fatty Acids

Fats and oils are both triglycerides. Their molecules contain three chains of carbon and hydrogen atoms called *fatty acids*. There are three main types of fatty acid: saturated fatty acids, monounsaturated fatty acids, and polyunsaturated fatty acids. All fats contain more than one type, but are categorized by the most prevalent type.

Saturated fatty acids (SFAs) contain as many hydrogen atoms as possible. Foods containing high levels of SFAs include meat, poultry, whole-milk dairy products, and the tropical oils—palm oil and palm kernel oil. These fats raise LDL cholesterol significantly and HDL cholesterol slightly. Consumption of high amounts of SFAs has been linked to an increased risk of heart disease.

Monounsaturated fatty acids (MUFAs) contain one fewer pair of hydrogen atoms than SFAs. Foods high in MUFAs include olives, olive oil, avocados, peanuts, peanut oil and canola oil. These fats lower LDL blood cholesterol and maintain HDL levels.

Polyunsaturated fatty acids (PUFAs) have the fewest pairs of hydrogen atoms. They are the main component of many vegetable oils. Omega-3 fatty acids are found in soybeans, walnuts, flax oil, and salmon. They raise your HDL blood cholesterol and lower your LDL blood cholesterol. Omega-6 fatty acids are found in sunflower oil and margarine. Your body can make most of the PUFAs it needs except for the essential fatty acids (EFAs) linoleic acid (an Omega-6 fatty acid) and linolenic acid (an Omega-3 fatty acid) (Powell, 2003). Both linoleic acid and linolenic acid lower your LDL blood cholesterol.

THINK CRITICALLY

1. What types of fatty acids were present in foods you have eaten in the past day?
2. Why should you limit the amount of saturated fat you consume even though it raises your HDL levels?

CASE STUDY

Hydrogenated and Fractionated Fatty Acids

In order to make an oil more solid at room temperature—for example, when manufacturing margarine—manufacturers saturate the oil by adding hydrogen atoms. This process is called hydrogenation. Trans fatty acids are a type of hydrogenated fatty acid. They raise LDL cholesterol, reduce HDL cholesterol, and are linked to an increased risk of heart disease. Manufacturers now offer some vegetable oils that have been converted to solid form using fractionation—a process that separates a mixture of chemical substances into its component parts—instead of hydrogenation. This method results in fewer trans fatty acids being formed, but raises saturated fat levels.

Question:

Find examples of trans fats and fractionated fats on nutrition labels. Explain why each product may contain these substances.

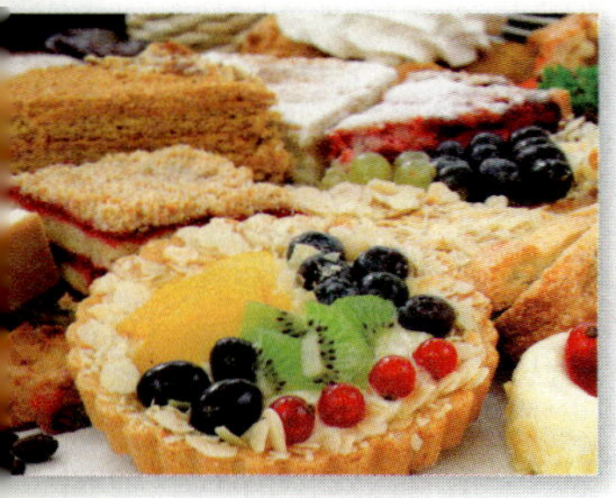

FIGURE 1.20 A diet high in saturated fats can increase the risk of illnesses such as heart disease, cancer, and obesity.

Daily Lipid Requirement

Health experts recommend that people ages four to 18 consume a range of 25 to 35 percent of their total calories from fat (Health Canada, 2007). *Eating Well with Canada's Food Guide* recommends that everyone should choose low-fat foods often and include a small amount—30 to 45 mL—of unsaturated fat each day to get the fat you need. Use of saturated fats should be limited.

Lipid Toxicity and Deficiency

A lipid deficiency can lead to a deficiency in the fat-soluble vitamins A, D, E, and K. It can also lead to a deficiency in the essential fatty acids linoleic acid and linolenic acid. As a result, production of hormones and other chemicals important for life may be compromised.

Some storage of fat is necessary to provide for growth and other increased energy demands. However, the typical Canadian diet includes more fats and oils than the body needs. The Canadian Community Health Survey conducted in 2004 found that approximately 13 percent of adolescents aged 14 to 18 consumed more than the recommended amount of Calories from total fat.

TIP for Healthy Living

Be cautious of ingredients used to replace fat when choosing low-fat food products. Sometimes sugar is added to compensate for the change in flavour and texture in low-fat products. Why is added sugar a concern in low-fat products?

THINK CRITICALLY

1. Which fat do you think is the healthier choice, butter or margarine? Why?
2. Describe some modifications that could be made to a diet to include fewer saturated fats and more monounsaturated and polyunsaturated fats.

Protein

Every living cell contains protein. You need protein to constantly repair, replace, and make new cells. For example, skin cells only live for about 25 days. Your body has to make a huge number of cells to replace the cells that die (Royston, 2011). Your body also uses protein to manufacture enzymes used in every cell process. However, if the carbohydrates and lipids in your diet do not provide the energy you need, your body will stop using protein for growth and repair and start using it to provide energy instead.

Complete and Incomplete Proteins

Proteins are made of chains of amino acids. Different proteins have different combinations of amino acids in their chains. Your body uses 20 amino acids in various combinations in order to synthesize thousands of types of protein. Your body can manufacture 11 amino acids, but nine amino acids are essential—your body cannot manufacture them so you need to obtain them from food.

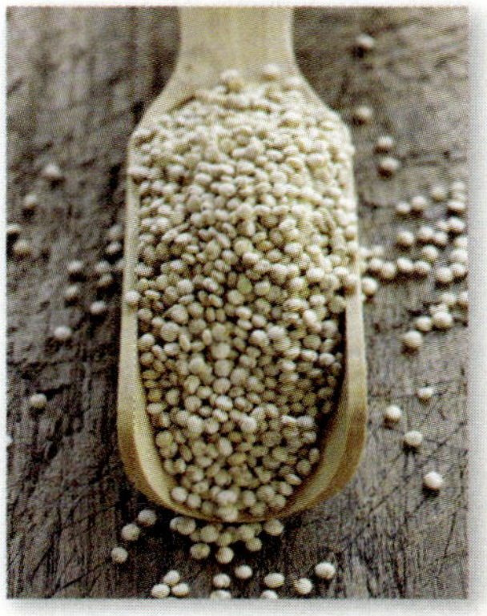

Figure 1.21 Soy products and this whole-grain quinoa are excellent sources of complete protein.

The proteins found in foods from animal sources such as beef, poultry, fish, and dairy products are complete proteins because they contain all nine essential amino acids. Proteins found in all plants, except in soy and quinoa (pronounced *keen-wah*), are incomplete proteins—they lack one or more essential amino acids. On their own, they would not provide adequate amounts of amino acids. However, two or more proteins that lack different amino acids are known as *complementary proteins*, and can be eaten together to provide a source of all nine essential amino acids. For example, you can form complete proteins by combining legumes with grains or nuts, or grains or nuts with dairy products. Complementary proteins do not have to be eaten at the same meal to have this effect, but within a few hours of one another. Eating a variety of foods containing protein will help ensure that you obtain all nine essential amino acids.

Daily Protein Requirement

Health experts recommend that people ages four to 18 consume 10 to 30 percent of their total Calories from protein. Eating two or three servings of meat and alternatives and three or four servings of milk and alternatives every day should provide you with enough protein in your diet. Athletes and those who want to increase muscle mass should consume around 20 grams of protein (for example, two cups of milk, one quarter cup of nuts, one hard boiled egg) after athletic activity for optimal gain in strength and muscle mass.

Figure 1.22 Each of these foods is an excellent source of protein.

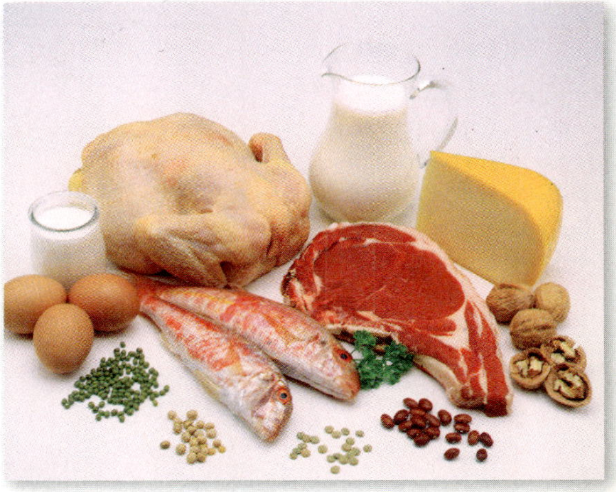

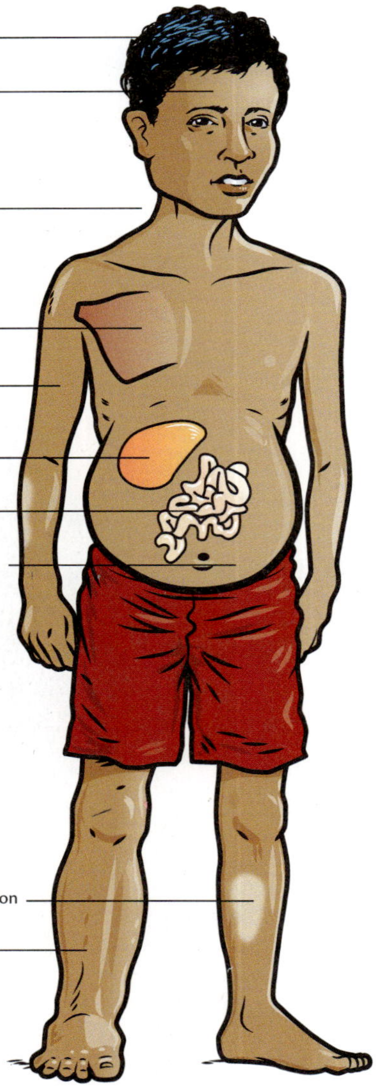

While some athletes who train heavily consume protein supplements in addition to the protein in the foods they eat, extra protein from protein shakes, powders and supplements does not have the added benefit of providing other essential nutrients and these supplelments often costly (Dietitians of Canada, 2012). For people who consume sufficient protein in their diets, additional protein will simply be used as energy or stored as fat. It will not result in additional muscle growth.

Protein Toxicity and Deficiency

Extra protein is not stored in the body like carbohydrates and fats. Instead, some extra protein is converted to glucose or glycogen by the liver and the rest is filtered by the kidneys and excreted. If there is a large amount of extra protein in the diet, the extra work required of the liver and kidneys can lead to tissue damage.

Most Canadians get enough protein in their diet. However, some conditions, such as eating disorders or economic issues, may cause a protein deficiency. Early signs of protein deficiency include muscle weakness and an inability to fight off illness. A severe lack of protein can lead to a disease called *kwashiorkor*. A swollen belly filled with liquid collected below the skin (not fat) is a common symptom of kwashiorkor.

FIGURE 1.23 Kwashiorkor is a form of protein deficiency. Although protein deficiency is uncommon in Canada, what group(s) of Canadians might be at increased risk of developing kwashiorkor?

TIP for Healthy Living

Eat a variety of protein-rich foods. If you haven't already, try a soy-based veggie burger, a falafel made with chickpeas, or sprinkling nuts on your breakfast cereal.

THINK CRITICALLY

1. How can you ensure that your diet includes high-quality proteins?
2. Plan a meal that includes appropriate amounts of carbohydrates and lipids, and combines two or more incomplete proteins to make a complete protein.

Water

Although water does not provide you with energy, it is essential for survival. Your body is 50 to 70 percent water. You can live for a few weeks without food but you can only live a few days without water. Water helps move nutrients and waste through your body, helps keep your blood pressure normal and helps regulate your body temperature (Royston, 2011).

The easiest way to quench your thirst is with water from your tap. Municipally treated tap water undergoes several processes to make it safe to drink. Chlorine is added to kill bacteria and in some places fluoride is added to help protect your teeth from tooth decay. Foods such as many fruits and vegetables are also good sources of water.

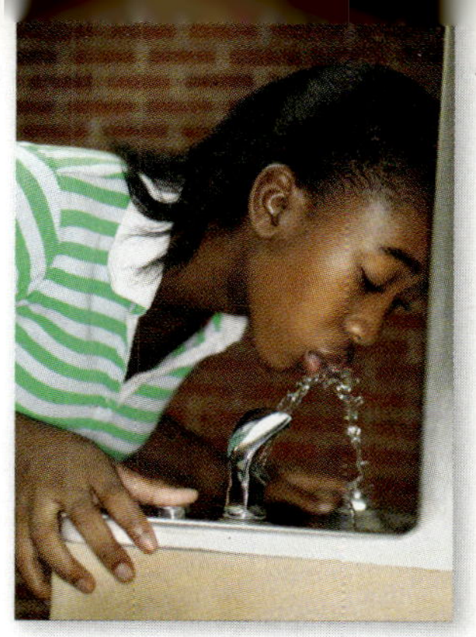

FIGURE 1.24 Get into the habit of drinking water throughout the day as your main fluid source without adding unnecessary calories.

Daily Water Requirement

The water in both beverages and foods contributes to your daily water intake. The amount of water you need to consume varies depending on your size, your diet (high-fibre diets increase fluid needs), your activity level, and the weather. During exercise your body releases heat by generating sweat. If you lose too much fluid in sweat, you become dehydrated, your muscles cannot function efficiently, and you become fatigued. You can use the colour of your urine as a guide to know if you are dehydrated. For adequate hydration, your urine should be light yellow.

OPEN FOR DEBATE

Debate this statement: "Since water is essential for health, schools should make bottled water available to students."

Water Toxicity and Deficiency

It is difficult to drink too much water, but it is possible. If you drink too much water too quickly, you may upset the balance of water and salt in your body. Water toxicity can cause fluid to collect in body tissues. This condition is called *edema*. It can lead to confusion, convulsions and in extreme and rare cases, death.

If you lose more fluid than you take in, you become dehydrated. Some signs of dehydration are thirst; headache; dry lips and mouth; dizziness and fainting; dark yellow, strong smelling urine; low blood pressure and increased heart rate.

You may be dehydrated even if you don't have any of these signs. When you feel thirsty, dehydration has already begun, so it is important to drink fluids often, even before you feel thirsty.

Pause and Think
How could drinking tap water and eating locally grown vegetables and fruits reduce your environmental footprint?

Micronutrients

Vitamins, minerals, and phytochemicals are micronutrients. They do not provide any energy, but they are necessary in small amounts to maintain health. Most people can get all the essential micronutrients simply by following *Eating Well with Canada's Food Guide* and by eating a variety of nutritious food. In cases where this is not possible, a health professional may recommend taking a supplement.

Vitamins

Vitamins regulate a variety of body functions and help carbohydrates, proteins, and fats extract energy from food. In addition, some vitamins, including vitamins A, C, and E, have antioxidant properties. Antioxidants are substances that can reduce the number of harmful **free radicals** in the body, by counteracting the effects of **oxidation.**

free radical:
a highly reactive substance, produced by oxidation, that can cause cell damage

oxidation:
the chemical combination of a substance with oxygen; in cells, oxidation causes damage and can lead to cancer, heart disease, and premature aging

Scientists have identified 15 different vitamins that you need in small amounts to maintain health. You obtain all of these vitamins from the foods you eat, with the exception of vitamin D, which is made by your body. Vitamins are classified into two groups: water-soluble vitamins and fat-soluble vitamins.

Water-Soluble Vitamins

Water-soluble vitamins are soluble in the watery parts of food and body tissue. They consist of

- Thiamine (vitamin B_1)
- Riboflavin (vitamin B_2)
- Niacin (vitamin B_3)
- Pantothenic acid (vitamin B_5)
- Vitamin B_6
- Biotin (vitamin B_7)
- Folic acid (vitamin B_9)
- Vitamin B_{12}
- Vitamin C

Most water-soluble vitamins are not stored in your body, so toxicity is rare, but the vitamins should be consumed daily.

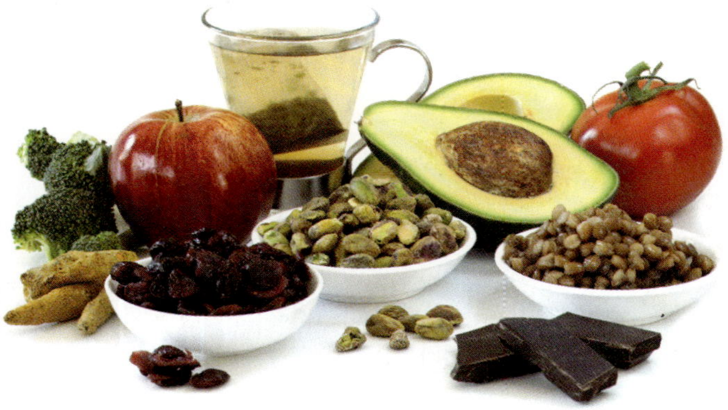

FIGURE 1.25 Most of the foods you eat contain vitamins. These foods have the added benefit of antioxidants to help neutralize the effect of free radicals. Which of these foods are part of your regular diet?

B Vitamins

All the B vitamins function as **coenzymes**, assisting in the activity of other important enzymes and allowing for energy-producing reactions to proceed effectively. As a result, any lack of water-soluble vitamins affects growing or rapidly metabolizing tissues such as skin, blood, the digestive tract, and the nervous system. With the exception of biotin (vitamin B_7) and vitamin B_{12}, the excess water-soluble vitamins not used by your body are excreted in your urine. For that reason, they must be replaced daily and they are not normally found in toxic amounts. Foods from all the four food groups contain B vitamins. For example, you can obtain thiamine (B_1), pantothenic acid (B_5) and vitamin B_6 from whole grains; riboflavin (B_2) from milk; niacin, biotin, and vitamin B_{12} from meats; and folic acid (B_9) from green leafy vegetables.

coenzyme: a vitamin that combines with another molecule to form an organic compound

Vitamin C (Ascorbic Acid)

Vitamin C helps maintain the integrity of the capillary blood vessels and promotes the formation of normal teeth and bones. Vitamin C helps your body heal wounds and resist infections. It also aids in the absorption of iron. Citrus fruits and tomatoes are excellent sources of vitamin C, as are strawberries, cabbage, spinach, and other green leafy vegetables. The potato is not a concentrated source of vitamin C, but because of the large quantities commonly consumed in Canada, it represents an important source of vitamin C in our diets.

A deficiency of vitamin C causes a disease called scurvy, resulting in a weakening of connective tissue in bone and muscle. It can also cause anemia because iron, which is critical to the transport of oxygen in the blood, cannot be utilized without vitamin C.

Pause and Think
Historically, scurvy was of serious concern for the traveller. Why has this changed?

POINT OF VIEW

Vitamin C and the Common Cold

Some studies suggest that vitamin C can reduce the severity of the symptoms and duration of a cold. The antioxidant properties of vitamin C offer additional benefit by protecting cells from weakening and breaking down (Daniel, 2012). Other studies have not found that vitamin C provides significant protection from symptoms of the common cold. While this is a controversial topic, vitamin C does have several confirmed health benefits.

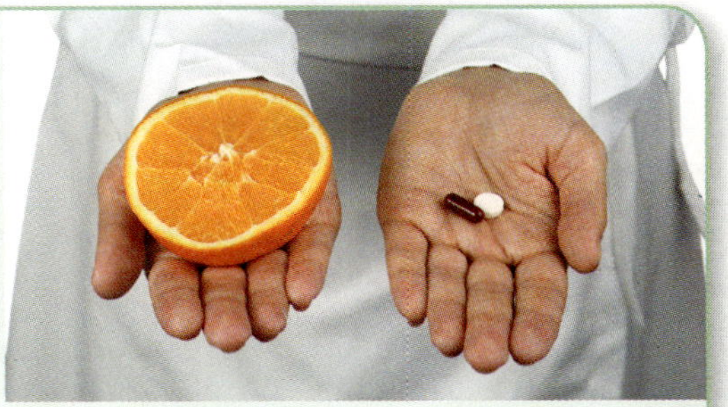

FIGURE 1.26 Oranges are good sources of vitamin C and may provide relief from the common cold. Try getting all your vitamin C requirements from food before resorting to supplements.

Nutrition Literacy

You can use this mnemonic (memory jogger) to remember these vitamins: "All Dogs Eat Kibble." In other words, the fat-soluble vitamins include vitamins A, D, E, and K.

Fat-Soluble Vitamins

Fat-soluble vitamins are soluble in the fatty parts of plants and animal tissue. Because these vitamins are stored in your fatty tissues, consuming too much of them can cause toxicity.

Vitamin A (Retinol)

Vitamin A helps protect you from infections; helps form and maintain healthy skin, hair, mucous membranes, bones, and teeth; and helps you see normally at night. Vitamin A is present in animal tissue, mainly in liver, fish oil, egg yolks, butter, and cheese. Plants do not contain vitamin A, but they do contain the antioxidant *beta-carotene*, which is converted to vitamin A in the intestine and then absorbed by the body.

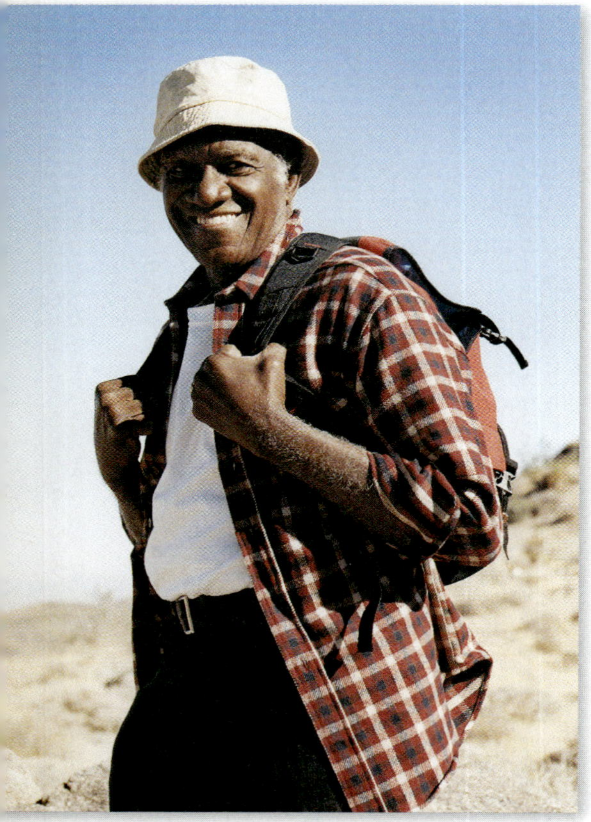

Figure 1.27 Older adults, people with dark skin, those who don't go outdoors often, and those who wear clothing that covers most of their skin should take vitamin D supplements year-round.

Vitamin D (Cholecalciferol)

Vitamin D helps your body use calcium and phosphorus to build strong healthy bones and teeth. Vitamin D is often called the sunshine vitamin. Your body produces it when compounds that occur naturally in your skin are exposed to sunlight. Because most Canadians do not produce adequate amounts of vitamin D on our own—especially in the winter months—we need to consume some vitamin D in our food. Fatty fish such as salmon and fortified milk are good sources of vitamin D. Some other foods contain small amounts of vitamin D.

Vitamin D deficiency causes a bone disease called *rickets* in children, resulting in weak muscles, delayed tooth development, and soft bones. Deficiency in adults causes fatigue, and a condition called *osteomalacia*, which makes bones soft and easy to break.

Vitamin E (Tocopherols)

Vitamin E works as an antioxidant, reducing numbers of free radicals to maintain a healthy reproductive system, nerves and muscles. Vitamin E is present in green leafy vegetables, wheat germ, and other plant oils such as sunflower oil.

Vitamin K (various, including Prothrombin)

Vitamin K is found in many plants (especially green leafy ones like spinach), in liver, and in the bacteria of the intestine. Vitamin K is vital to the formation of prothrombin—one of the chemicals necessary for blood clotting—found in the liver, and is also involved in bone metabolism.

POINT/COUNTERPOINT

Vitamin Supplements

In addition to obtaining vitamins from foods, many people take vitamin supplements. They may take them because they believe their diet is not supplying vitamins in the quantities they need, because vitamin supplements have been prescribed by a health professional, or simply for insurance. Some people believe that large amounts of a vitamin will have medicinal effects. The following points explore the opposing viewpoints about the question, "Are vitamin supplements beneficial?"

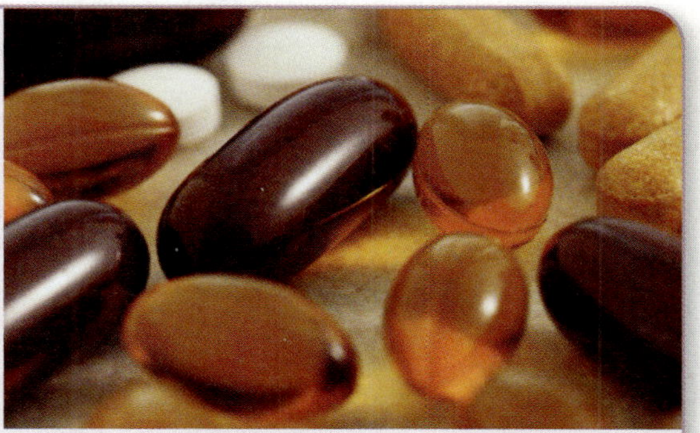

FIGURE 1.28 Canadians spend billions of dollars every year on vitamin supplements.

Yes	No
Jonny Bowden is a certified nutrition specialist who argues that • the North American diet does not supply the essential vitamins and minerals needed for good health • vitamin supplements are essential to maintaining good health and avoiding disease • supplements strengthen the immune system, improve memory and brain function, protect the liver, and reduce the risk of cancer • health experts recommend daily nutrient intake on the basis of avoiding disease rather than optimizing health	Colin Brennan is a medical journalist who argues that • most people who eat a balanced diet do not need to take vitamin supplements • most people eating a lot of fruit and vegetables will receive all the vitamins and minerals necessary to maintain good health • whole foods provide nutrients that cannot be made into pills, such as phytochemicals • megadoses of some vitamins can have toxic effects • only people with special needs, such as dieters and elite or professional athletes, require the added vitamins and minerals found in supplements

Questions:

1. According to Bowden, why should our diets include nutrient supplements?
2. According to Brennan, why should our nutrients come from food?
3. With whose argument do you most agree? What is it about that person's argument that makes it more believable?
4. Who do you think should take vitamin supplements? Why?

Minerals

You obtain minerals from the foods you eat and the water you drink. Most minerals that you consume become a part of your body. For example, calcium becomes part of your teeth and bones, and iron becomes part of your red blood cells. Some body processes require several minerals to work together. For example, calcium, magnesium, and phosphorus are all important for the formation and maintenance of healthy bones. In some cases, minerals compete with each other for absorption, and interact with other nutrients. This can affect their **bioavailability**. Minerals can be divided into three groups: major minerals, electrolytes, and trace minerals.

bioavailability: the degree to which the amount of an ingested nutrient is absorbed and available to the body

Major Minerals

Major minerals are needed in relatively large amounts. These include calcium, phosphorus, magnesium, and sulfur.

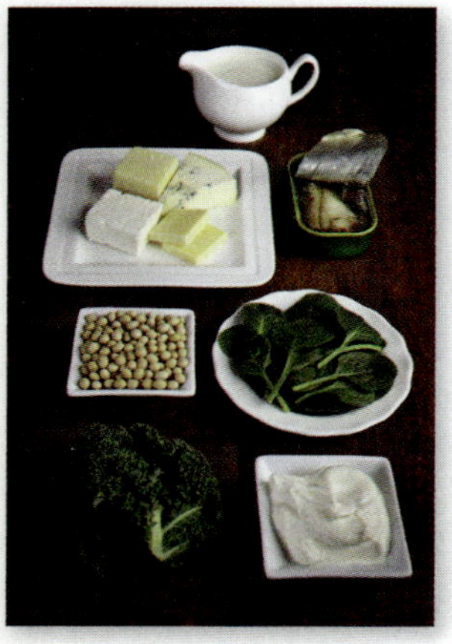

FIGURE 1.29 These foods are all rich in calcium. Calcium from green leafy vegetables can often be absorbed better in the presence of vitamin D.

Calcium and phosphorous play important structural roles in building bones and maintaining bone strength. Consuming adequate amounts of calcium throughout your lifespan can help to prevent osteoporosis, a condition in which bones become weak and fragile. Calcium also helps regulate blood clotting, nerve activity, and other body processes such as muscle contractions, including the heart. Organic acids such as oxalic and phytic acid can lower calcium absorption in foods such as spinach.

Magnesium helps build bones and manufacture proteins, and helps nerves and muscles function normally. The best sources of magnesium are whole grains and green leafy vegetables.

Sulfur helps the body to digest carbohydrates, fats and some vitamins. It is also used to make the hormone *insulin*, the keratin that makes up your hair, and the collagen that holds your body together. Onions, garlic, egg yolks, and sunflower seeds are good sources of sulfur.

Electrolytes

Electrolytes work together to maintain the body's fluid balance. They include potassium, sodium, and chloride. Sodium helps muscles and nerves function, and regulates blood pressure. Chloride helps transmit nerve signals. Table salt is a good source of both sodium and chloride. The body is very efficient in maintaining sodium levels in the body, so deficiency normally doesn't occur even when sodium is scarce. However, certain conditions like extreme sweating, chronic diarrhea, and vomiting can lead to the inability to retain sodium.

Potassium helps regulate the heartbeat, helps muscles and nerves function, and helps maintain normal blood pressure. Good sources of potassium include fruits such as bananas and oranges, vegetables, meat, poultry, fish, legumes and peas, and milk products.

TIP for Healthy Living

On average, Canadians consume well over the recommended upper intake level of sodium per day. Sodium intake can be reduced by eating fewer restaurant and fast-food meals and using herbs and spices to flavour foods instead of salt.

Trace Minerals

Trace minerals are needed in very small amounts, but they are just as important as other nutrients. They include iron, copper, zinc, iodine, and selenium.

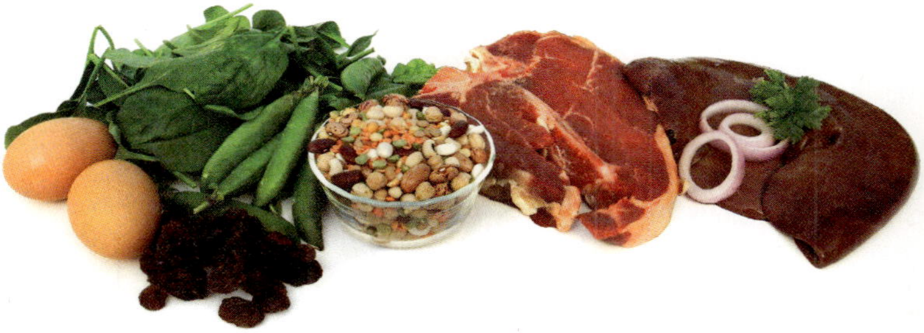

FIGURE 1.30 These foods are rich in iron. How can you improve the bioavailability of iron in some of these foods?

Iron deficiency is the most common nutrient deficiency in Canada and around the world (Center for Science in the Public Interest, 2012). Iron is an important component of the hemoglobin in red blood cells that transports oxygen to the body's tissues. The best sources of iron are meat (especially liver), and egg yolk. The body can absorb iron from these animal sources much better than the iron found in plant food such as grains, dried fruit and green vegetables, supplements, and fortified foods. For this reason, the requirement for iron is 1.8 times higher for vegetarians than it is for non-vegetarians. Vitamin C can enhance the absorption of iron from plant sources.

Iron deficiency can cause **anemia** and is usually due to blood loss, infections, diets low in iron, or diets high in iron inhibitors.

anemia: a lack of healthy red blood cells; symptoms can include weakness, fatigue, trouble concentrating, and shortness of breath

Phytochemicals

Phytochemicals give plants their colour, flavour, and odour, and provide us with benefits beyond basic nutrients. So far, scientists have discovered over a thousand phytochemicals including *lycopene* in tomatoes, *allicin* in garlic, and *isoflavones* in soybeans. Known phytochemicals have a broad range of protective benefits, from reducing inflammation to speeding healing, preventing infection, and curbing cancer. Since there are so many different kinds, the best way to ensure you obtain important phytochemicals is to eat a wide variety of foods.

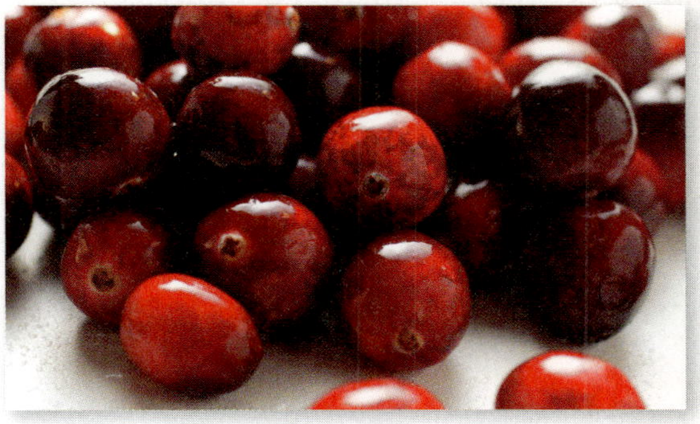

FIGURE 1.31 The phytochemical *anthocyanin* is found in cranberries and can help treat and prevent urinary tract infections. It is also a powerful antioxidant.

THINK CRITICALLY

1. Why is it important for Canadians to reduce their salt intake? How can they achieve this goal?
2. Why is it important to understand bioavailability?
3. People with what conditions should not add table salt to their prepared meals?

SAFETY AND SANITATION

Allergen Labelling

You can develop a food allergy at any point in your life. Be aware of the following common allergens. Manufacturers must clearly identify whether these may be present in the food at the end of the list of ingredients:

Peanuts	Eggs
Milk	Tree Nuts
Wheat	Soy
Sesame Seeds	Seafood
Sulphites	

(Health Canada, 2012)

Food Labelling

Food packaging includes a lot of information. This information can help you make decisions to get the most out of the foods you eat. Health Canada and the Canadian Food Inspection Agency (CFIA) share responsibility for food labelling policies in Canada. The CFIA verifies that the information consumers see on labels is truthful and not misleading. It does this by enforcing Canada's packaging, labelling, and advertising laws. However, it is important to know that CFIA allows for the nutrients in the food to vary by up to 20 percent from the nutrition information found on food labels (CFIA, 2010).

You should be able to find these items on every Canadian food label:

❶ **The common name of a food**. The correct common name is displayed in both French and English. For example, orange drink must be described as orange drink and not orange juice.

❷ **The net quantity**. The quantity of the food product is declared in metric units in both French and English.

❸ **The name and address**. The manufacturer's name and address is provided in either French or English.

❹ **Ingredients**. The common names of the ingredients are listed, and their components are listed by mass from greatest to least. For example: enriched flour (wheat)(niacin, thiamine, riboflavin, iron).

❺ **Durable life date ("best-before" date)**. You will find a best-before date on prepackaged foods with a durable life of 90 days or less.

❻ **The Nutrition Facts table**. The Nutrition Facts table provides information on energy (Calories) and 13 nutrients, based on the stated serving size.

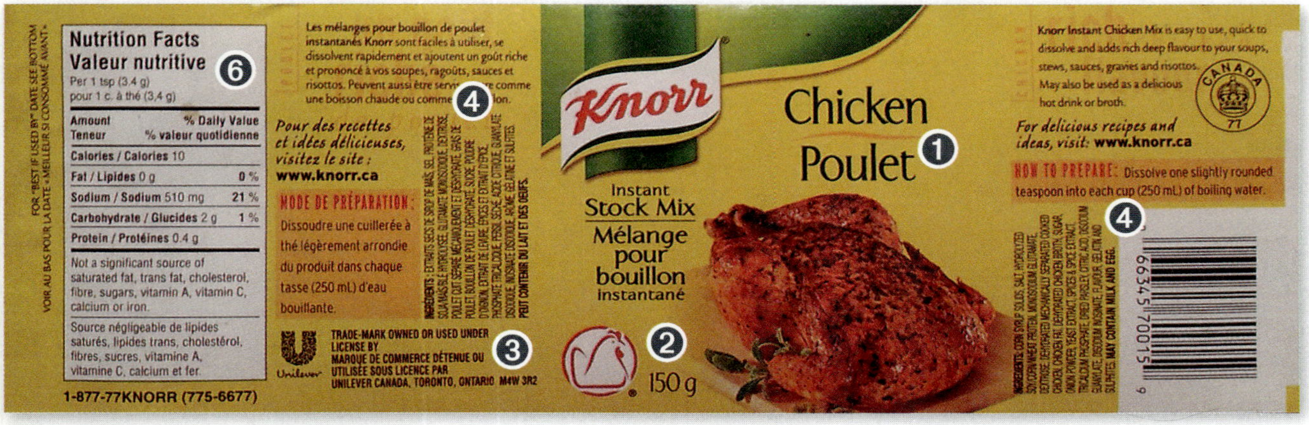

FIGURE 1.32 A typical Canadian food label.

IN FOCUS

Using the Nutrition Facts Table

The Nutrition Facts table on food labels gives you information about calories and 13 core nutrients. Follow these three steps to use it:

1. Look at the amount of food. Compare this to the amount you actually eat.
2. Read the *% Daily Value*. If the *% Daily Value* for a nutrient is 15 percent or greater, this food provides a large amount of the nutrient. If the *% Daily Value* for a nutrient is 5 percent or less, this food provides a small amount.
3. Use the information to choose healthy foods. You may want to choose foods with small amounts of fat, saturated and trans fats, and sodium or large amounts of fibre, vitamin A, calcium, and iron.

Nutrition Facts Valeur nutritive Per 1/5 of package (91 g) / pour 1/5 au paquet (91 g)	
Amount **Teneur**	**% Daily Value** **% valeur quotidienne**
Calories / Calories 330	
Fat / Lipides 2 g	**3** %
Saturates / saturés 0.5 g + Trans / trans 0 g	**3** %
Cholesterol / Cholestérol 0 mg	
Sodium / Sodium 2 mg	**1** %
Carbohydrate / Glucides 65 g	**22** %
Fibre / Fibres 9 g	**36** %
Sugars / Sucres 3 g	
Protein / Protéines 13 g	
Vitamin A / Vitamine A	0 %
Vitamin C / Vitamine C	0 %
Calcium / Calcium	2 %
Iron / Fer	50 %

Questions:

1. What type of product is this label likely to be from? How do you know?
2. Is this product likely to contribute to a healthy diet? Why or why not?

CASE STUDY

Making an Informed Choice

John is shopping for crackers and picks up two types from the grocery store shelf. He is most interested in the information on fat, fibre and salt. The wheat cracker lists boldly on the front of the package: "low fat" and "a source of dietary fibre." The vegetable-type cracker makes no claims. So John looks to the Nutrition Facts tables to get the details:

Wheat Cracker per 4 crackers (20 g)	
Fat	5%
Saturated + Trans	4%
Fibre	8%
Sodium	4%

Vegetable-Type Cracker per 13 crackers (20 g)	
Fat	8%
Saturated + Trans	8%
Fibre	4%
Sodium	6%

Because the Nutrition Facts are based on the same amounts of food for both types of cracker (20 grams), John can compare the % Daily Values of the crackers without calculations.

Questions:

1. Which cracker would you choose to buy? Why?
2. If you bought the least nutritious cracker, what could you do to make it part of a healthy diet?

THINK CRITICALLY

1. Why would a manufacturer choose to make a nutrition claim?
2. How might restaurant menus that include calories, salt, sugar, and fat information affect your diet?

CHAPTER 1 REVIEW

Chapter Review

Knowledge and Understanding/Thinking

1. What is the difference between essential and non-essential nutrients?
2. What are some of the most significant ways that nutrients support good health?
3. What is the difference between a saturated and unsaturated fat?
4. What are the differences in the uses and health effects of trans fats and monounsaturated fatty acids?
5. What is an incomplete protein?
6. Explain why you can eat only incomplete proteins, and still end up with all the essential amino acids.
7. Why is fat-soluble vitamin toxicity more common than water-soluble vitamin toxicity?
8. How can you use the % Daily Value on a Nutrition Facts label to improve your diet?

Thinking/Communication

9. Why is it challenging for Canadians to consume enough fibre in their diets?
10. Create a poster that explains the glycemic index and how teens can incorporate low-GI foods in their diet.
11. Sammy is making brownies for a school assignment. The recipe requires butter as an ingredient. How can Sammy replace the fat used in the recipe with another fat that maintains the integrity of the recipe and makes it healthier?
12. Explain how you could compare the nutritional information for two foods that had different serving sizes.

Test Your Nutrient IQ (page 9) **Answers:**

1. False—amounts of other nutrients also influence a food's healthiness.
2. False—there is no significant nutritional difference between honey and sugar.
3. True—baked potato: 7 g fibre; bread: 4 g fibre.
4. True—6 mg vitamin E per 30 mL sunflower oil vs. 1.9 mg vitamin E per 30 mL olive oil.
5. False—the best sources of magnesium are leafy greens, beans, nuts, and whole grains.
6. False—all beverages except alcoholic drinks count.
7. False—approximately 830 mg sodium in the potatoes vs. 1200 mg in the French fries.
8. False—they tell you what amount is in one serving of the food.
9. False—celery provides small amounts of vitamin A, folate, calcium, potassium, and fibre.
10. True.
11. False—soy *milk* is a good substitute for milk because it has added calcium.
12. True.
13. False—other sources include dark green leafy vegetables, tofu, sesame seeds, and almonds.
14. False—*apple juice*, however, has had vitamin C added to it.

Communication/Application

13. Create a public-service announcement about the importance of bone health and nutrition for teens.
14. Many people are interested in adopting a healthy diet. Find or create recipes that are nutrient dense and compile them in a recipe book.
15. Create a multimedia display or a bulletin-board display to show relationships between nutrition and disease.
16. Research 10 phytochemicals, their sources in foods, and their functions in the human body. Create a table to communicate your results.
17. Revise a commonly eaten fast-food recipe to make it healthier and more nutritionally dense. Prepare the food item for your class to try and explain the changes that you made.
18. Bring a food to class in its natural and processed state (oats and a cereal bar, for example). Compare the nutritional content of both food items and explain their value in a healthy diet.

Putting It All Together

In this chapter, you have studied

- the food sources and functions of carbohydrates, lipids, proteins, water, vitamins, and minerals
- the effects of consuming too many or too few nutrients
- how to read food and nutrition labels

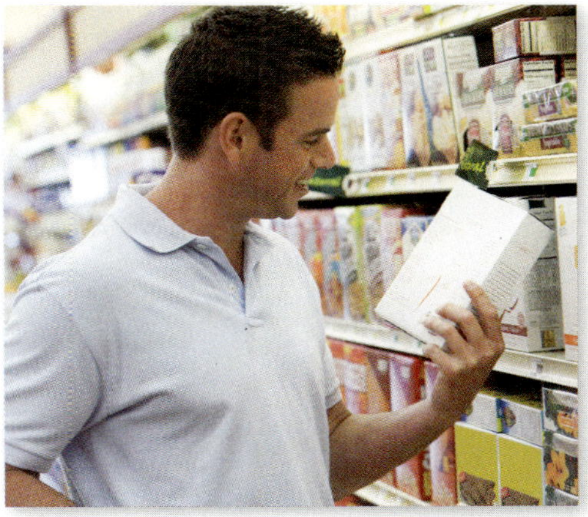

Summarize what you know by selecting a package of food and making notes about each nutrient that appears on its Nutrition Facts label. Include common food sources of the nutrient, its functions, information about deficiencies or toxicities, and an evaluation of the amount of this nutrient that the food contains. You can create a table to record your summary.

Chapter 2

Food Guidelines: Eat Well—Be Healthy

Key Terms

energy dense

percentage daily value

pulses

Recommended Dietary Allowance

Research and Inquiry Skills

- Collect primary data
- Evaluate information: checking for bias

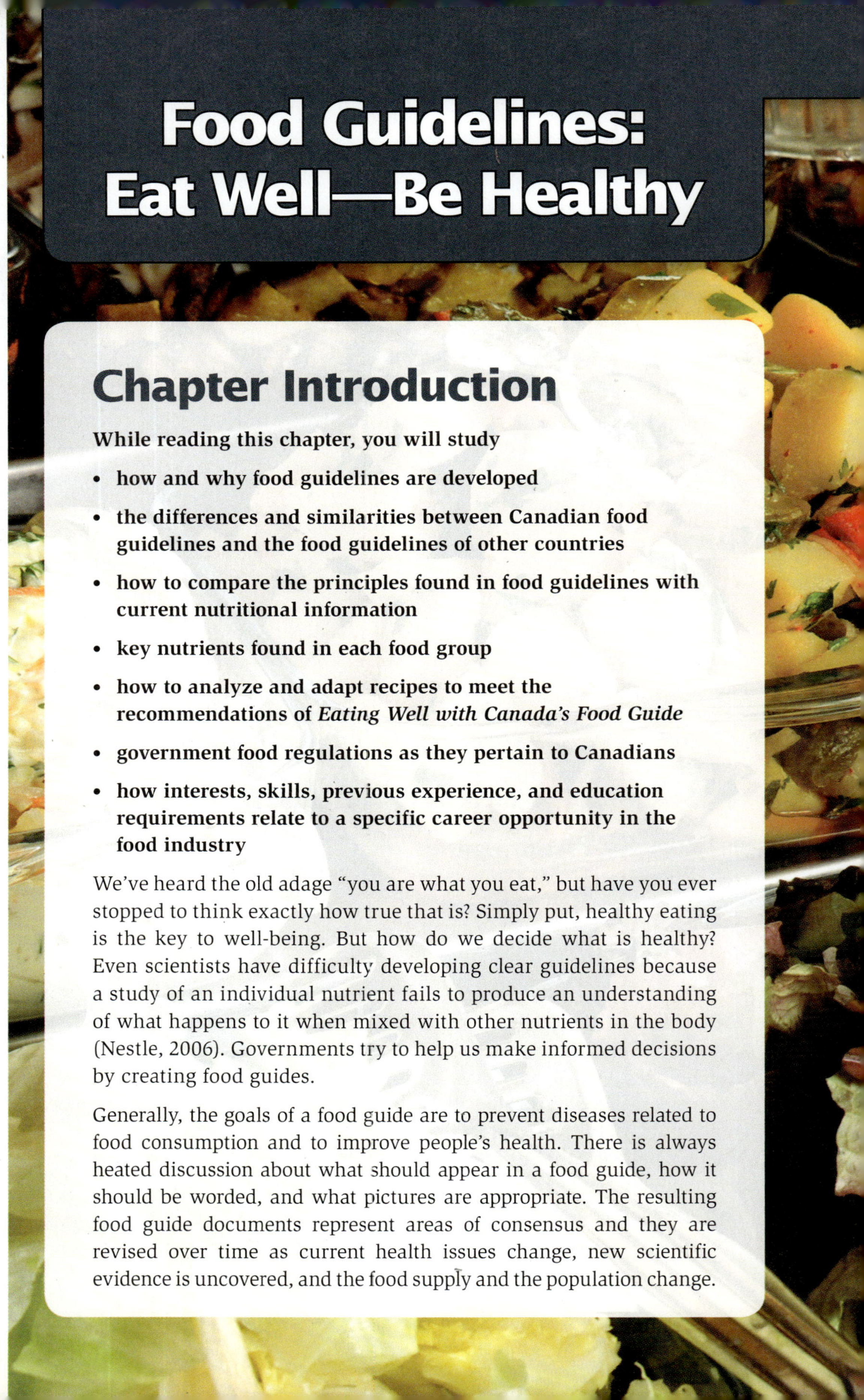

Figure 2.1 How can people make wise food choices when there are so many foods to choose from?

Chapter Introduction

While reading this chapter, you will study

- **how and why food guidelines are developed**
- **the differences and similarities between Canadian food guidelines and the food guidelines of other countries**
- **how to compare the principles found in food guidelines with current nutritional information**
- **key nutrients found in each food group**
- **how to analyze and adapt recipes to meet the recommendations of *Eating Well with Canada's Food Guide***
- **government food regulations as they pertain to Canadians**
- **how interests, skills, previous experience, and education requirements relate to a specific career opportunity in the food industry**

We've heard the old adage "you are what you eat," but have you ever stopped to think exactly how true that is? Simply put, healthy eating is the key to well-being. But how do we decide what is healthy? Even scientists have difficulty developing clear guidelines because a study of an individual nutrient fails to produce an understanding of what happens to it when mixed with other nutrients in the body (Nestle, 2006). Governments try to help us make informed decisions by creating food guides.

Generally, the goals of a food guide are to prevent diseases related to food consumption and to improve people's health. There is always heated discussion about what should appear in a food guide, how it should be worded, and what pictures are appropriate. The resulting food guide documents represent areas of consensus and they are revised over time as current health issues change, new scientific evidence is uncovered, and the food supply and the population change.

Spotlight On...

Making Sense of Nutrition Information

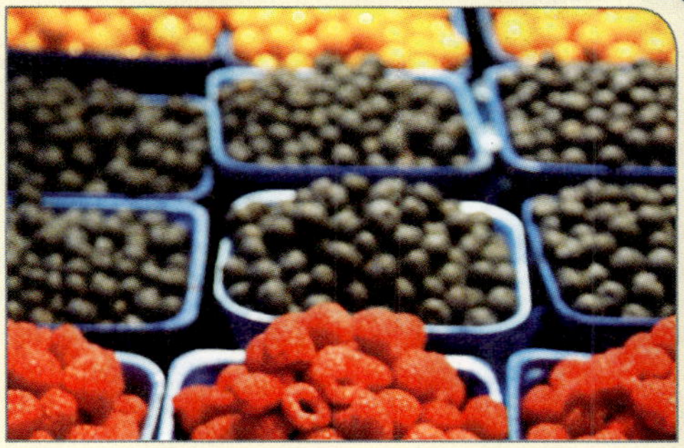

FIGURE 2.2 Berries like these are considered by some to be "superfoods." What is a superfood? Who determines whether or not a food qualifies?

We receive nutrition information from a variety of sources. Research shows that the most common sources are "... food product labels (68% of people); the Internet (51%); and magazines, newspapers and books (46%)" (Canadian Council of Food and Nutrition, 2008). However, not all advice is reliable. While some sources of nutritional advice have thoroughly researched their material to reach their conclusion, others will have little to no evidence for their claim. With such a wide variety of information and advice, some contradictory, how are we to evaluate the credibility of what we read? The Dietitians of Canada have developed five questions to help distinguish reliable information from nutrition misinformation pitfalls. The next time you read or hear nutrition news, ask yourself these questions:

1. Are testimonials used as the basis for the recommendation? One person feeling better after taking a treatment or remedy doesn't necessarily mean that it works for everyone. Many other factors could be at play.
2. Does the statement sound too good? If a claim sounds too good to be true, it probably is. Some claims are made based on testimonials or on studies that have been neither peer-reviewed nor published in respected journals.
3. Does it involve purchasing special products or services? Many theories are promoted in order to gain profit from the sale of products of questionable value, and may have no basis in fact.
4. Does the claim promise a miracle or an instant cure? Miraculous promises and claims do sound appealing, but don't be fooled by their charm.
5. Does the advice contradict researched and accepted nutrition advice? Be wary of such advice. For example, some food combination diets claim that the body cannot digest protein and starch at the same time. This claim has no scientific basis. Although you may lose weight on these diets, the weight loss will occur because you are eating fewer Calories, not because of the odd food combinations.

Activity:

Read these five statements about nutrition. Use what you know about common nutrition misinformation pitfalls to determine the credibility of each claim.

1. Eat these "superfoods" to stay healthy.
2. Pasteurization destroys the flavour and vitamins in milk.
3. Drink eight glasses of water a day for optimum health.
4. Organic food is healthier than conventionally raised food.
5. Detox diets flush toxins and fat out of your body.

Research and Inquiry Skills

Evaluating Information for Bias

Even when nutritional advice is based on research, it is important to evaluate the research to determine if the results are credible and unbiased. When reviewing research, examine the researchers' methods, results, and discussion, looking for instances of bias. While all research will have some elements of bias (Abdoler, Emanuel, & Stunkel, n.d.), it is important that researchers remove as much as possible.

First, consider whether the research is based on opinion or fact.

- Have the scientists referenced others' work to help prove their statements? If so, have they referenced peer-reviewed journals or special interest groups, whose methods may not be as rigorous?
- What evidence have they used to support their conclusions? Anecdotal evidence, or descriptions of one person's experience, can be a part of research, but should not be used exclusively. In most credible research, conclusions are drawn at least partly from experimental observations.

Then consider who participated in the research.

- Is the sample of participants large and diverse enough to reflect the population at large?
- Have observations been gathered from people of only one gender, cultural, or age group?
- What barriers might have been in place that dissuaded a segment of the population from participating in the study? For example, Fröding, Elander, and Eriksson (2011) found that participants in neighbourhood public-health initiatives are more likely to be born inside the country and less likely to be immigrants. When a segment of the population is excluded from a study, important information may be missed.

Read the following description of a research study (Wansink & Park, 2001).

> In this study, researchers wanted to compare the influence of the taste of a food on the amount eaten and the influence of container size on the amount eaten. They hypothesized that the amount of food eaten would be affected by both variables.
>
> To test their hypothesis, 151 people attending two matinee performances of the same action movie were randomly given either a medium or a large container of fresh or stale popcorn. The containers were collected at the end of the movie so that the researchers could determine how much popcorn had been eaten.

In addition, the research subjects were given a questionnaire to complete that asked whether they liked the popcorn, how much of it they believed they ate, and whether they believed the popcorn was healthy, as well as demographic information such as gender, age, and whether they attended the movie alone.

As expected, moviegoers who enjoyed the taste of the popcorn ate more than those who did not enjoy the popcorn. In addition, among moviegoers who did not enjoy the taste of the popcorn, those given a large container ate 61 percent more. Among moviegoers who did enjoy the taste of the popcorn, those given a large container ate 49 percent more. Men and those who ate their food with others also consumed more popcorn than other groups. Research subjects given medium containers were more likely to believe the popcorn was healthy than research subjects who were given large containers.

The researchers concluded that the amount eaten is influenced by taste, but is also influenced by serving size, as well as other factors.

Activities:

1. Do you think the sample in Wansink and Park's study was representative of the entire population? If not, what groups may not have been adequately represented? Why?
2. Describe factors other than those listed that may have affected how much popcorn the research subjects consumed during the study.
3. Apply the questions on page 33 to this research. Evaluate the credibility of the results.
4. How might other researchers use the results of this study?
5. What are the implications of this research for food companies? What are the implications for consumers?

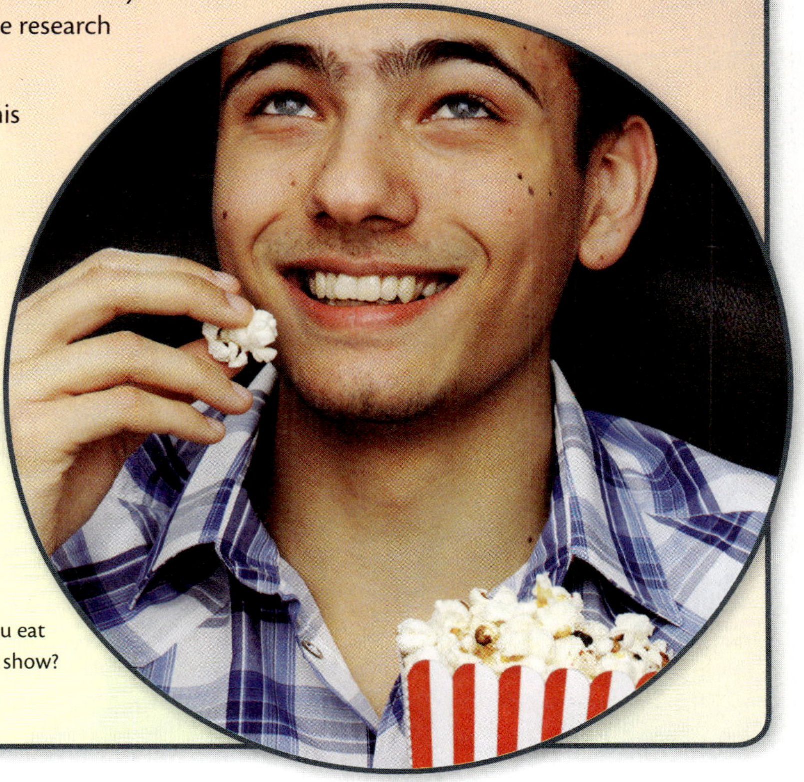

FIGURE 2.3 Popcorn and the movies are a well-known combination. What have you observed about how much you eat while watching a movie or TV show?

Canada's Food Guidelines

Health Canada is a government agency charged with the promotion and protection of the health of Canadian citizens. Like other government agencies around the world, Health Canada created and maintains a nutrition guide to help Canadians make healthy food choices. Governments work with researchers and dietitians to create guides to healthy eating because they have a vested interest in the health of their citizens.

History of Canada's Food Guidelines

"Let food be your medicine, and medicine be your food."
– Hippocrates

The government created Canada's *Official Food Rules* in 1942 to help Canadians make nutritious food choices. Because many Canadians were unsure how to prevent nutritional deficiencies during the food shortages that occurred during the Second World War, it was important for Health Canada to create a tool that Canadians could use to make healthy food choices. The food guide has been revised many times since 1942. The most recent revision, *Eating Well with Canada's Food Guide*, was published in 2007.

1940s–1960s

First published during the Second World War, at a time when Canadians were undergoing rationing of food, the *Official Food Rules* aimed to help Canadians derive the most benefits from the food that they could access. The *Official Food Rules* included six food groups organized by the nutrients the foods provide: Milk; Fruit; Vegetables; Cereals and Breads; Meat, Fish, etc.; and Egg. Called *Health Protective Foods*, a minimum number of servings was recommended for each group. People were also encouraged to eat at least one serving a week of organ meats, and to take fish oil (a source of vitamin D) as a supplement. The *Official Food Rules* did not suggest specific serving sizes of any foods, other than the milk group.

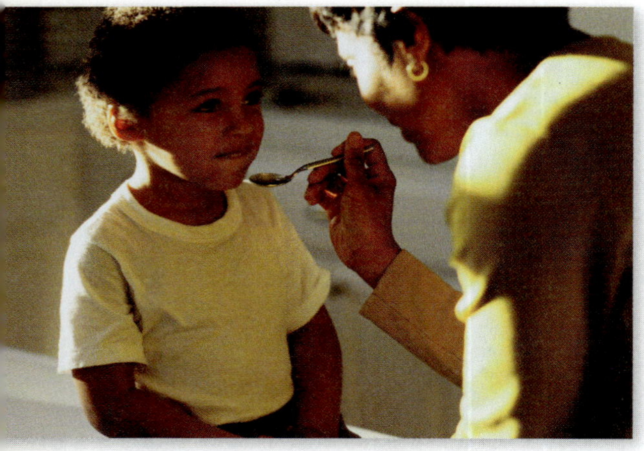

FIGURE 2.4 The levels of vitamin D recommended by Health Canada have recently been increased. What are some barriers Canadians may face in getting adequate amounts of this vitamin?

In 1944, the *Official Food Rules* were revised. Changes included removing the suggestion to eat organ meat, and including eggs and cheese in the Meat and Fish group. When the guide was revised again in 1949, the recommendation to take a vitamin D supplement was made more specific, and wording was changed to reflect the understanding that more wasn't always better. After 1949, no changes were made until 1961, when *Canada's Food Guide*, as it was then known, was published. In *Canada's Food Guide*, alternatives to meat, such as eggs and legumes, were included in the meat food group.

1970s–2000s

In 1977, *Canada's Food Guide* was published, including the familiar four food groups: Breads and Cereals, Fruits and Vegetables, Milk and Milk Products, and Meat and Alternatives. In this version, specific serving sizes were included, helping Canadians to determine how large a serving was. Very few changes were made to the food groups in 1982, but a more significant change was included: encouraging Canadians to limit the amount of fat, sugar, salt, and alcohol they consumed, and to balance the energy they consumed with their activity levels. Up to this time, the focus had been on preventing nutrition deficiencies; this food guide marked a change in focus to reducing chronic diseases.

In 1992, the guide was renamed *Canada's Food Guide to Healthy Eating*. The wheel that had been used to represent all food groups was changed to a rainbow. Canadians were encouraged to eat more servings from the food group with the longest band of colour in the rainbow and fewer servings from each subsequent group. The guide also included a new group, called Other Foods, which included foods and beverages that would not have normally been included in any other food group (e.g., condiments and high-Calorie or high-fat baked products).

The latest update was released in 2007 and renamed *Eating Well with Canada's Food Guide*. This current guide has moved vegetables and fruit to the top of the rainbow and reduced the number of servings of grain products, highlighting an increased understanding of the role that fibre, vitamins, and minerals play in our health. The group Other Foods has been eliminated, and Health Canada produced both print and electronic versions of the food guide.

TIP for Healthy Living

With new technology and ongoing research, our understanding of food and nutrition continues to grow. Canada's current guidelines will change in the future. When you hear about new discoveries related to nutrition, use the questions on page 33 to help you evaluate their credibility and decide whether to make lifestyle changes.

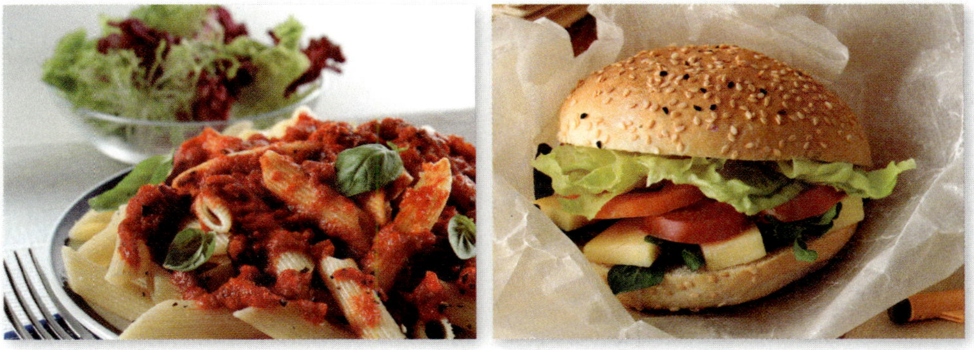

FIGURE 2.5 Each meal pictured includes foods from more than one food group. Which food groups does each meal represent in different editions of *Canada's Food Guide*?

THINK CRITICALLY

1. Summarize the major changes that have occurred between the first edition of *Canada's Food Guide* and the most current.
2. What do you believe was the most significant change that took place? Why was that change the most significant?

Career Connection

Dietitian and Health Care Manager

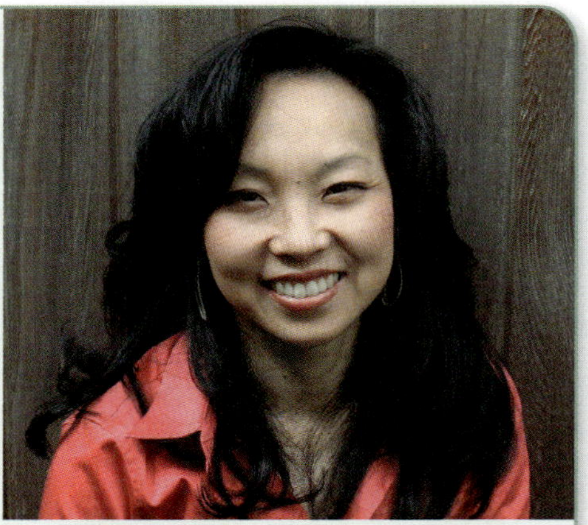

Figure 2.6 Melodie Yong uses her training as a dietitian in a variety of creative ways.

Melodie Yong became a dietitian because she loved food—and because she wanted a practical career where she could apply her knowledge to help the public. Melodie realized a career as a dietitian would fulfill her needs, and enrolled to study dietetics at The University of British Columbia. After graduating, she became a registered dietitian.

Melodie has wide-ranging interests, and her work allows her to perform a variety of roles. Her main position is as an Operations Leader for Cardiac Ambulatory Clinics at St. Paul's Hospital in Vancouver. There, she oversees the hospital's cardiac clinics. She has worked in a range of areas at the hospital, including renal, diabetes, and nutritional support. In addition, Melodie is a distance-course supervisor for nutrition courses in the Department of Biomedical, Physiology, and Kinesiology at Simon Fraser University. She also consults with personal and corporate clients and has worked in research and in clinical trials.

Working with media allows Melodie the opportunity to reach an even broader audience. She hosts a regular nutrition segment on a television newscast. In addition, she is a dietitian spokesperson for Healthy Families BC, an initiative of the provincial government that aims to reduce levels of chronic disease and encourage families to make healthy choices in their daily lives. While she finds that people have more access to nutrition information than ever before, Melodie wants to help ensure that they are able to make sense of what they read and hear. Through her many roles and responsibilities, she hopes to "inspire somebody out there to make a healthier choice about what they are going to eat" and likes that she is able to "present nutrition information in a really practical yet informative way." Canadians agree—dietitians are rated as the most credible source of nutrition information (Canadian Council of Food and Nutrition, 2008).

She is able to combine clinical work and working with the public, and has been able to transfer the skills she uses as a dietitian to her current position as a health care manager.

As the mother of two energetic children, the flexibility and variety of roles available to Melodie make it possible for her to achieve a balance between work and family life. After 15 years, Melodie is still encountering new opportunities and challenges. She believes the three keys to success are taking risks, being open to trying new things, and taking advantage of working with mentors.

Questions:

1. In addition to a love of food and a desire to help the public, why might a person want to pursue a career in dietetics?
2. What skills would a dietitian possess that are transferrable to other professions?
3. Other than dietetics, what fields of study could lead to a career in health care management?

Eating Well with Canada's Food Guide

Eating Well with Canada's Food Guide emphasizes making healthy food choices. It also promotes physical activity. It continues to stress that a variety of foods should be eaten. Fats and oils, as well as beverages, while not food groups, earn special mention in the guide. In addition to English and French, the guide has been translated into 10 different languages, making it more accessible to Canadians.

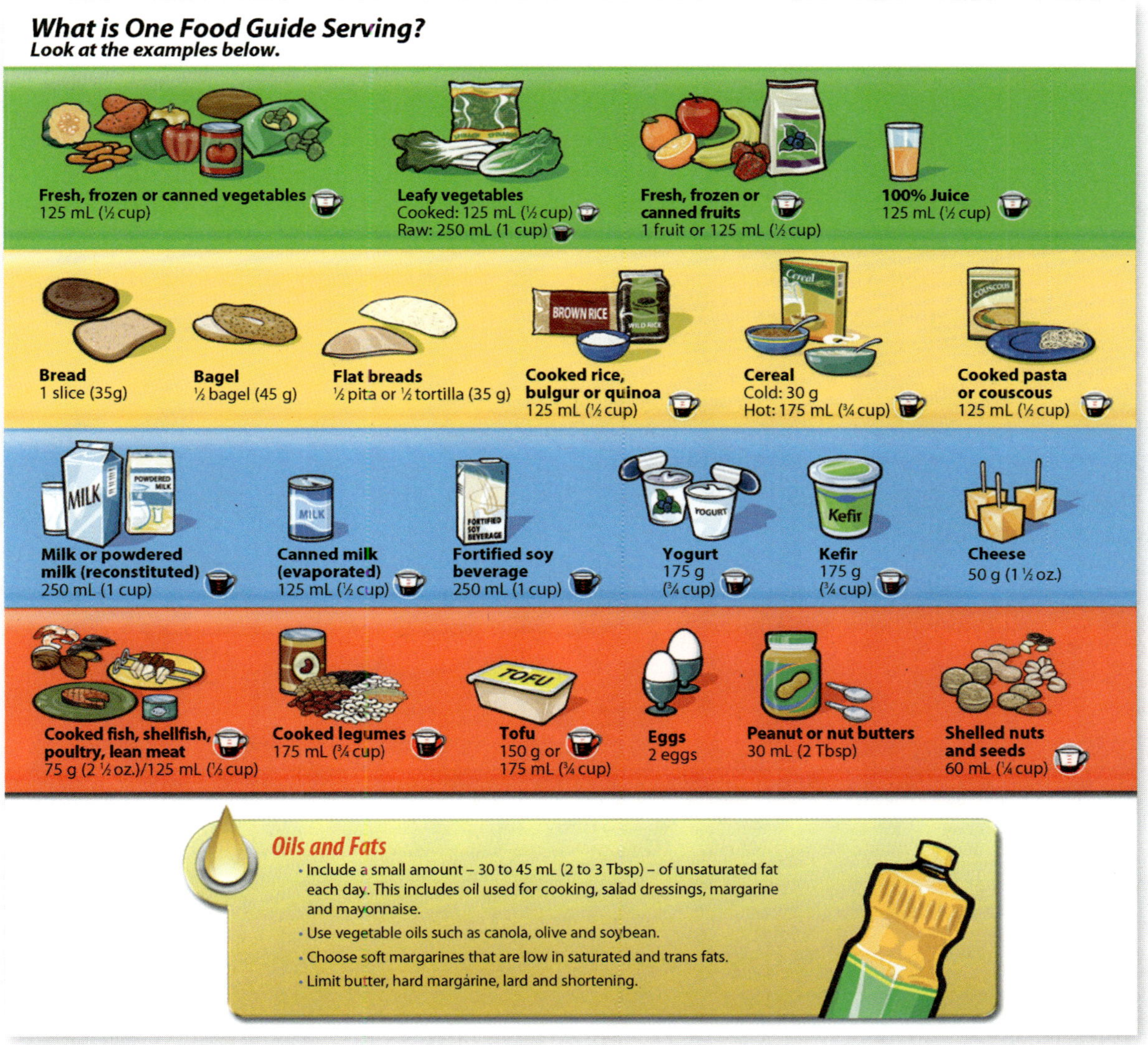

FIGURE 2.7 An excerpt from *Eating Well with Canada's Food Guide.*

Pause and Think

Examine a copy of *Eating Well with Canada's Food Guide*, or the excerpt above. Which features make it easy to use? Which features make it more challenging?

Eating Well with Canada's Food Guide—First Nations, Inuit, and Métis

When *Eating Well with Canada's Food Guide* was released, an Aboriginal version called *Eating Well with Canada's Food Guide—First Nations, Inuit, and Métis* was also released. With previous versions of *Canada's Food Guide*, regional editions of Aboriginal food guides were created. However, *Eating Well with Canada's Food Guide—First Nations, Inuit, and Métis* is a national food guide. Along with English and French, it is also available in Inuktitut, Ojibwe, Plains Cree, and Woods Cree, which are the most common Aboriginal languages in Canada.

Foods commonly eaten by Aboriginal people are an important part of this guide. For example, the Vegetables and Fruit food group includes berries and fiddleheads, and the Grain Products group includes wild rice and bannock. Traditionally eaten meats such as elk, caribou, deer, seal, and other wild game are also included. *Eating Well with Canada's Food Guide—First Nations, Inuit, and Métis* incorporates non-traditional foods that are currently available for purchase as well.

FIGURE 2.8 An excerpt from *Eating Well with Canada's Food Guide—First Nations, Inuit, and Métis.* Explain the importance of a distinct food guide for Canada's Aboriginal population

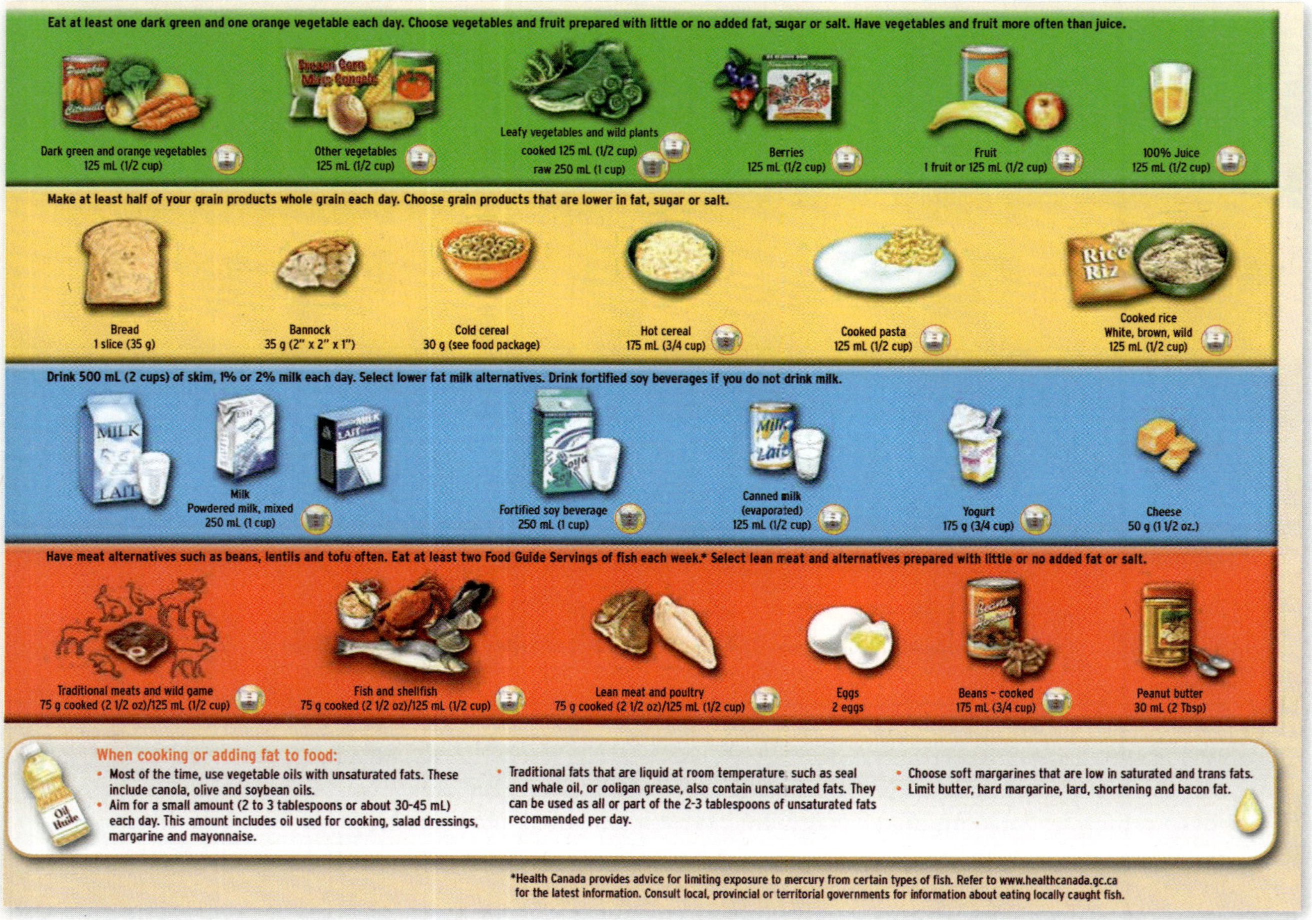

This version of *Eating Well with Canada's Food Guide* includes other unique features. As milk products were not part of the traditional Aboriginal diet, special attention has been given to foods such as bannock, fish bones, and wild plants that allow people to gain nutrients such as calcium and protein. Canned and powdered milk are included as they are often the only milk source available to people in some isolated communities. While the low-fat content of many game meats is beneficial from a health point of view, it can create some difficulty when it comes to preparing these foods. Therefore, the guide discusses methods to cook low-fat meats. It includes information about the benefits of traditionally used fats, such as ooligan grease and seal fat, and suggestions for incorporating them into the diet.

Pause and Think

What are the benefits of creating a national version of *Eating Well with Canada's Food Guide—First Nations, Inuit, and Métis*, rather than regional guides? What are the problems with creating a national version?

Bannock

Yield: 4 servings

There are countless recipes for bannock. This one features lard and the addition of dried fruit. To "plump" dried fruit such as currants, cover fruit with hot water and allow to stand for 5–10 minutes. Drain well and proceed with the recipe.

Ingredients

- 500 mL (2 c) flour
- 15 mL (1 tbsp) baking powder
- 5 mL (1 tsp) salt
- 50 mL (c) lard
- 200 mL (c) currants
- 250 mL (1 c) water

Method

1. Preheat oven to 220 °C (425 °F).
2. Lightly grease a baking sheet.
3. Measure flour, baking powder and salt into a medium sized mixing bowl. Stir well using a fork.
4. Using a pastry blender, cut in lard until it is the size of small peas.
5. Stir in currants, tossing lightly.
6. Add water and stir just until all ingredients are well combined. The dough will be very soft.
7. Turn dough onto a floured board. Knead lightly to form a 20 cm round disc. Place on baking sheet.
8. Bake in a hot oven for 15–20 minutes

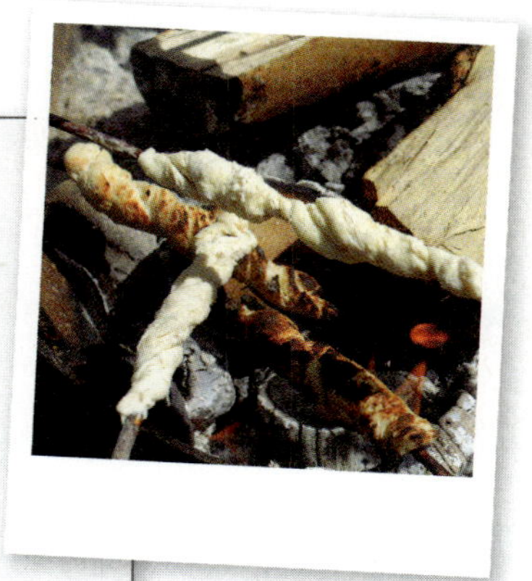

FIGURE 2.9 Try this recipe over an open campfire. Divide dough into two portions. Roll each into a thick rope. Wrap each rope around a long stick. Prop over the fire until browned.

Nunavut Food Guide

"When you eat packaged foods, two hours later you get cold. If you eat Inuit food, you stay warm."
– Inuit elder

The government of Nunavut has created a food guide that is more specific to the territory, highlighting traditionally eaten foods. In addition to English, it is available in Inuktitut, the most commonly spoken language in Nunavut. While the guide is based on similar principles of healthy eating, serving sizes are illustrated using hands rather than a specific amount of food. For example, a meal may consist of two handfuls of vegetables and fruit, one handful of meats or alternatives, and one handful of grain products. The guide emphasizes the sharing of meals, as it helps strengthen relationships and gives youth an opportunity to learn from their elders about traditional ways of harvesting, preparing, and storing food.

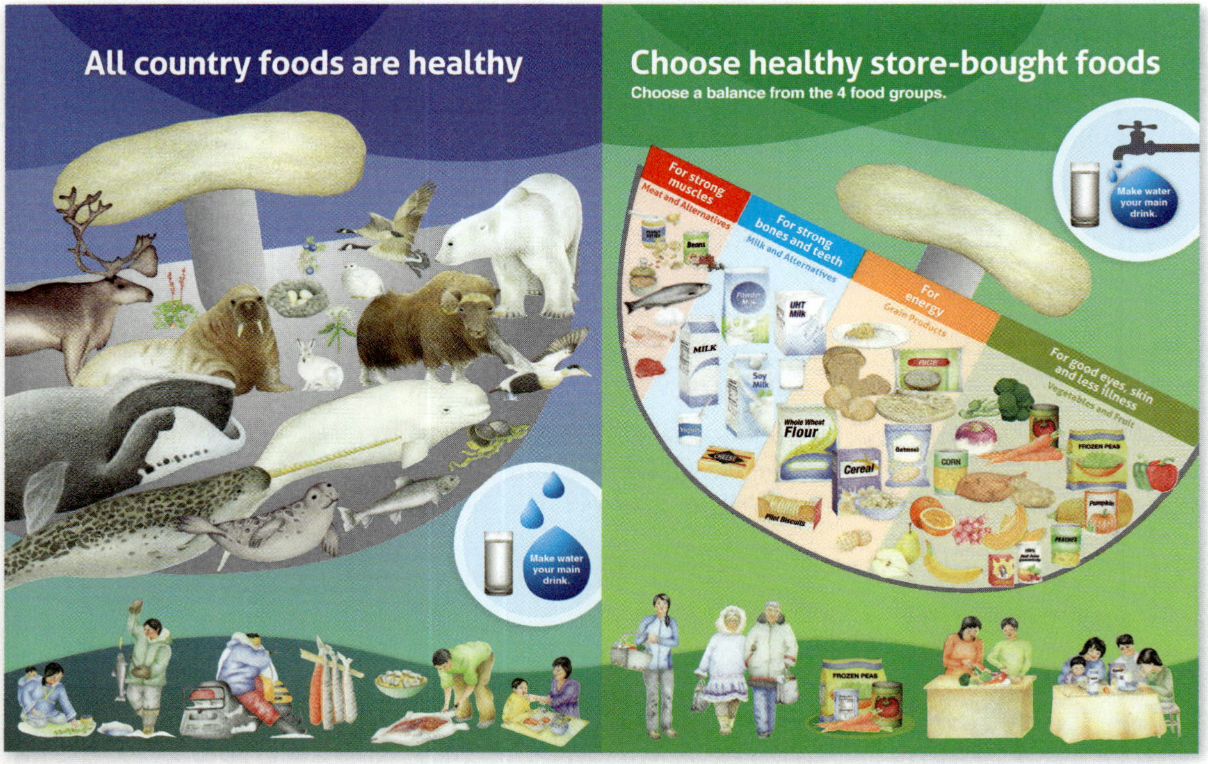

Figure 2.10 An excerpt from the *Nunavut Food Guide*. What features make this guide an effective educational tool for people living in Nunavut?

THINK CRITICALLY

1. How is the nutrition advice in the *Nunavut Food Guide* presented differently from that in *Eating Well with Canada's Food Guide—First Nations, Inuit, and Métis*?
2. The *Nunavut Food Guide* states that "country food is always a good choice." What are the benefits of promoting the consumption of country food? What problems might be associated with this?
3. Examine the illustrations at the bottom left of the *Nunavut Food Guide*. Describe their significance and explain why they would be included.

Access to Food in Remote Communities

How do people in isolated communities access perishable food? Many members of northern communities hunt to provide for their families. In addition, through a federal government program called Nutrition North Canada, as well as some provincial programs, people in northern and more isolated parts of Canada are able to receive food at a subsidized cost. Nutrition North Canada makes fresh foods available to communities who would otherwise not have access to them, especially during the winter. As the cost of transporting food makes the price substantially higher in the North, the aim of the program is to reduce food costs. In the Nutrition North Canada program, retailers receive a subsidy on the shipment of a selection of foods, which can then be passed on to the consumer as lower prices.

FINANCIAL LITERACY

The Canadian Nurses Association reports that in 2010 the monthly cost of feeding a family of four in Ottawa was $724. The monthly cost of feeding a family of four in Rankin Inlet, Nunavut, was $1803. What other expenses might a family reduce if food is expensive?

Food Guides Around the World

Canada is not the only nation to create a food guide for its citizens. Many countries have produced similar guides, emphasizing foods traditionally eaten in the country and reflecting both current nutritional concerns and governmental initiatives. In some countries, such as Canada and the United States, food guides tend to promote a diet that prevents chronic diseases like diabetes or heart disease. In some other countries, food guides promote a diet that provides nutrients to safeguard against malnutrition.

All food guides use symbols and graphics to communicate nutrition information in a consumer-friendly way. Graphics such as stars, squares, wheels, pyramids, or, as in Canada's case, a rainbow are used to make complex nutritional information clear and understandable to all readers, with the ultimate goal of promoting eating habits that provide essential nutrients and protect against chronic illnesses. In all food guides, a great amount of information must be summarized in few words or symbols. Depending on the culture and the literacy rate of the country, words and symbols are selected so that all citizens, regardless of socio-economic status and education level, can identify with and easily use the food guide. The placement of the least desirable foods is influenced by cultural values; for example, a pyramid graphic often puts the least desirable food at the top of the food guide, but in some cultures whatever is at the top has the most status so a different image is used. While some specific information differs, most food guides are similar in their recommendations, encouraging people to

- eat more vegetables, fruits, legumes, and whole-grain products
- limit the consumption of meats, fats, salt, and added sugar
- drink more water and fewer sweetened beverages
- use appropriate serving sizes

Some, but not all, food guides also emphasize the importance of exercise.

Case Study

Comparing Food Guidelines and Dietary Models

Governments are not the only bodies to create food guidelines. Health professionals, health organizations, community groups, and laypersons have published guides to healthy eating. Guidelines may be created for the general public, or targeted to a specific section of a community. For example, while many countries produce a general food guide for the entire population, a community organization may take the nutritional information found in *Eating Well with Canada's Food Guide* and tailor it to a specific ethnic community. Most national food guidelines are created by people with expertise in nutrition.

Creators of other dietary models have varied backgrounds. While some may have extensive training in nutrition, others with little to no formal education may create a guideline or dietary model to promote their own beliefs about making sound food choices.

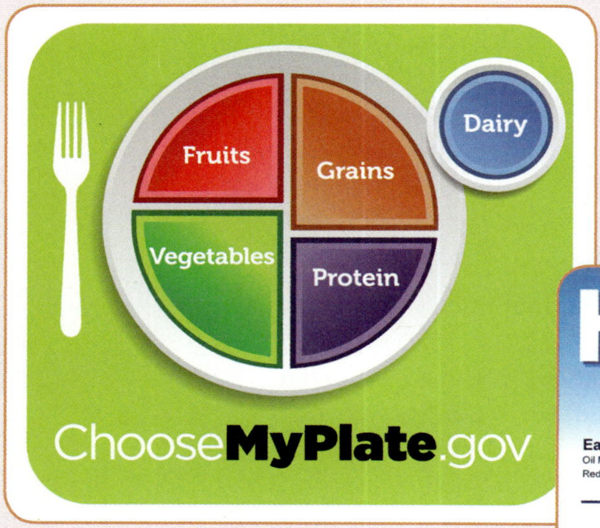

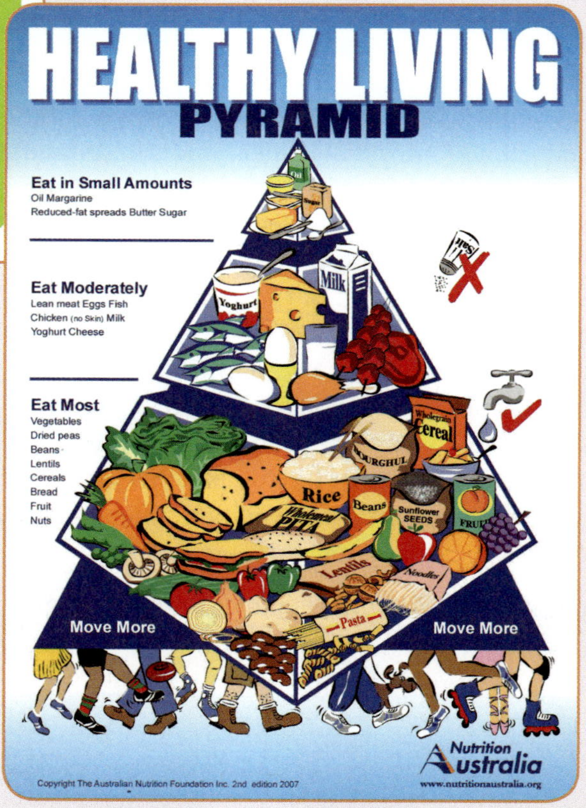

Figure 2.11 *MyPlate*, from the United States, and Australia's *Healthy Living Pyramid*. What similarities and differences do you notice in these food guides? What features make each graphic—plate, pyramid, or Canada's rainbow—effective at transmitting the message of healthy eating? Which graphic does the best job, in your opinion?

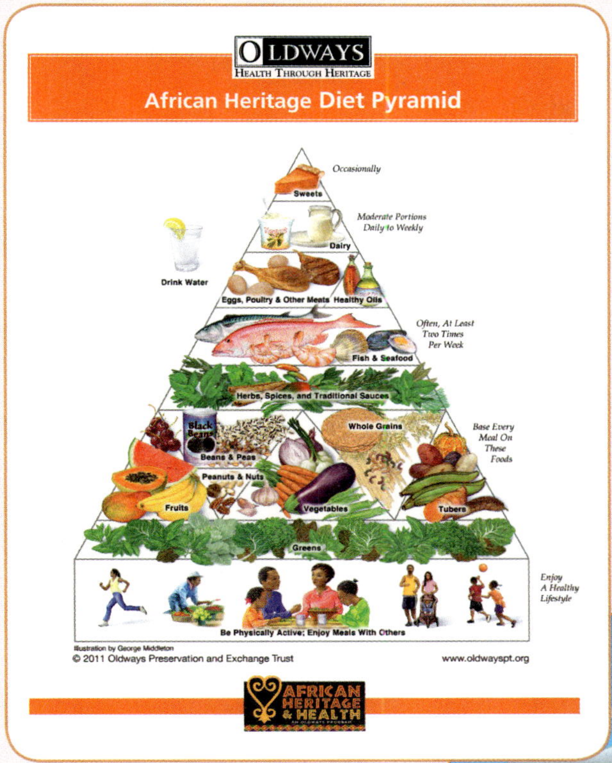

FIGURE 2.12 Compare the *African Heritage Diet Pyramid* and *The Vegan Food Pyramid.* How is each guide similar to, and different from, *Canada's Food Guide*?

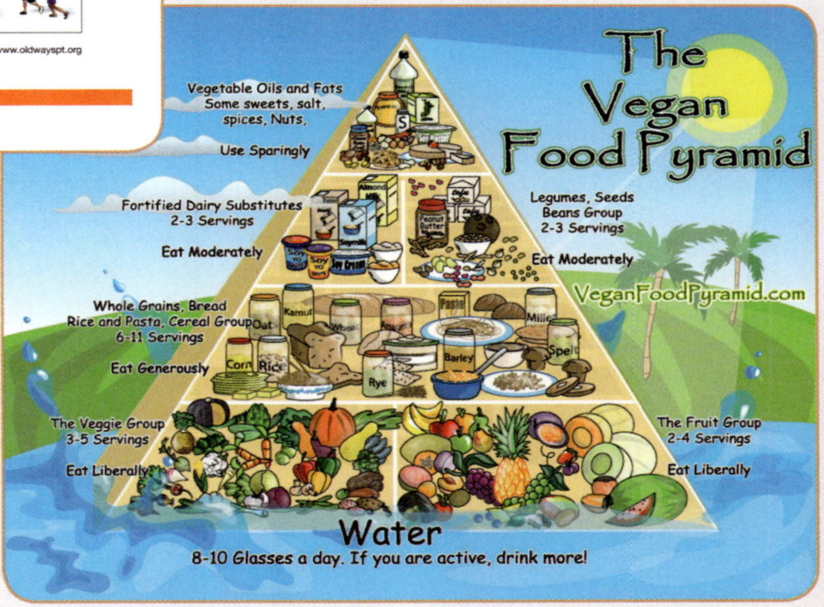

Questions:

1. Compare and contrast the food guidelines produced by the United States, Australia, and Canada. Identify strengths and weaknesses of each guideline.
2. Look at *Spotlight On...* on page 33. What questions could you ask to evaluate the reliability of each guideline pictured above?

NUTRITION LITERACY

Health Canada has developed a detailed list of nutrients in hundreds of common foods. You can download *Nutrient Value of Some Common Foods*, or order a print copy.

Nutrition Messages Found in Food Guidelines

Eating Well with Canada's Food Guide includes many important nutrition messages. These include the nutrients found in various types of foods, as well as recommendations for choosing healthy foods and healthy amounts of foods.

Nutrients

Foods are classified into groups based on the nutrients that those foods provide, as well as how the food has traditionally been classified. Since no single food group provides all the nutrients the body needs, it is important that people eat a variety of foods from each food group every day. However, the foods in each food group tend to supply some similar key nutrients. **Figure 2.15** shows which major nutrients are found in significant amounts in each food group.

Even within a food group, some foods are a better choice than others. Foods that are nutrient dense are higher in a variety of nutrients, while relatively lower in Calories. Health Canada recommends that nutrient-dense foods should be eaten more often. In practice, this can mean choosing whole grains instead of refined grains and whole fruits instead of fruit juice. Other foods are **energy dense**. These foods provide a lot of Calories (energy) relative to their size. Fats and refined grains are energy dense. While they do supply some nutrients, consuming large quantities of them may lead to weight gain and/ or nutrient deficiencies. By eating foods that are less energy dense and more nutrient dense, people can obtain all the nutrients they need and eat a larger volume of food, but consume fewer total Calories. For example, for roughly the same number of Calories, a person could choose a burger or vegetable soup and a turkey sandwich. Some foods are considered empty-Calorie foods. These foods include no significant nutrients other than fat, sodium, and sugar, and often contain a high number of calories. The consumption of empty-Calorie foods should be limited.

energy dense: describes the relationship between the caloric value of a food and its size, weight, or volume. A food that is energy dense will have a larger Calorie content, while a food that is not energy dense will have fewer Calories relative to the amount of food.

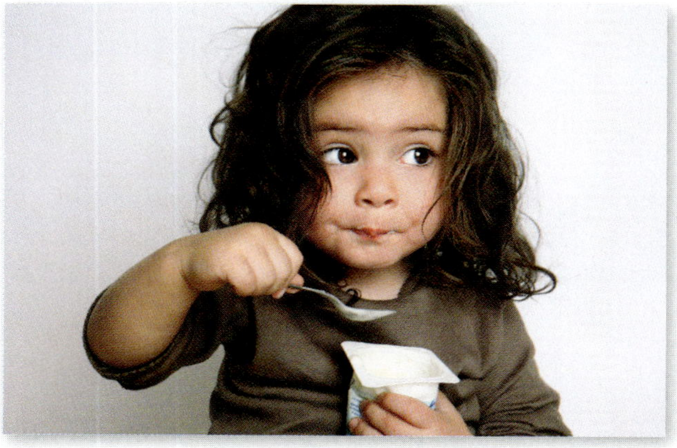

FIGURE 2.13 While all foods provide nutrients, they can be classified as nutrient dense, energy dense, or empty Calorie. How would you categorize this yogurt? Why?

Nutrients in Significant Amounts in Each Food Group

Nutrient	Vegetables and Fruit	Grain Products	Milk and Alternatives	Meat and Alternatives
Carbohydrates	X	X		
Fibre	X	X		
Protein			X	X
Fat			X	X
Vitamin A	X		X	
Vitamin B — Niacin		X		X
Thiamine		X		
Riboflavin		X	X	X
Folacin/Folic Acid	X	X		X
Vitamin B_6	X			X
Vitamin B_{12}			X	X
Vitamin C	X			
Vitamin D	X		X	
Calcium			X	
Iron		X		X
Magnesium	X	X	X	X
Potassium	X	X	X	X
Zinc		X	X	X

FIGURE 2.14 How can you use the information in this table to plan healthy meals?

THINK CRITICALLY

1. What types of carbohydrates are likely to be supplied by the Vegetables and Fruits group?
2. Categorize each food listed below as nutrient dense, energy dense, or empty Calorie. Discuss your answers with the class and compare results.

Raisins	Cheddar cheese	Salami
Salad	Apple juice	Granola
Rye bread	Chocolate bar	Olive oil

3. List three commonly available empty-Calorie foods.

TIP for Healthy Living

When choosing a breakfast cereal, look for one that is high in fibre, but low in added sugar. If you want it to be sweeter, add nutrient-dense fruit.

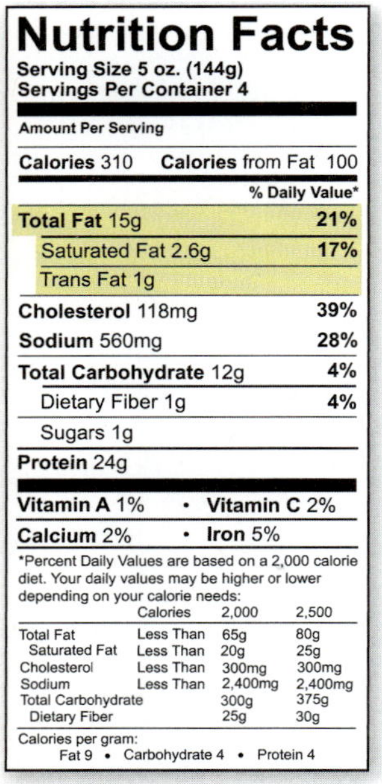

FIGURE 2.15 You can use the information on Nutrition Facts labels to control your intake of saturated and trans fats. What advice would you give to a friend who is using a nutrition label to determine whether a food is healthy?

percentage daily value (% daily value): listed on nutrient fact labels, it provides the percent of an average daily healthy diet that a particular nutrient provides

Other Recommendations

While selecting foods from all four food groups is important, other habits also play a significant role in health. For example, the way you prepare a food can make it more or less nutritious. *Eating Well with Canada's Food Guide* makes several recommendations that will help you maintain good health.

Choose Oils and Fats Carefully

As you have previously learned, fat is a nutrient, and an essential part of our daily diet. Approximately 25 percent of Canadians have a higher fat intake than is recommended (Health Canada, 2011). *Eating Well with Canada's Food Guide* advises people to limit the amount of oils and fats they consume each day, and, wherever possible, to choose unsaturated fats, such as canola, olive, and soybean oils. Unsaturated fats promote a healthy heart, optimal cholesterol levels, and general good health. Even though Canadians are encouraged to consume some unsaturated fats, they are cautioned to limit the amount they consume. Health Canada's recommendation is to consume no more than 30–45 mL (2–3 tbsp) of added fat per day used in the preparation and serving of food.

As you have learned in Chapter 1, by reading labels on packaged food, it is possible to determine the **percentage daily value (% daily value)** of the various types of fats, as well as other nutrients, in a food product. The Heart and Stroke Foundation recommends that approximately 20 percent to 35 percent of your daily Calories should come from fat. For an adult female, this means 45–75 g of fat per day. For a male, this means 60–105 g per day. Health Canada recommends keeping consumption of saturated fats as low as possible and limiting trans fat consumption to no more than one percent of total daily Calories.

Limit Consumption of Certain Beverages

Many people associate Calories only with food, and forget that they can drink their Calories as well. Studies show that between the ages of one and 18, children consume up to 20 percent of their daily Calories in liquid form (Statistics Canada, 2004a). The percent for adults is only slightly less (Statistics Canada, 2004b). Health professionals, however, suggest that no more than 10 percent of our daily Calories should come from beverages (Popkin et al., 2006). In fact, researchers have found that the greater the percent of daily Calories a person consumed in beverages, the more likely that person was to gain weight (Malik, Schulze, & Hu, 2006). They theorize that people's bodies do not recognize Calories in beverages in the same way that they recognize Calories from solid food. If a person eats more food than usual, he or she usually compensates by eating less food later in the day. However, if a person consumes more Calories through beverages, he or she does not make the same adjustment, leading to the consumption of more total Calories, and ultimately resulting in weight gain.

Because of this, *Eating Well with Canada's Food Guide*, like most other food guides, emphasizes that water is often the best beverage choice, but recognizes that low-fat milk products, in moderation, can also be healthy choices. It cautions people to limit consumption of sweetened hot and cold drinks, sports drinks, and alcohol, since these are much higher in Calories.

Energy Drinks

Energy drinks, which frequently contain significant levels of caffeine and sugar, are marketed as convenient ways to increase or maintain energy that can be used for studying, sports, or a late night. Since these products contain more caffeine than is recommended for youth, and since they have been linked with health risks including seizures and heart problems, health professionals have issued frequent warnings about the safety of these beverages for young people (Seifert, Schaechter, Hershorin, & Lipshultz, 2011). Due to the fact that adolescents' bodies are changing rapidly and not everyone is the same size, it becomes difficult to determine how much or how little of an energy drink is safe for young people to consume. Another major concern is the combination of energy drinks with alcohol. The energy drink may mask the effect of the alcohol, preventing people from realizing how intoxicated they really are. As a result of these concerns, some health professionals have called for the sale of energy drinks to be regulated for adults, and banned for children and adolescents.

In Canada, these drinks are not banned for youth. Instead, they are now classified as food products, which means that their ingredients and nutrition information must be listed on the container. Maximum allowable limits of caffeine have been imposed—100 mg per 250 mL of energy drink—and limits have been placed on the amount of vitamins and minerals that can be added to a beverage. Manufacturers are now required to state on the label that the drinks should not be combined with alcohol and include warnings cautioning children and pregnant women not to consume energy drinks.

OPEN FOR DEBATE

Debate in class the following statement: "The sale of energy drinks to adolescents and children should be banned."

Be Active

While it is important to eat a balanced diet, it is also important to couple food intake with exercise. Physical activity helps to

- maintain an appropriate weight
- build and maintain strong muscles and bones
- reduce risk of disease, including type 2 diabetes, cardiovascular disease, and certain cancers
- maintain mental health

(Downs & Ashton, 2011)

"Those who think they have not time for bodily exercise will sooner or later have to find time for illness."

– Edward Stanley, Third Earl of Derby

Recommendations for being active are an important part of *Eating Well with Canada's Food Guide*. People of all ages are encouraged to exercise daily. Ideally, adults should get between 30 and 60 minutes of moderate to vigorous exercise per day, while children should have at least 60 minutes per day. As with food intake, people are encouraged to incorporate a variety of physical activities into their lives.

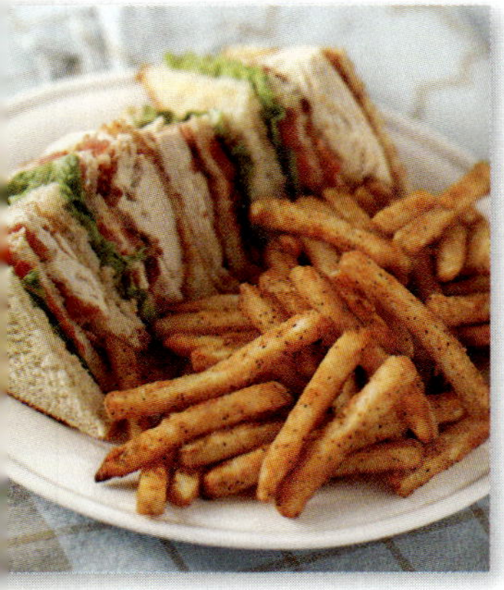

FIGURE 2.16 Are these serving sizes appropriate? How can people learn about appropriate serving and portion sizes of the food they consume?

Be Aware of Serving Size

Portion sizes of foods vary considerably, but average portion sizes have increased in the past 20 years (Alpert, 2012). As a result, many people are unaware of what an accurate serving size is. They are eating more food than they may realize, consuming more Calories, and gaining weight. The serving sizes recommended by Health Canada may seem small to some, but they reflect the number of Calories and amounts of nutrients needed for optimal health and weight control. Too often, portion sizes served at restaurants and in homes are much larger than the sizes Health Canada recommends. In addition, people may read a nutrition label and assume that it is for the entire package of food, not realizing that the package may contain more than one serving. This leads to confusion about the amount of food eaten, and people often end up eating more food than they believe they are eating.

Use Healthy Methods to Prepare Food

While an individual ingredient or food may be considered "healthy," the way it is prepared or served can diminish its healthiness. If a food is prepared with large amounts of fat by breading or frying, or served with large amounts of sodium in the form of prepared sauces or garnishes, it is not as healthy as it looks. By changing cooking methods and altering recipes, the nutritional value of foods can be improved.

NUTRITION LITERACY

Develop personal benchmarks for appropriate portion sizes. For example, one serving of meat is about the size of a deck of cards. One serving of fruit is a little smaller than your fist. You can use these benchmarks to monitor portion sizes.

THINK CRITICALLY

1. Jarred buys an iced coffee every morning. He is a long-distance runner so he feels he can justify consuming the extra Calories and fat. Is his reasoning sound? Why or why not?
2. Although French fries and potato chips are made of potatoes, most food guides do not count one serving of French fries as a serving of vegetables. Why?
3. Using secondary sources, describe the healthiest ways to cook a chicken. Describe methods that can be used to cook a whole chicken, and also to cook its various parts (e.g., breast, thighs, drumsticks, and organ meats). Explain why you chose each method.

Active Learning

Determining the Healthiest Beverage

The consumption of some beverages is related to weight gain. Below are five beverages along with their nutrition information.

Nutrition Information for Five Popular Beverages

Figure 2.17 These beverages contain widely different amounts and combinations of nutrients.	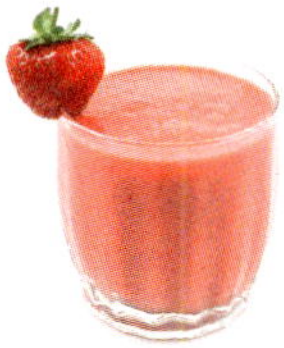 Banana-berry smoothie (250 mL)	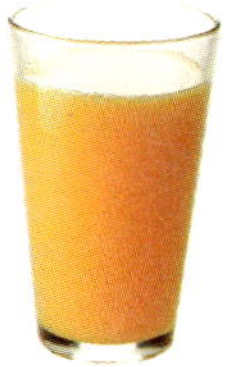 Orange juice (250 mL)	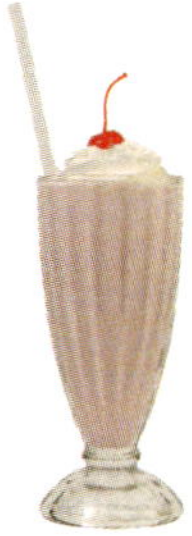 Strawberry milkshake (400 mL)	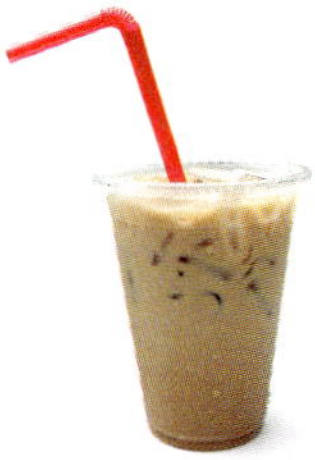 Iced coffee (350 mL)	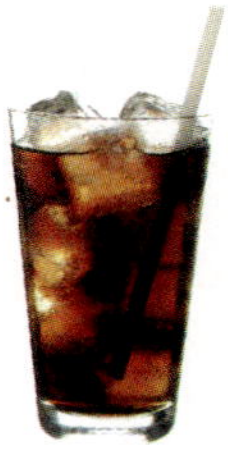 Cola (355 mL)
Calories	180	112	560	120	136
Carbohydrate	42 g	26 g	79 g	16 g	35 g
Fibre	0 g	0 g	0 g	0 g	0 g
Protein	2 g	2 g	10 g	1 g	0 g
Lipids	1 g	0 g	26 g	6 g	0 g
Saturated fat	0 g	0 g	16 g	4 g	0 g
Unsaturated fat	0 g	0 g	10 g	0 g	0 g
Trans fat	0 g	0 g	0 g	0 g	0 g
Vitamin A	55 IU	496 IU	500 IU	260 IU	0 g
Vitamin C	6 mg	224 mg	0 g	0 g	0 g
Calcium	68 mg	27 mg	350 mg	20 mg	7 mg
Sodium	55 mg	2 mg	250 mg	35 mg	15 mg

Activities:

1. As a class, determine criteria that you can use to determine which beverage is the healthiest (for example, Calories, fat, sugar, or other nutrients).
2. On your own, use the information provided to determine which beverage is the healthiest. Be prepared to justify your choice. For which beverage did you find the results most surprising?

TIP for Healthy Living

In some cases, an easy way to modify the nutritional content of a meal is to serve a smaller portion of an energy-dense food, with an accompaniment that includes missing nutrients. For example, you can serve a small portion of lasagna with a large salad (with light dressing) and fruit.

FINANCIAL LITERACY

Determine the total cost and per-serving cost of The lasagna recipe on page 53. If you managed a restaurant, what price would you charge per portion for this lasagna, considering that food costs typically make up 30 percent of the price of an item on a menu? Do you think people would pay more for a healthier food choice?

pulses:
dried seeds from certain pod-bearing plants, such as lentils, kidney beans, and chickpeas

Adapting and Revising Recipes

By modifying ingredients, cooking methods, and serving sizes, many recipes can be adapted to better fit within the recommendations of *Eating Well with Canada's Food Guide*. When modifying recipes, remember that ingredients have a culinary purpose, so simply reducing amounts or omitting ingredients from a recipe may not result in the desired outcome. Therefore, recipes should be tested to assess any modifications made.

These tips can help you modify recipes successfully:

To reduce fat

- reduce the amount of added fat in recipes, especially butter and oils for cooking
- use reduced-fat versions of ingredients such as milk and cheese
- trim visible fats from meats, and choose lower-fat meat options such as extra-lean ground beef or ground turkey
- replace high-fat cooking methods such as frying and deep-frying with methods such as baking, grilling, and poaching

To reduce salt

- replace salt with herbs, spices, and other seasonings
- use lower-sodium versions of processed foods

To reduce sugar

- reduce the sugar content slightly
- replace up to one quarter of the sugar with applesauce or other fruit purée when baking

To increase fibre

- replace some or all flour with whole-grain flour
- use brown rice and whole-wheat or other whole-grain pasta
- add vegetables, fruit, **pulses** and whole grains to recipes

To decrease caloric value

- reduce serving size
- reduce amounts of high-Calorie ingredients such as meat and milk products in recipe

ACTIVE LEARNING

Adapt a Recipe

You can use the recommendations in *Eating Well with Canada's Food Guide* to make recipes healthier without significantly changing the taste of the product.

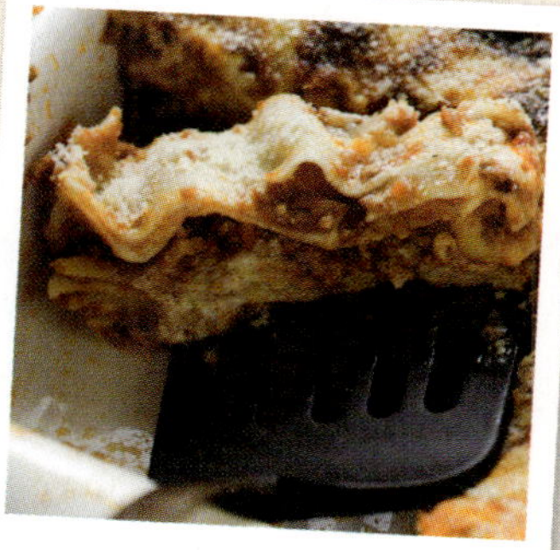

FIGURE 2.18 Beef and pork ragù lasagna

Beef and Pork Ragù Lasagna

Yield: 4–6 servings

Ingredients

1 recipe ragù sauce

1 recipe cream sauce

150 g oven ready lasagna pasta

125 mL (½ c) grated Parmesan cheese

Ragù Sauce

45 mL (4 tbsp) butter or margarine

30 mL (2 tbsp) olive or vegetable oil

1 medium celery stalk, finely chopped

1 medium carrot, peeled and finely chopped

1 small yellow onion, finely chopped

500 g (1 lb) ground meat (beef, pork, lamb, chicken, turkey)

250 mL (1 c) broth (beef, chicken, vegetable) (first amount)

125 mL (½ c) tomato sauce

250 mL (1 c) broth (beef, chicken, vegetable) (second amount)

125 mL (½ c) milk

Salt and Pepper

Method

1. Melt butter or margarine in a large, heavy saucepan over medium heat. Add oil.
2. Add celery, carrots, and onions, coating the vegetables with the fats. Stir occasionally, until softened and lightly golden, about 10–15 min.
3. Add the ground meat, breaking up the meat using a wooden spoon. Stir frequently until the meat is well cooked, 6–8 min.
4. Stir in the broth (first amount) and the tomato sauce. Simmer uncovered over medium heat until the liquid has almost evaporated, 10–15 min.
5. Reduce the heat to low.
6. Add the second amount of broth and the milk. Stir well. Simmer gently to produce a rich sauce, approximately 1 h. Stir well occasionally, adding more liquid, if needed, to prevent scorching.
7. Season with salt and pepper.
8. Skim fat, if necessary.

Recipe continues on next page.

continued from previous page

Beef and Pork Ragù Lasagna

Cream Sauce

15 mL (1 tbsp) butter or margarine
15 mL (1 tbsp) all-purpose flour
250 mL (1 c) milk, warmed
1 mL (¼ tsp) salt
pinch black pepper
pinch nutmeg

Method

1. Melt butter or margarine in a medium-sized saucepan over medium-low heat. Add the flour and cook, stirring constantly with a small whisk for 1–2 min.
2. Slowly whisk in the warmed milk. Whisk frequently until the sauce has thickened, 6–8 min.
3. Remove from heat and whisk in salt, pepper, and nutmeg.

To Assemble

1. Heat oven to 350 °F (180 °C).
2. Grease a 23 x 30 cm (9 x 12") baking dish.
3. Spread a thin layer of ragù sauce on the bottom of the baking dish.
4. Cover with a layer of lasagna pasta.
5. Spread about one-third of the remaining ragù sauce over the pasta.
6. Drizzle about one-third of the cream sauce over the ragù sauce. Sprinkle with Parmesan cheese.
7. Add a new layer of lasagna pasta and repeat with layers of the ragù sauce, cream sauce and Parmesan. There should be about three layers, in total.
8. Cover tightly with tin foil. Place baking dish on a baking sheet. Bake for about 45 minutes or until pasta is cooked and sauces are bubbling at the edges.
9. Remove from the oven and let rest 10–15 minutes before serving.

Adapt a Recipe

1. Using the tips on page 52 as a guideline, adapt the recipe for beef and pork ragù lasagna so that it better supports the recommendations of *Eating Well with Canada's Food Guide*. Fully justify the decisions that you have made.
2. As an extension, you may choose to prepare the recipe, making adjustments as necessary.

Working with Food Guides

The **RDA (Recommended Dietary Allowance)** refers to dietary reference intake, the minimum levels of nutrients needed daily to satisfy health requirements. These allowances are different for each nutrient and vary among age and gender groups, so *Eating Well with Canada's Food Guide* recommends different numbers of servings for different population groups. Because it is difficult for the average Canadian to calculate the amount of every nutrient consumed each day, *Eating Well with Canada's Food Guide* uses food groups and serving sizes to provide an easier way to make healthy food choices.

RDA (Recommended Dietary Allowance): the minimum levels of nutrients needed daily by different groups to satisfy health requirements

Making Changes to Canada's Food Guide

As researchers learn more about nutrients and their role in health, RDAs are updated and *Canada's Food Guide* is revised. Current scientific knowledge and stakeholder feedback are both used to make and change recommendations to the number of servings, suggested food choices, and other food and activity recommendations in *Eating Well with Canada's Food Guide*. A wide variety of stakeholders are consulted in order to revise *Eating Well with Canada's Food Guide*, including health professionals, educators, the food industry, and the general public. Health Canada analyzes and evaluates the input from all of these groups before revising the guide.

Pause and Think
How has the current edition of *Eating Well with Canada's Food Guide* incorporated and highlighted new knowledge about fat, fibre, sodium, and sugar?

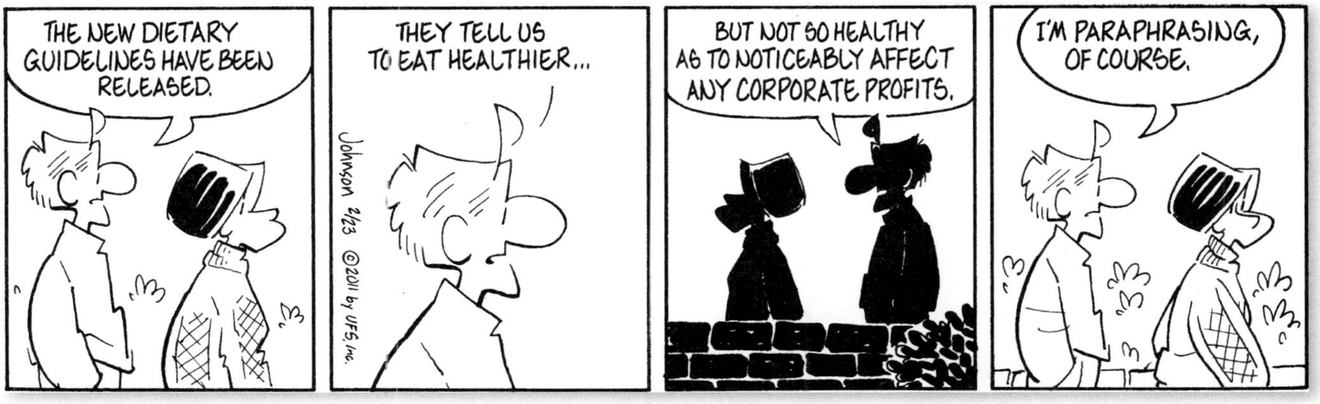

FIGURE 2.19 Analyze this cartoon. Why might some people believe that food industry groups do not want the public to eat too healthily?

Trends and Change

Which salt is healthier?

Many types of salt are available to us. While different salts might come from different sources, salts are generally a combination of two minerals: sodium and chloride. These minerals form the chemical compound *sodium chloride*. Salt may also contain some trace minerals, depending on where it was obtained. As we focus more and more on the sodium content of food, it is reasonable to ask: is there a type of salt that is a healthier choice?

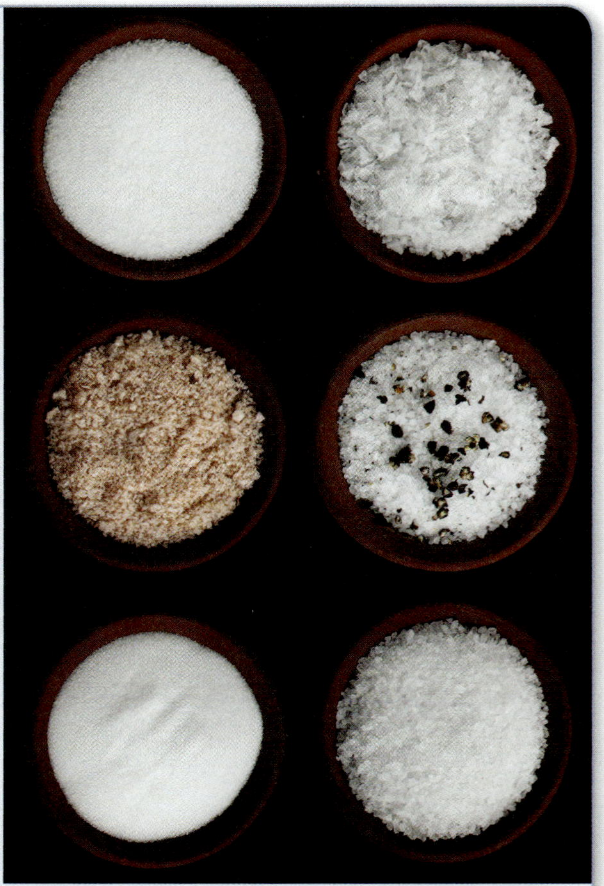

Figure 2.20 Various types of salt: sea salt, smoked sea salt, and table salt. Canadians consume twice the recommended intake of salt. Which foods do you eat that are high in salt?

Types of Salt

Table salt is a fine-grained salt that comes from salt mines. The mineral iodine was added to table salt in the 1920s to prevent goitre (an enlarged thyroid gland), which was a health concern in parts of North America. Even though iodine deficiency is no longer a problem, the majority of table salt is still iodized. Table salt is almost completely sodium chloride.

Sea salt is made from evaporated seawater. Unrefined sea salt contains mostly sodium chloride and a small amount of trace minerals. These minerals can lend distinctive flavours and textures to sea salt, and differ depending on the source of the seawater.

Kosher salt has a coarser grain than table salt and is unrefined. It is normally not iodized. Kosher salt is used to prepare meat according to Jewish dietary regulations, and also in other applications.

Pickling salt is used for brines to make pickled foods. While it has a similar texture to table salt, it doesn't contain iodine or preservatives, which could make a brine cloudy.

As all the salts listed above contain the same amount of sodium, about 2300 mg per teaspoon, no one type is healthier than another. A healthy adult requires only 1500 mg of sodium per day.

Questions:

1. For what applications might people use sea salt?
2. For what applications might a coarse-grained salt be preferable?

Promoting Food Guides

Since the goal of food guides is to help people make healthy food decisions, people need to be able to access the guides easily. Creators make food guides available in a variety of ways. For example, Health Canada has translated *Eating Well with Canada's Food Guide* into 10 languages in addition to English and French, so that more people are able to access the content of the guide. Health Canada has included foods commonly eaten by some ethnic groups in the guide, and has made free print copies of the guide available to Canadians. As a result, *Eating Well with Canada's Food Guide* is Canada's second most requested government document.

Those responsible for educating others about nutrition, including dietitians, teachers, and community-based or other educators, also have access to a wide variety of teaching materials. Health Canada provides visuals and lessons that they can use to help teach groups about making healthy food choices, in addition to teaching groups about *Eating Well with Canada's Food Guide*, *Eating Well with Canada's Food Guide—First Nations, Inuit, and Métis*, and the *Nunavut Food Guide*. Provincial health agencies have also created age-appropriate educational materials and lesson plans targeted to various age groups.

Technology plays an important role in the promotion of food guides. In addition to print copies, many countries have posted their food guides online, thus making them available not just to people within their country, but to those in other locations as well. Some countries have also created computer-based programs that allow consumers to interact with their food guides so that they can see accurate serving sizes and create personalized versions of the food guide. As you have seen, non-governmental groups produce food guides as well. While print copies of non-governmental guides may only be available for purchase, online versions are often free. As these guides may be specifically targeted to a segment of the population (for example, vegetarians), creators may need to work directly with their intended audience in order to promote their guides.

Skills Focus

Check the questions you develop for your survey in *Active Learning* to make sure the answers will provide specific information that you can analyze and use. Focussed questions like "How many servings of fruits and vegetables should you eat every day?" generally provide more useful data than open-ended questions like "How can you choose a balanced diet?" Then check them again to make sure they are free of bias—that is, that they don't seem to favour one answer over another.

Active Learning

Developing a Marketing Strategy

Good advertising messages are well researched in order to reach their intended audience. In order to determine how to sell an idea or product, advertisers first need to investigate the needs of their intended audience. They then use the results of their research to effectively create a marketing strategy targeted to their audience. Following the strategies on the next page, conduct research to create a strategy to market *Eating Well with Canada's Food Guide* to adolescents. Then you will carry out your marketing strategy and evaluate it.

continued on next page

continued from previous page

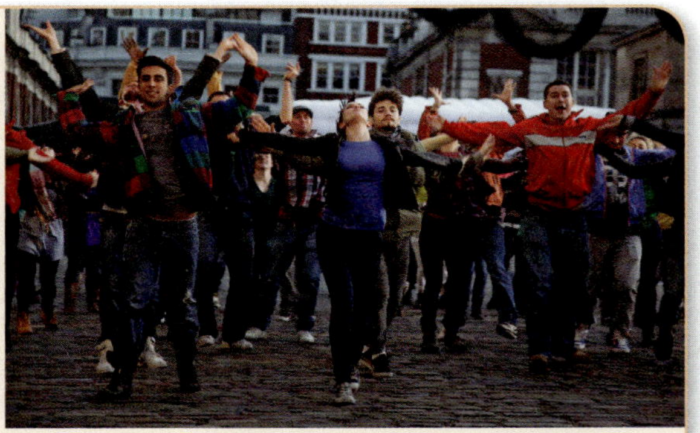

FIGURE 2.21 Social media has become an important part of marketing. How can social media be used to market *Eating Well with Canada's Food Guide*?

Step One: Survey the Intended Audience Surveys or questionnaires are quick ways to determine what knowledge a population has about an idea, product, or service. Within your school or another population, survey adolescents to determine what they know about the recommendations in *Eating Well with Canada's Food Guide*. You may choose to conduct your survey online or face-to-face.

Determine Appropriate Questions for Survey

Include questions in your survey that will help reveal what adolescents do and don't know about the food guide, as well as revealing their perceptions or beliefs about it.

Develop your Marketing Message

From the data you collect, establish the important and unique messages about *Eating Well with Canada's Food Guide* that need to be conveyed to your target group.

Step Two: Study your Target Market As a group, what do adolescents enjoy? How do they learn about things? Focus on marketing techniques that would be most appropriate and effective for teenagers. For example, would adolescents be more likely to listen to a spokesperson, or is a word-of-mouth campaign a better way to spread your message? Would technology help to spread your message, or would a different approach be more successful?

Step Three: Create a Marketing Strategy Choose a strategy, develop the materials you will need, and use the strategy for a specific period of time (e.g., one week, one month). You may use more than one communication technique. Examples of marketing techniques include the following:

Broadcast commercials or advertorials
Graphics such as posters
Parties or other gatherings
Flash mobs or other performances
Contests
Apps or other technological tools

Step Four: Test your Strategy and Elicit Feedback from your Target Audience Was your strategy successful? In what ways has your audience's understanding of healthy eating increased?

Questions:

1. Consider what you discovered adolescents know and do not know about *Eating Well with Canada's Food Guide*. How can you use this information to plan an effective marketing strategy?
2. How effective was your marketing strategy? What would you change to more effectively promote the strategies for healthy eating in *Eating Well with Canada's Food Guide*?

Regulations

Federal and provincial governments have passed regulations for food products. Regulations help protect consumers, and help combat health issues such as obesity. For example, the Canadian Food Inspection Agency has regulations about the composition of food (for example, what can and cannot be included in salad dressing). The government also has detailed regulations about how food can be marketed and advertised, including the use of terms such as *organic* and *natural*. You will learn more about how these terms can be used in Chapter 6. These regulations may change with time: as new information about the role of nutrients in the body becomes available, and as new health concerns are raised by health professionals and the public, new regulations may be passed and existing regulations may be amended. Food manufacturers, packagers, and marketers must be sure they understand the current regulations and follow them.

Trans Fat Recommendations

While the amount of fat that people consume has increased over time, the type of fat in foods has also changed. Trans fats are modified fats that are used to give processed foods certain desirable characteristics. However, trans fats play a negative role in our health, increasing the risk of coronary heart disease and raising insulin resistance. As a result, all nutrition labels must state the amount of trans fat in the food. The federal government created a Trans Fat Task Force to examine how to reduce and eventually eliminate the trans fats in foods. In 2007, the Minister of Health adopted two recommendations of the Trans Fat Task Force: that companies limit to two percent the total amount of trans fat in margarines, oils, and spreads; and limit trans fat to five percent in other foods. These recommendations apply not only to foods available at stores, but also to foods served in restaurants and other food service establishments. These trans fat limits are not regulations; they are only recommendations. The government has set up a monitoring program to monitor how well these recommendations are being followed. Nutrition Facts on labels must also indicate the amount of trans fat in a food product. British Columbia has developed provincial regulations to enforce the trans fat limits described above.

TIP for Healthy Living

To limit trans fats when you eat in a restaurant, avoid appetizers such as chicken wings and cheese sticks, any foods that are fried in shortening or margarine, and pastries.

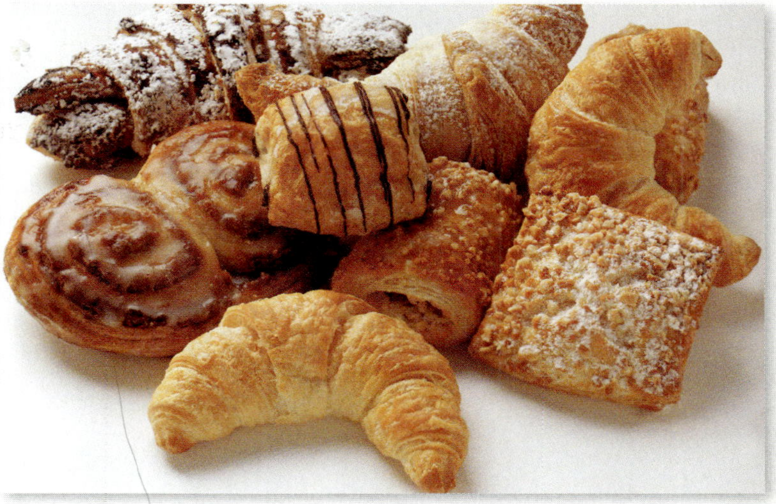

FIGURE 2.22 Trans fats can make baked goods more tender and flaky, and help preserve shelf life.

School Nutrition Policies

Studies have shown that students who have healthy diets have improved brain function, are more able to concentrate, and are better able to learn (Alaimo, Olson, & Frongillo, 2001). Schools often provide meals for students at lunch, and often breakfast as well. For some students, school meals are the only meals they eat. For other students, school meals are the only healthy meals that they eat in a day.

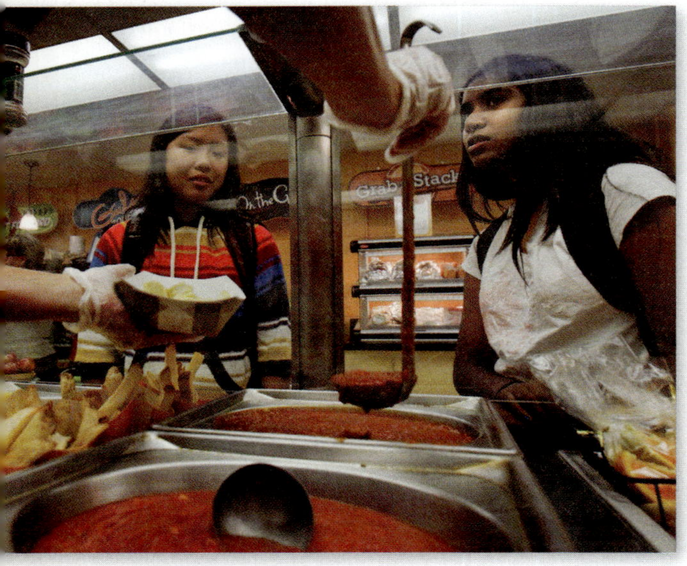

FIGURE 2.23 Some schools in other countries require that all students eat lunch prepared by the school. Do you believe this would help or hinder students' access to nutritious food?

As schools often have limited funds for feeding students, cost may receive more attention than nutrition. In addition, to raise funds, many schools have entered into contracts with snack-food providers, who insist that their brands of often-unhealthy drinks and snacks be available to students in vending machines and in cafeterias. Educators, nutritionists, and the public increasingly believe that schools should be required to provide healthy food choices for students. Schools are under increasing pressure to ensure that healthy options are made available.

Many provinces have now enacted school nutrition guidelines created in consultation with nutrition and health professionals, and are based on *Eating Well with Canada's Food Guide* as well as the Trans Fat Task Force recommendations. In British Columbia, school food guidelines are mandatory.

School nutrition policies often share the following goals:

- Increase amounts of fibre and reduce amounts of processed grains
- Increase amounts of vegetables and fruit
- Reduce amount of fat, especially trans fat; some provinces, such as Ontario, have banned trans fat in foods sold in schools
- Promote water as a preferred beverage
- Reduce added sugar, salt, and caffeine
- Increase attention to serving sizes

"More must be done to invest in an all-round food education for our kids—one that includes learning about where food comes from and how it's grown as well as the hands-on experience of cooking in the classroom."

– Jamie Oliver
(*Feed Me Even Better*, 2011)

THINK CRITICALLY

1. What healthy options are available to you for lunch at school?
2. What healthy options are available for lunch at home?
3. How often do you choose the options you listed in Questions 1 and 2?

POINT OF VIEW

Advertising Food and Beverages to Children

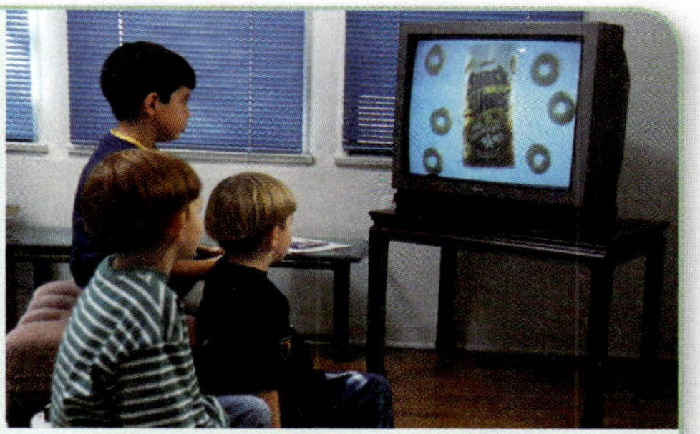

FIGURE 2.24 Children are more vulnerable to marketing messages than adults. To what extent should governments play a role in determining what advertising is acceptable for children?

Advertising directly to children is a controversial topic. Advertisers and marketers know that in later life, people adhere to brand choices they made as children, so they have strong incentive to market food products to young people. Food companies sometimes give away toys and cartoon figures, and have even created their own television programs to help get the message out about their food products to children. Meanwhile, psychologists know that many children cannot tell the difference between what is real life and what is an advertising pitch.

Canada has regulations about advertising food and making health claims related to food, both in Health Canada's *Food and Drugs Act* and in the Canadian Food Inspection Agency's *Guide to Food Labelling and Advertising*, However, Canada currently has no laws about advertising food products directly to children. In 2007, a group of food and beverage companies created a voluntary set of guidelines aimed at protecting children. Called the Canadian Children's Food and Beverage Advertising Initiative, these guidelines aim to ensure that children are being informed about healthy food and beverage options. These voluntary guidelines apply to all traditional forms of media (television, print, and radio), as well as to video/computer games, mobile applications, and company Web sites.

According to these voluntary guidelines, all foods and beverages advertised directly to children must be healthy choices. To be considered healthy, the food or beverage must meet and follow the principles of *Eating Well with Canada's Food Guide* or the Canadian Heart and Stroke Foundation's Health Check™ program. Unhealthy foods can still be advertised, but not to children. Furthermore, foods and beverages cannot be advertised in elementary schools. Each year, the Initiative publishes a compliance report, detailing to what extent the guidelines are being followed by each company that is a part of the Initiative.

Questions:

1. What would be some benefits and drawbacks of an industry choosing to self-regulate, rather than follow government-imposed regulations?
2. How could a company work around the guidelines if it wanted to advertise unhealthy food and beverages to children?
3. What are the consequences if a company does not follow the guidelines? What do you believe the consequences should be?
4. Do you believe that these guidelines will be effective in helping children to make healthier food choices? Fully explain your answer.
5. The province of Québec, through its 1980 Consumer Protection Act, has had a legislated ban on all advertising directed at children under the age of 13. However, it only covers advertising that was developed in Québec, and excludes advertising that is broadcast from outside the province. Should Québec's model be adopted nationally?

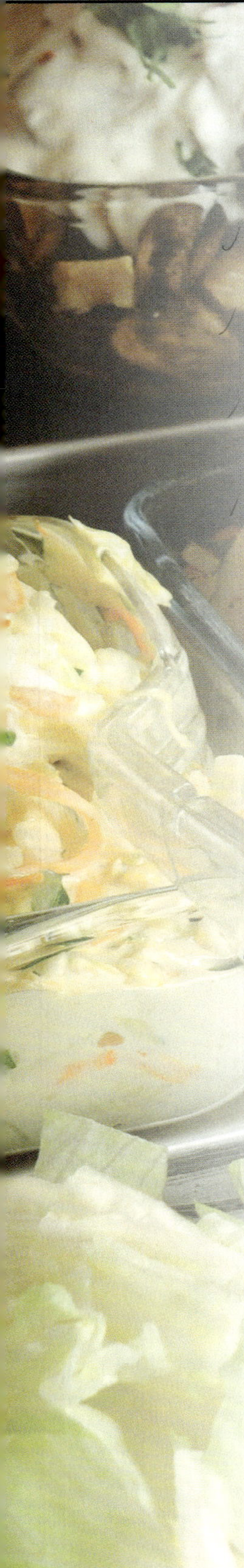

CHAPTER 2 REVIEW

Chapter Review

Knowledge and Understanding/Thinking

1. Your friend believes that everyone should eliminate wheat from his or her diet. Describe the response that you would give to your friend.
2. Why do governments have a vested interest in the health of their citizens? Where should the role of governments end in encouraging healthy diets?
3. In addition to soy products, what other foods are suitable choices for the Milk and Alternatives food group? What qualities make them an appropriate choice for the Milk and Alternatives food group?
4. Why are fish bones given as an example in the Aboriginal food guide? What nutrient do they supply?
5. Identify at least three foods that are not part of the Meat and Alternatives food group that contain iron.
6. You have been told by a health professional that your iron level is low. What foods would help you increase your level of this nutrient?
7. Describe a salmon sandwich that might be considered energy dense. Explain how it could be modified to no longer be energy dense.
8. You would like to revise a recipe for a chocolate cake in order to make it healthier. Explain the factors that you would need to consider when deciding how to revise the recipe.

Thinking/Communication

9. Research some traditional Aboriginal foods in your area. How was each food prepared traditionally? How are these foods prepared now?
10. Plan a menu for yourself for three days that follows *Eating Well with Canada's Food Guide*. Compare this with a menu that follows one of the guidelines shown on pages 44 and 45. Which guideline would you find easier to follow? With which did you feel you were better able to create a balanced and varied menu?
11. Investigate other non-governmental food guides. Compare and contrast them with *Eating Well with Canada's Food Guide*. Include details about key similarities and differences.
12. Research criticisms to *Eating Well with Canada's Food Guide*. Summarize the concerns, and evaluate whether they are credible.

13. Research the symbol used in the background of the *Nunavut Food Guide*. Explain its importance and why it would be used as a graphic on this publication.

14. Compare the rainbow used to represent food groups in *Canada's Food Guide* and the plate used to represent food groups in the United States' *MyPlate* food guide. What are the advantages of each? What are the disadvantages of each? Why might one be more effective than the other?

Communication/Application

15. Create a display to show the difference between portion sizes reflected in *Eating Well with Canada's Food Guide* and common portion sizes seen in restaurants and other food products.

16. Produce an awareness campaign in your school about the levels of sugar or salt in a group of related products (for example, breakfast cereals, packaged soups, beverages, or instant noodles).

17. Investigate to find the food- and beverage-sales guidelines for schools in your province or territory. Plan foods that would be appropriate for a school fundraiser and fit within the guidelines.

18. Find a recipe that would be considered "not recommended" for your province or territory's guidelines for food and beverage sales in schools. Adapt the recipe so that it would be allowed for sale in schools. Test the recipe, commenting on the results of your changes.

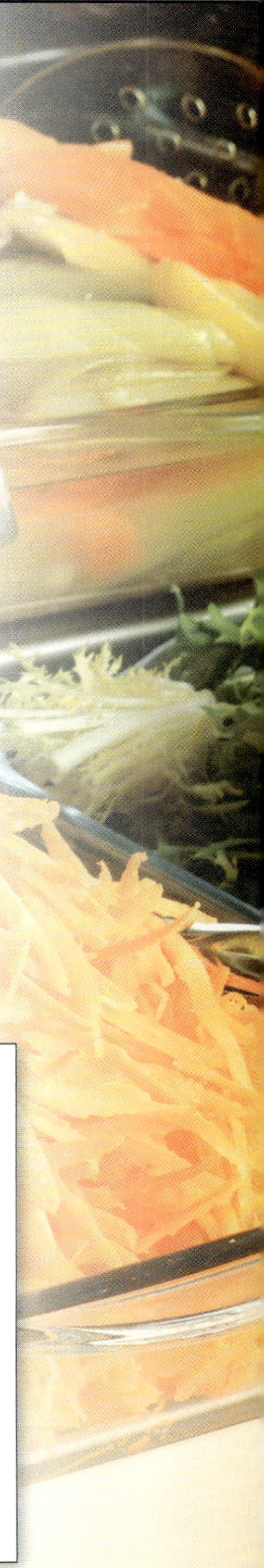

Putting It All Together

In this chapter, you have

- read why food guidelines are developed, and how they are used
- compared a variety of food guidelines
- identified the key nutrients in each food group
- used food guidelines to modify a recipe
- promoted key messages in *Eating Well with Canada's Food Guide* in your school

Create a new food guide that you believe would be an effective resource for Canadians. Describe your model and explain how your features, design, and content will be useful.

Chapter

3

Balanced Eating

Key Terms

absorption
basal metabolic rate
basal metabolism
digestion
gastrointestinal (GI) tract
insulin resistance
intrinsic factor
lipid
peristalsis
portion distortion
sedentary
starvation mode

Research and Inquiry Skills

- Take notes during research

Chapter Introduction

While reading this chapter, you will study

- **the process of digestion, absorption, and metabolism of food**
- **the relationships among macronutrient intake, energy expenditure, and energy balance**
- **various ways of regulating energy balance to achieve and maintain healthy body weight**
- **personal nutrient intake, as it compares to the nutritional status of Canadians**
- **how interests, skills, previous experience, and education requirements relate to a specific career opportunity in the food industry**

The relationships among the energy content of food, physical activity, metabolic processes, and body weight have long been of interest to the public and health experts. During adolescence, energy requirements increase to accommodate growth, but that increased demand slows down as growth slows down. As adolescents approach the end of their growing years and enter their adult lives, they need to consider how their eating habits will affect their energy balance. When people consume a healthy diet that corresponds with their activity levels, or adopt activity levels that correspond to their diets, they can achieve and maintain a healthy weight throughout their lives. In this chapter, you will learn the details of balancing energy intake with energy use.

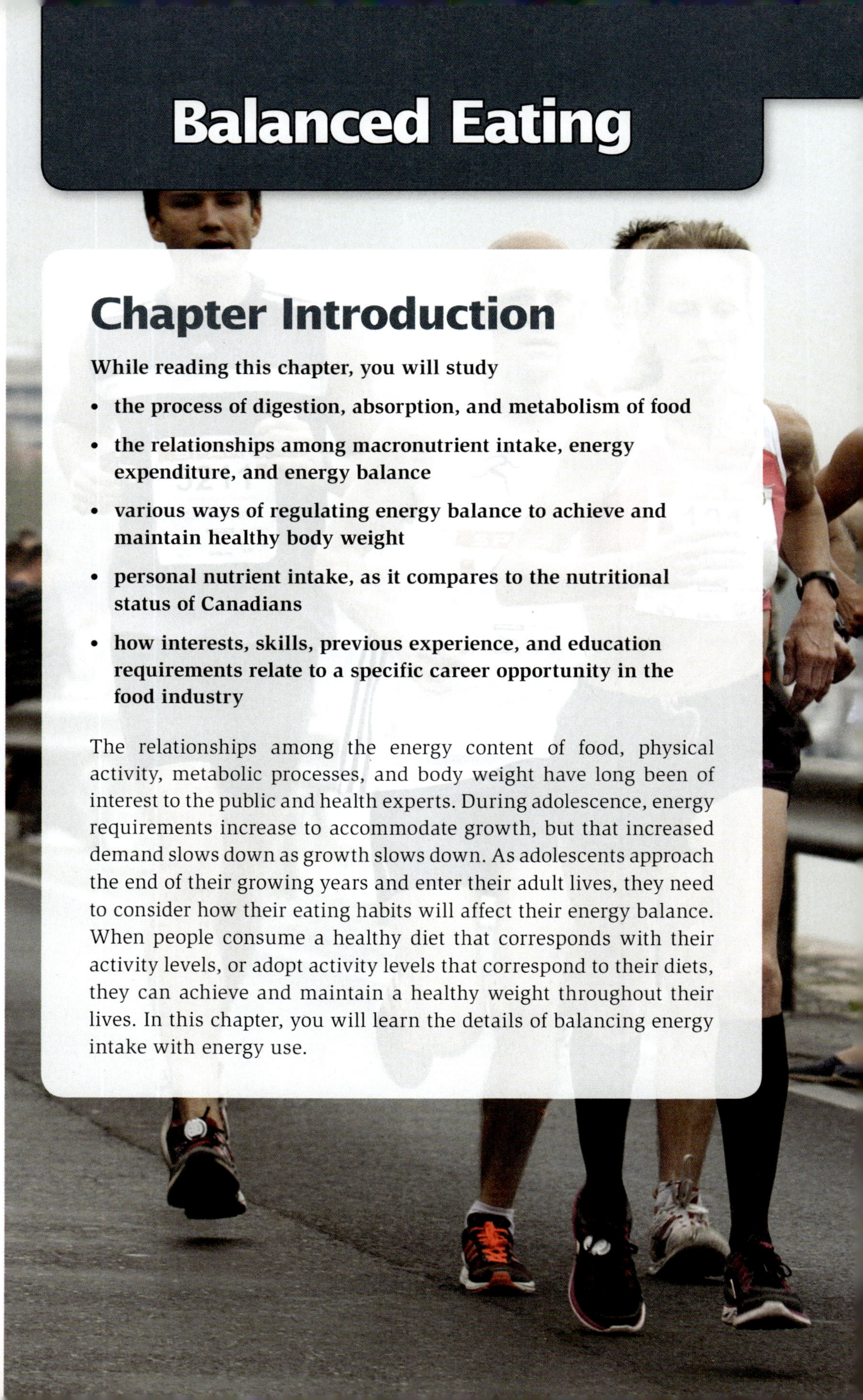

Figure 3.1 Different people have different energy needs. What factors can affect energy balance?

Spotlight On...

Calorie-Restricted Diets

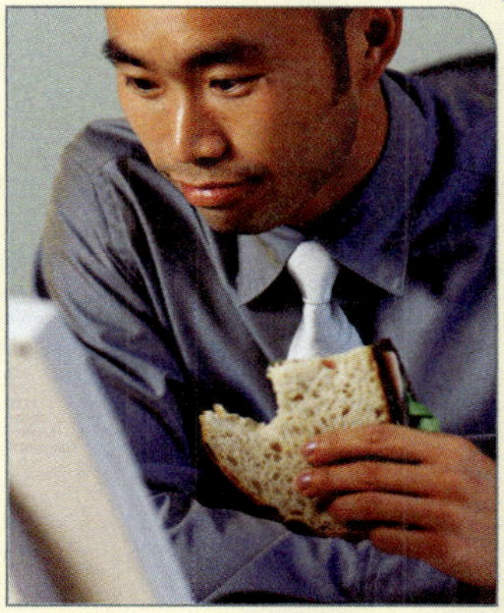

FIGURE 3.2 Learning to pay attention to the body's hunger signals can help achieve energy balance.

Balancing energy consumption and energy use is an important part of healthy eating and of maintaining a healthy weight. People who have been consuming more energy than they use often try to regain a healthy weight by eating a Calorie-restricted diet for a period of time. While most dieters try to eat less, it doesn't always work out that way. Studies have shown that when placed in situations of stress, fatigue, depression, or even exposure to foods not allowed on the diet, people on diets often eat more than non-dieters do. Studies show that dieters also tend to eat more snacks (McCabe, 2012).

One study of men on extremely low-Calorie diets found that they were more likely than the general population to develop behaviours associated with eating disorders, including binge eating. These behaviours persisted even after the diet had ended.

The sad truth is that most dieters eventually regain the weight they lost while on the diet, and even more!

Why does this happen? While no one knows for sure, one area of speculation is that the body attempts to compensate for the period of insufficient energy intake (during the diet) by storing energy in case of famine (EatRight Ontario, 2012). Another possible explanation is that dieters deliberately do not eat when they are hungry, but instead eat when (and how much) they think is appropriate. They teach themselves to use conscious thought to control their eating, rather than feelings of hunger. This allows other thoughts (of anger, boredom, or even simple temptation) to interfere with their good intentions. Overriding the body's natural hunger signals with conscious thought may interfere with the body's ability to sense hunger after the period of dieting is over, helping to explain the weight that is commonly regained.

Today, most health professionals prefer to help people control their food intake by helping them focus on signals of hunger and satiety that their body is sending and teaching them how to respond appropriately, for example by choosing foods that will satisfy their hunger and provide the nutrients they need. There is also a very healthy trend to accepting our bodies and caring for them—by eating healthy foods and being physically active, because these activities both promote health—but not torturing ourselves to be any particular size or shape. Healthy bodies come in a variety of shapes and sizes.

Activities:

1. List reasons why focussing on eating healthy foods and being physically active might be a more successful strategy to develop and maintain a healthy body than dieting would be.
2. Brainstorm reasons why people may go on diets even if they do not result in long-term weight loss.
3. Speculate about what events may work together to cause the phenomenon known as *yo-yo dieting* (a cycle of dieting to lose weight and regaining the weight that was lost). You may wish to present your ideas as a flowchart or web.

Research and Inquiry Skills

Taking Notes During Research—Record, Relate, Reflect

As researchers gather data about a topic, their goal is to learn as much as they can, then draw conclusions from what they have learned. By taking notes in an organized format as they research, they develop notes that they can analyze more effectively, which helps the researchers draw more reliable conclusions. In addition to these important goals, taking notes in an organized way can also help you

- focus on what you are reading or learning; by recording key points, you pay attention to what you are reading
- keep track of sources of information; by recording the sources of your information in a systematic way, you make the job of preparing a bibliography much easier
- assess when your question has been answered; a quick review of organized notes will tell you if you have enough information to answer your research question
- decide whether to revise your research question or add a supplementary question; notes can indicate surprising trends that you may want to investigate further

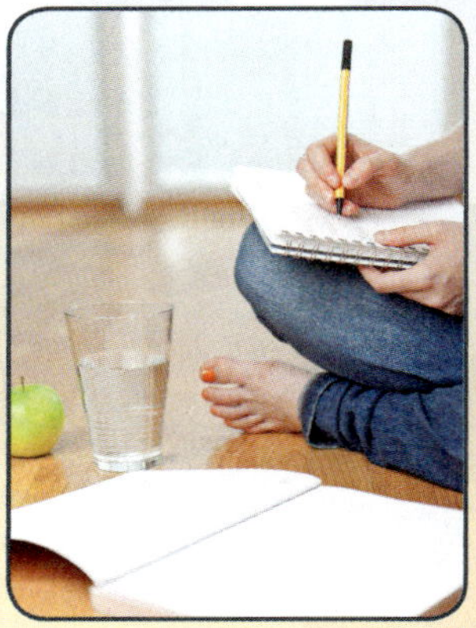

FIGURE 3.3 Efficient note taking will help you understand your research on food and nutrition. What foods might help you stay focussed while you do your research?

The format you use to take notes will depend on the purpose of your research, the types of sources you are consulting, whether you are using your notes to gather information or to organize it, and your personal style and preferences.

Journals can be useful for recording personal observations over time. For example, a person who suspected that they had a food allergy might record their response to the foods they eat every day in a journal.

Logs consist of many short entries. They are often used to record actions that were taken and the times they were taken. For example, if an experiment takes several weeks, a log can be used to record what was done each day.

Report outlines provide a template to ensure that your research addresses all sections of the report. After you have conducted some research and you have a general idea of what you will say in a report, it can be helpful to draft an outline of your report, then take notes from your original research for each section of the outline. Later, you can smooth and edit your notes into a formal report.

Note-making formats can help organize the information you gather. These can be set up so that you write information from the source in the left column and your own thoughts about it, or about how it might relate to other information you have gathered, in the right column. Many people find it effective to take notes by writing a main point at the left of a page, and indenting supporting points slightly.

Graphic organizers such as flowcharts, concept maps, and Venn diagrams are often useful for making sense of information you find in research. They can help you identify connections and relationships as you analyze the data. (Graphic organizers can help you review your notes from class for the same reasons.)

As you continue to develop your food and nutrition knowledge, learning to take good notes will help you record the most important information in a way that you will understand. Use these tips to manage your research notes:

1. **Record**. Whatever tool you use to take notes—sticky notes, index cards, electronic organizers, notebooks or any other method—document all source information needed for a reference list while you complete your research. This makes it easier to refer back to your sources, if necessary.
2. **Relate**. As you take notes, begin to make connections between the information you are collecting from different sources. Look for any similarities or differences in the information collected, relationships, patterns, or contradictions.
3. **Reflect**. Keep all of your notes in one location for easy access. Look at them from time to time to plan your next steps, whether those are further research or drawing conclusions. Ask yourself if you have enough information to use as evidence to support your opinion or answer your questions. Reflecting on your notes may lead to new questions, ideas, conclusions, and more research.

Questions:

1. Think about a note-taking style you have used. Create a T-chart to record the advantages and disadvantages of taking notes that way.
2. Choose a section or a feature of this textbook that interests you. Look at the headings and decide what question(s) you expect it to answer. Choose an appropriate method of making organized notes and gather information from the section.
3. Review your notes. What questions do you still have about the topic?

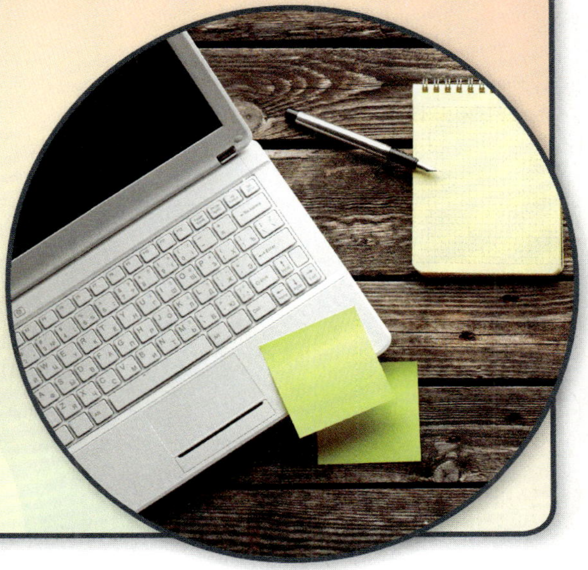

FIGURE 3.4 What tools do you use to keep your notes organized?

TIP for Healthy Living

Eating slowly can help you avoid overeating by giving the brain time to register that your hunger has been satisfied.

The Body Obtains Energy from Food

As you have previously learned, the food you consume provides you with energy and nutrients. The body then uses the energy it obtains from food to perform many functions. To be able to balance your energy consumption and expenditure, it is important to understand how your body breaks down and uses the energy obtained from food.

Hunger and Appetite

When and how much we eat is regulated partly by hunger and appetite. When the body's blood-glucose levels drop, we experience hunger. The contractions of an empty stomach can also cause feelings of hunger. Appetite, in contrast, can be caused by a variety of stimuli, including seeing or smelling foods we like, being in social situations, and even boredom.

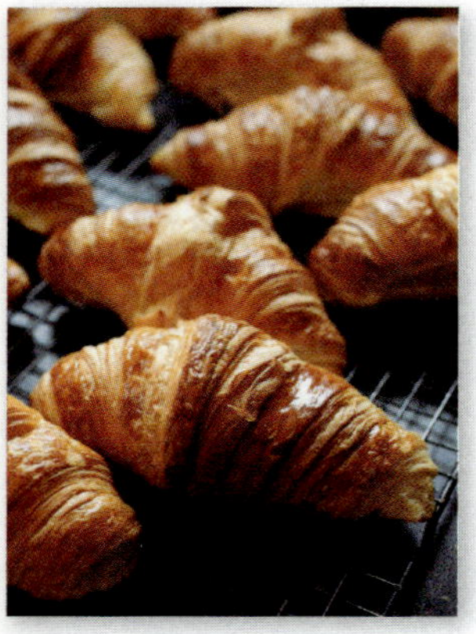

FIGURE 3.5 Smelling freshly baked bread, hearing the school lunch-bell ring, or seeing a juicy hamburger on television can stimulate your appetite. What sights, sounds, or smells stimulate your appetite?

Ingestion and Digestion

The first step in nourishing the body is eating, or ingesting, food. When food is eaten, blood-glucose levels rise, causing hunger to subside. It takes around 20 minutes after ingesting food for your brain to register that you are no longer hungry.

Before the cells of the body can use food, it must undergo many changes to convert its nutrients to forms that can be absorbed through the intestinal wall. This process of **digestion** occurs in the organs of the **gastrointestinal (GI) tract**: the mouth, esophagus, stomach, small intestine, and large intestine. In addition, the pancreas and liver secrete important enzymes and chemicals into the intestine to aid digestion. Food travels through the GI tract from the time it is swallowed until any undigested residue is excreted in the feces. Until the food is absorbed through the walls of the digestive tract and into the blood, it cannot be used by the cells. The cells lining the digestive tract control not only the form in which nutrients enter the body, but also the amounts of nutrients that enter.

digestion: the process by which the body breaks food down to its component nutrients

gastrointestinal (GI) tract: a tubular passage of specialized mucous membrane and muscle from mouth to anus that carries out the processes of digestion and excretion

Mechanical digestion is the first step in breaking down the food you eat. As food is chewed, the salivary glands secrete saliva to lubricate the food bolus (soft mass) so it can easily pass through a large, muscular tube called the *esophagus* to the stomach. Saliva contains digestive enzymes that begin the process of chemical digestion. Tasting, or even smelling or seeing food can cause saliva to be secreted in the mouth.

When you swallow, gravity and **peristalsis** propel the food downward. The epiglottis (a flap) closes the trachea (windpipe) so the food flows down and through the esophageal sphincter into the stomach instead of the lungs.

peristalsis: a wave-like movement in the esophagus created by muscle contraction and relaxation

Pause and Think
How is it possible for astronauts in space to eat normally?

The Stomach

Although we often think of the stomach as the major organ in the digestive process, it actually plays a relatively minor role. The stomach can hold around 1 L of food and slowly empties into the intestine 5 mL to 15 mL at a time (Fessler, 2010). The churning of the stomach combined with the mixture of hydrochloric acid, **intrinsic factor**, and pepsinogen—a digestive enzyme secreted by the stomach wall—liquefies the food. The hydrochloric acid has several functions including destroying ingested bacteria, and converting pepsinogen into its active form, pepsin, in order to initiate the digestion of protein.

intrinsic factor: a substance that binds with vitamin B_{12} in food so that the nutrient can be absorbed

The resulting mixture of gastric juices and food is called *chyme*, and is very acidic. In fact, the stomach wall secretes mucous to form a protective coat over the stomach lining, or mucosa. Slowly, the chyme passes through the pyloric sphincter into the duodenum, the first portion of the small intestine. The emptying of the stomach takes an average of two to six hours, depending on the type of food being digested. The stomach empties fluids more rapidly than solids. Carbohydrates are emptied before proteins, which are emptied before fats.

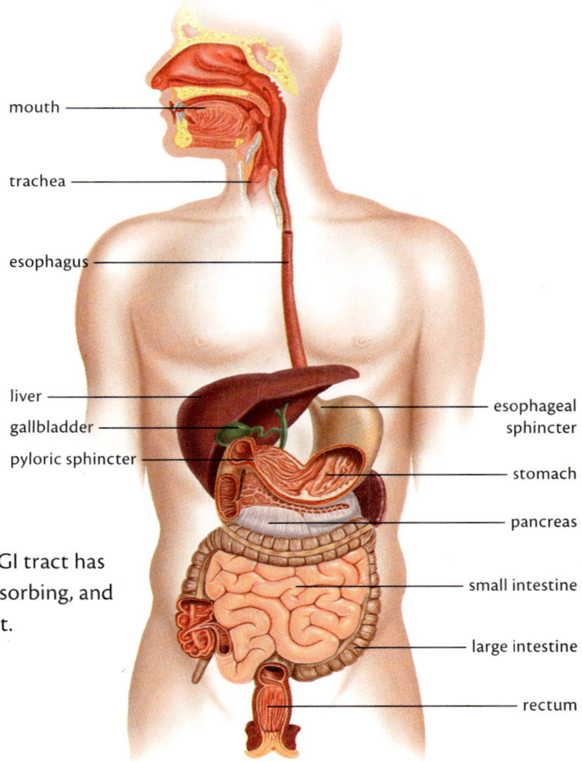

FIGURE 3.6 Each part of the GI tract has a specific role in digesting, absorbing, and metabolizing the food you eat.

Pause and Think
Dinner is not for three hours and you need a snack. What types of food are most likely to keep you from feeling hungry until dinnertime? Why?

Career Connection

Educating Communities about Healthy Eating

Public health departments employ nutritionists, dietitians, community nutrition assistants, and public health nurses to inform and support communities in all areas related to health. May Hughes is a public health nurse. She says the most enjoyable part of her job is working with a team of experts in diverse areas to achieve a common goal: promoting health.

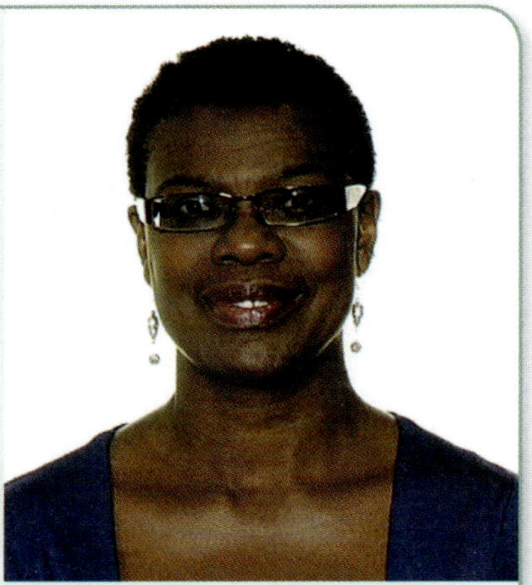

Figure 3.7 May Hughes, a public health nurse.

Monotony is certainly not part of a public health nurse's job description. Public health nurses provide services in diverse program areas including immunization, sexual health, communicable diseases, healthy development of babies and children, family health, chronic disease prevention and management, injury prevention, and substance abuse prevention. Every day can bring a different set of challenges and May's enthusiasm is still present after over 15 years in the field.

May's degrees in nursing and education provided her with a solid foundation for her career as a public health nurse. Effective training along with experience over time helped her to develop the skills necessary to function in her role. Along with the rewards of the job come challenges. May says, "One of the challenges is the broad knowledge required to function in the role and the need to be aware of the current and evidence-based information. One needs to adopt and enjoy life-long learning principles to keep abreast with learning needs."

The following skills and work habits are important for a public health nurse:

- an ability to handle challenging assignments in a high-profile professional and political environment
- excellent interpersonal and public-relations skills
- an ability to work independently and as part of a diverse team
- an ability to provide appropriate services to diverse clients and communities
- leadership skills
- organizational skills
- oral and written communication skills
- skills in counselling, advocacy, program planning, social marketing, facilitation and presentation, policy development, mentorship, and emergency response

Questions:

1. Categorize each of the skills and work habits listed above as primarily an attitude, an interest, a result of education, and/or a result of experience. Some items may fit in more than one category.
2. What aspects of a public health nurse's role could a background in nutrition—especially as it pertains to energy balance—help with?

The Small Intestine

Despite the name *small*, the small intestine is the longest (670 cm to 760 cm) and most important organ of digestion. The name *small* refers to its diameter (about 3 cm to 4 cm) in comparison to the diameter of the large intestine. Most of the **absorption** from the gastrointestinal (GI) tract occurs in the small intestine, whose mucosal surface is highly specialized for this absorptive process. The small intestine is divided into three sections: the duodenum, the jejunum, and the ileum.

absorption: the movement of nutrients through the walls of the intestine into the bloodstream

The small intestine contains the enzymes needed to complete the breakdown of large carbohydrate, **lipid**, and protein molecules into units small enough to move through the intestinal wall. Bile, produced in the liver and stored in the gallbladder, is secreted into the duodenum to aid lipid digestion by breaking fat into small particles. The pancreas secretes digestive enzymes that aid in protein, lipid, and carbohydrate digestion. It also secretes sodium bicarbonate, an alkali that neutralizes the hydrochloric acid in chyme. This, in turn, brings the intestinal contents to the optimal pH for the intestinal digestive enzymes to work. Once they are broken down, most nutrients pass out of the GI tract into the cells lining it and from these cells into the blood, where they travel to the liver for further processing.

lipid: a nutrient in foods; fats, oils, and cholesterol are lipids

Skills Focus

Create a flowchart to take notes about how food passes through the digestive system.

The surface area of the small intestine is approximately 4500 square metres—the size of a tennis court! This vast surface area, especially in the duodenum and jejunum, is made possible by intricate folds. Densely packed, small, finger-like projections called *villi* line the inner intestinal surface. The villi are covered with even smaller projections called *microvilli*. Enzymes embedded in the microvilli carry out the final stages of digestion before nutrients are absorbed through the villi. The cell membrane acts as a selective barrier that regulates the rate at which nutrients enter the blood; many minerals and vitamins are absorbed into the blood at a greater or lesser rate depending on the body's need for them at that time.

Pancreatic enzymes are secreted into the duodenum to aid with digestion. Peristalsis moves the chyme into the jejunum, where the bulk of digested carbohydrates, protein, water, water-soluble vitamins, electrolytes, and minerals are absorbed. Remaining nutrients are propelled to the last third of the small intestine, the ileum. There, fat, the fat-soluble vitamins (A, D, E, and K), vitamin B_{12}, and bile salts are absorbed.

Figure 3.8 Microvilli enlarge the surface area of the villi in the small intestine, while keeping the intestine compact. What would happen if the microvilli or villi were damaged?

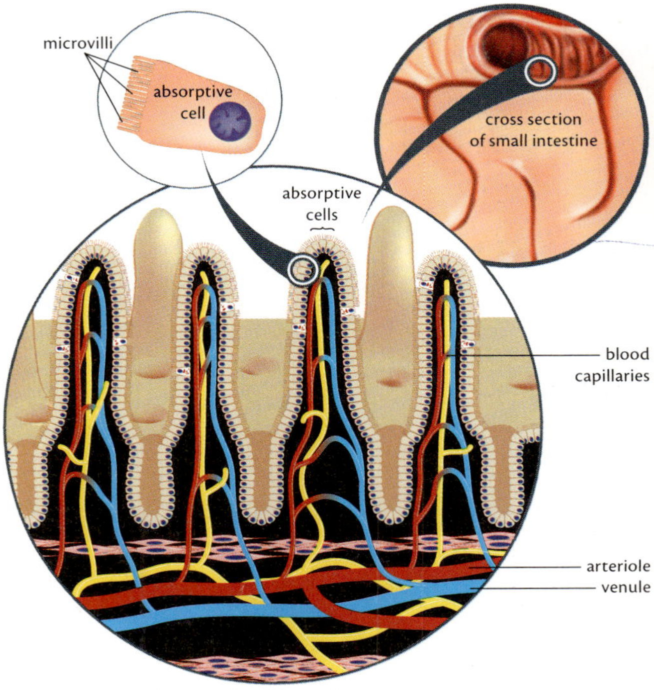

Absorption of Carbohydrates, Lipids, and Protein

Digestible carbohydrates include sugars and starches. Sugars can be absorbed from the intestine into the bloodstream as they are. Starch molecules are long chains of sugar molecules. Starches need to be broken down into sugars (monosaccharides or disaccharides) in order to be absorbed. Carbohydrates that are not digestible by humans, such as cellulose, are called *dietary fibre*.

Some Carbohydrate Digestive Enzymes and their Products

Source	Enzyme	Products
Salivary glands	Salivary amylase	Begins to break down starch to maltose
Pancreas	Pancreatic amylase	Completes the breakdown of starch to maltose
Intestinal mucosa	Maltase	Breaks down maltose to glucose
	Lactase	Breaks down lactose to galactose and glucose
	Sucrase	Breaks down sucrose to glucose and fructose

FIGURE 3.9 What might happen if a person was unable to produce certain digestive enzymes?

NUTRITION LITERACY

An inability to produce lactase in sufficient quantities causes lactose intolerance. People who have lactose intolerance are unable to digest milk products properly, and often experience discomfort if they drink more than a small amount of milk.

Saturated and polyunsaturated fats need to be broken down into fatty acids in order to be absorbed. Bile emulsifies, or coats, fats in the duodenum to enable the enzyme *lipase* to access the lipid molecules and break them down. Lipase is found in the stomach and secreted by the pancreas into the small intestine.

Proteins are too large to pass through the intestinal wall and must be broken down into amino acids before absorption. Protein digestion is initiated in the stomach by acid and pepsin secretion. In the small intestine, the pancreatic enzyme *trypsin* breaks most of the undigested proteins down.

Excretion

By the time chyme passes into the large intestine or colon, most nutrients have been absorbed. No further digestion occurs in the large intestine, but the action of bacteria on the remaining mass can generate gases. Additional water is extracted, potassium is excreted, and the chyme is thickened to form stool. As the mass continues through the large intestine, water continues to be absorbed into the body. The solid mass that reaches the anus is a semisolid fecal matter, or feces. This is propelled by peristalsis into the rectum for evacuation. Stool consists mainly of micro-organisms, dietary fibre, and water. The more dietary fibre in the stool, the more water is retained.

THINK CRITICALLY

1. Explain why some people who have a small portion of their intestine removed can still digest most foods with few problems.
2. How would a diet low in insoluble fibre affect the digestive process?

ACTIVE LEARNING

Analyze Your Nutrient Intake

Health Canada (2012) has analyzed the nutrient intakes of Canadian adults. Some of the things they learned may surprise you:

- 70% of men and 50% of women had energy intakes greater than their energy expenditures. (Since this is difficult to measure, it was determined using an estimate of the amount of fat people had in their bodies, on the assumption that excess energy taken in had been stored as fat.)
- 32% of men and 21% of women had carbohydrate intakes below their acceptable macronutrient distribution range (AMDR).
- Almost 100% of men and women had adequate protein intakes.
- 25% of men and 23% of women had fat intakes above their AMDR and saturated fat levels above those modelled by *Eating Well with Canada's Food Guide*.
- Canadians consumed adequate amounts of most vitamins and minerals, but many consumed inadequate amounts of magnesium, calcium, vitamin A, vitamin D, and potassium.
- Many Canadians seemed to consume inadequate amounts of fibre, although data were inconclusive.
- Most Canadians consumed more sodium than the recommended maximum intake.

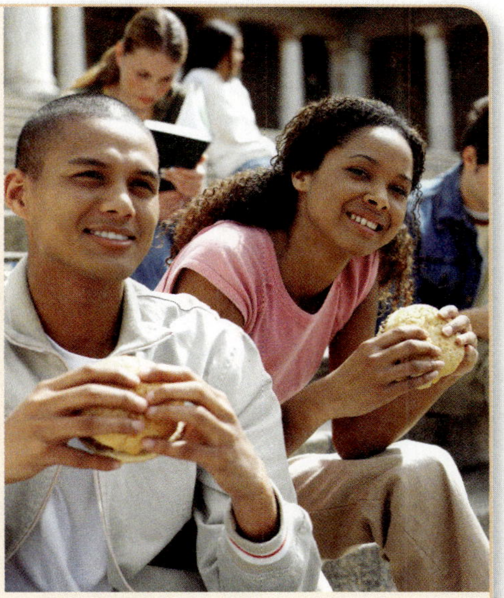

FIGURE 3.10 How does the average nutritional status of Canadians compare to your own?

Data like these help health organizations and dietitians identify areas where improvements to our diet could be made. Once nutritional gaps are identified, education programs can be put in place, regulations about food ingredients can be developed, and other strategies can be introduced to improve our diets.

Questions:

1. Write a paragraph or create a graphic organizer to summarize the nutritional status of Canadians based on this research.
2. What surprised you most about the nutrient intake of Canadians?
3. Create a table that you can use to record your nutrient intake. Include a column for each of the four food groups. Include rows to record food items and the servings of each. Use *Eating Well with Canada's Food Guide* to help you estimate numbers of servings. You will use this log for your own research. It is not to share.
4. Record every item you eat for a typical week in your log. If you forget to record for a while, do your best to remember.
5. Use what you know about the foods in each food group to estimate your consumption of macronutrients and major micronutrients. How does your estimated nutrient intake compare to the nutrient intake of Canadians, as determined by Health Canada?
6. What difficulties did you encounter in this research? What errors are likely to occur in any study of nutrient intake?

Using Energy

The amount of energy a person uses depends on several factors, including their age, body size, gender, and activity level. In general, infants and children use the most energy per kilogram of body mass, and adults use less. If all other factors are equal, a larger person always requires more energy than a smaller person. In general, the amount of energy used in a day, or total daily energy expenditure (TDEE), is a combination of the **basal metabolism**, the energy used by physical activities, and the energy used by the thermic effect of food. The amount of energy used for basal metabolism is often expressed as the **basal metabolic rate (BMR)**.

basal metabolism: the chemical processes by which the body uses energy to carry out functions necessary to sustain life; does not include energy used for daily activities

basal metabolic rate (BMR): the amount of energy used *per kilogram of body mass* to carry out basal metabolic functions

TIP for Healthy Living

People who consume as many Calories as they use will neither lose nor gain weight.

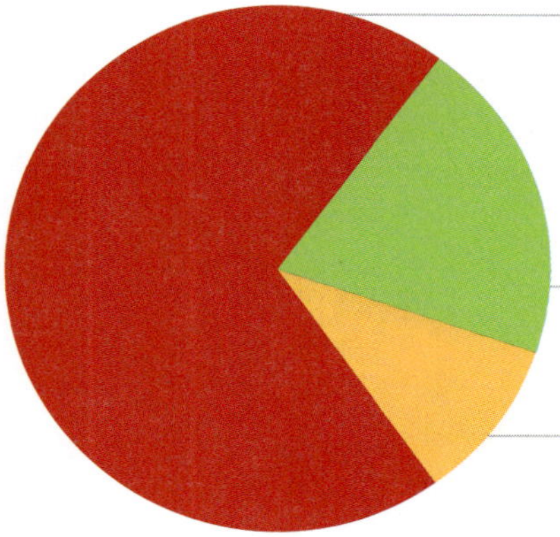

Basal metabolism includes all the essential metabolic processes your body carries out even while you are resting. Between 50 and 80 percent of your TDEE is used for basic metabolic processes such as breathing, circulating blood, and staying warm. Organs such as the liver, brain, heart, and kidney have the highest energy needs while the body is at rest.

Physical activities that require muscle movements such as exercise, maintaining posture, and even reading account for 30 to 40 percent of your TDEE. This percent may be higher in very active people.

The thermic effect of food—or the additional energy used after eating a meal to digest, absorb, store, and use the nutrients in the food—accounts for five to 15 percent of your TDEE.

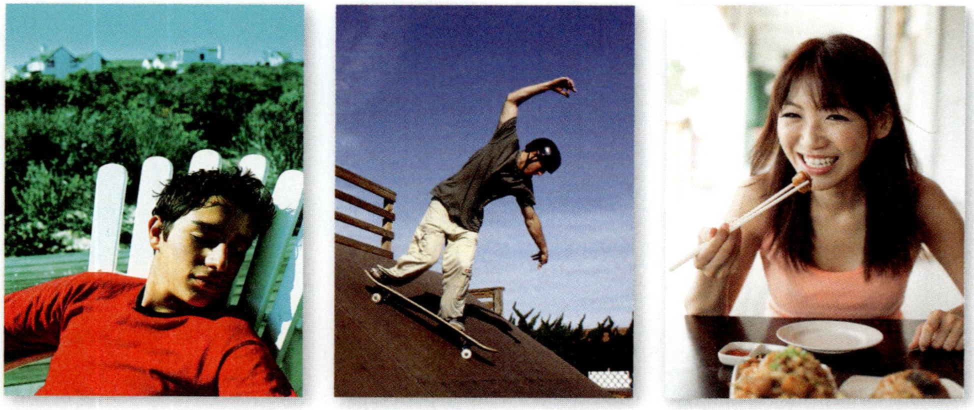

FIGURE 3.11 The human body uses energy for three types of work.

Pause and Think

List as many processes as you can that would be part of your basal metabolism.

Factors Affecting BMR

All body tissues are metabolically active; they are constantly maintained, degraded, and resynthesized. But not all body tissues use energy at the same rate. It takes more energy to maintain muscle tissue than it does to maintain fat or bone tissue. Since men typically have a higher percent of muscle than women do, their BMR is usually higher than that of women. For this reason, men require more energy per kilogram of body weight to sustain basic body functions. Since people tend to lose muscle mass as they age, older adults tend to have a lower BMR than young adults do and require less energy per kilogram of body weight to sustain basic body functions.

Hormones also have a significant effect on BMR. Secretions from the adrenal and thyroid glands have a stimulating effect on metabolism. For example, the hormone *epinephrine* (adrenaline) is produced in response to intense emotional stimuli such as anger or fear, and increases metabolism for two or three hours. Oversecretion (hyperthyroidism) or undersecretion (hypothyroidism) of the thyroid hormone *thyroxin* can significantly increase or decrease the BMR. Despite these metabolic differences, a fairly accurate estimate of most people's energy needs for basal metabolism can be made based only on body weight.

Nutrition Literacy

An average 19-year-old female might have a BMR of approximately 1450 Calories. As you have seen, an individual's BMR can differ depending on size, muscle mass, gender, and other factors.

Pause and Think
Why is weight an important factor in determining basal energy needs?

Factors Affecting Basal Metabolism

Factors that Increase Basal Metabolism	Factors that Decrease Basal Metabolism
High percent of body mass is muscle	High percent of body mass is fat
Good physical condition	Poor physical condition
Being male	Being female
Hyperthyroidism	Hypothyroidism
Pregnancy	Sleep
Puberty	Aging
Extremes of environmental temperature	Undernutrition

Figure 3.12 Suppose two men are the same age, height, and weight, but one is a construction worker and the other is an accountant. What can you predict about their BMR? What factors might cause your prediction to be incorrect?

> **Skills Focus**
>
> Record all your physical activity for five days in a log. Include every episode of activity longer than 10 minutes. Then use your log to compare your activity levels at different times of day. At what time of day do you typically use the most energy?

Energy Used for Activity

Your body uses energy to power muscular movement, and to increase heart rate and breathing rate during strenuous activity. The more active you are, the more energy you use. An athlete who trains every day may use thousands of Calories of energy for physical activities alone.

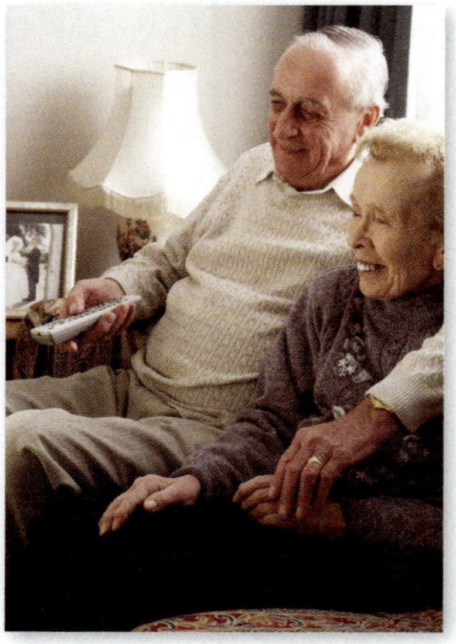

Figure 3.13 Someone who spends much of the day in sedentary activities will not use much more energy than that required for basal metabolism.

THINK CRITICALLY

1. Using what you know about basal metabolism, why might a person recovering from an illness have an increased BMR?
2. Lily has joined the school swim team and practises with them three mornings a week. Describe all the ways you can think of that this might affect her energy needs.

Life Connection

Getting Active

Physical activity is important for many reasons. Not only does it help you achieve an energy balance, it also builds muscle, strengthens bones, improves the health of your circulatory system, improves posture, reduces stress, and reduces the risk of some diseases. Physical activity even improves brain function and helps you concentrate.

Every step counts. The Public Health Agency of Canada recommends that adults

- take part in at least 2.5 hours of moderate to vigorous aerobic physical activity every week
- perform activities to build strong muscles and bones two days a week (CSEP, 2012)

Guidelines for Physical Activity

Type of Physical Activity	Description	Examples
Moderate aerobic activity	You breathe harder and your heart beats faster. You can talk but not sing.	walking quickly, skating, riding a bike, downhill skiing
Vigorous aerobic activity	You breathe even harder. You can speak a few words, then need to catch a breath.	running, playing basketball or soccer, cross-country skiing
Bone-strengthening activity	Your muscles become tired after a few minutes of focussed activity.	doing push-ups, lifting weights, climbing stairs, riding a bike uphill

FIGURE 3.14 All three types of physical activity shown here help to maintain good health.

To be successful, choose activities that you enjoy and that fit your lifestyle:

- Walk, run, or bike instead of getting a ride.
- Do something fun: run, jump, swim, skateboard, snowboard, ski, skate, toboggan, or dance.
- Rake the leaves, shovel snow, or carry groceries home.
- Join a team at your school.
- Set physical activity goals with your friends and family.

To make time for physical activity, and to encourage an active lifestyle, reduce screen time (time spent using the phone, computer, or television) to no more than two hours a day.

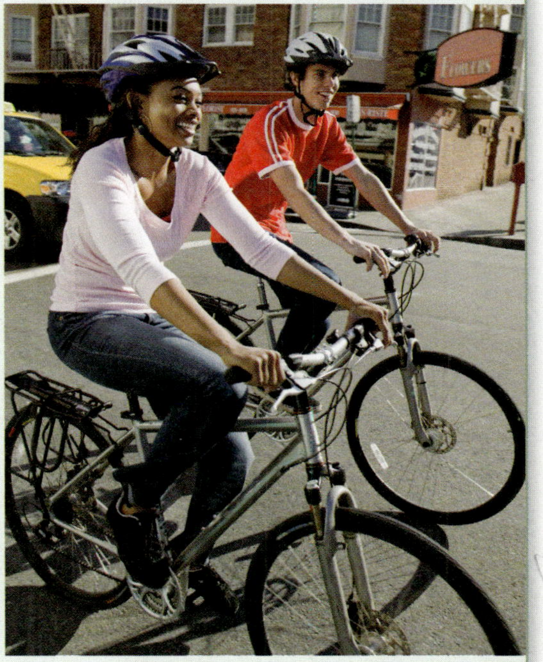

FIGURE 3.15 Experts recommend including moderate activity, vigorous activity, and bone-strengthening activity in your lifestyle.

Questions:

1. Why are both aerobic activities and bone-strengthening activities recommended every week?
2. How can reducing screen time to two hours a day improve your physical activity?
3. Analyze your own physical activity levels for a week. What changes could you make to improve your health?

Balancing Energy

As you have seen, the body breaks down nutrients in foods so that it can use the energy in them. It does this in a process known as *catabolism*. The body also builds and restores its own cells in a process known as *anabolism*. These processes of anabolism and catabolism together make up *metabolism*. When the energy the body obtains from foods is equal to the energy the body uses, the body neither gains nor loses weight. When the body takes in more energy than it uses, it stores the extra energy, and gains weight. When the body uses more energy than it takes in, it catabolizes its own cells to obtain the energy it needs.

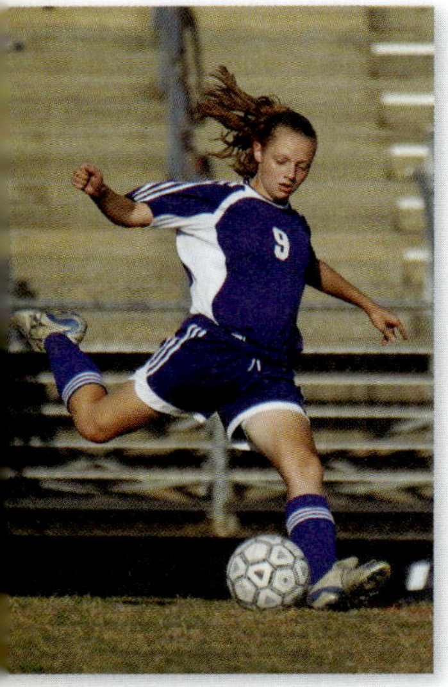

FIGURE 3.16 Unused energy is converted and stored by our body most often as fat in adipose tissue. Why is having some adipose tissue important for good health?

Storing Energy

During digestion, macronutrients in foods are broken down into simple sugars (from carbohydrates), fatty acids (from lipids), and amino acids (from proteins).

Simple sugars can be used directly for energy by all tissues. Excess sugars are taken up by the liver, and converted into larger glycogen molecules or fat for storage.

Fatty acids are also used for energy as well as becoming building blocks for several important biological chemicals such as hormones. Excess fatty acids are stored in adipose tissue, which is found most prominently beneath the skin, in the abdomen, and in the buttocks.

Amino acids become building blocks for protein in body tissues. Amino acids in excess of the body's requirements can be used for energy, and metabolized to glycogen or fat and stored for future needs.

The Risks of Too Much Adipose Tissue

While our bodies need some stored energy, too much can cause health risks. The extra weight of large amounts of adipose tissue can put unnecessary strain on the heart and joints. There are other risks as well, including:

- increased risk of coronary heart disease and stroke
- increased risk of type 2 diabetes
- increased risk of some cancers (endometrial, breast, and colon)
- increased risk of hypertension (high blood pressure)
- increased risk of high levels of cholesterol and fats in blood
- increased risk of liver and gallbladder disease
- increased risk of sleep apnea and respiratory problems
- increased risk of gynaecological problems for women (abnormal menstrual periods and infertility)

These conditions can affect people of any weight, and have other risk factors as well. For example, smokers have an increased risk of coronary heart disease, **sedentary** people have an increased risk of hypertension, and some cancers have genetic components.

sedentary: not engaging in physical activity

Metabolic Syndrome

Metabolic syndrome is not a disease itself, but a combination of factors that has been shown to correlate to increased risk of heart disease, type 2 diabetes, stroke, and kidney disease. It includes a combination of several of these factors: a large waist circumference, low HDL cholesterol, elevated blood sugar, elevated levels of fat in blood, and elevated blood pressure.

One in five Canadian adults are affected by metabolic syndrome. Just a generation ago, type 2 diabetes was unheard of in people under the age of 35; now, even teenagers are showing early signs of type 2 diabetes and heart disease. Excess adipose tissue in the abdomen seems to be directly related to metabolic syndrome. This visceral fat increases inflammation and risk of heart disease, and produces a protein that increases **insulin resistance**, causing high blood-glucose levels, and possibly type 2 diabetes. Since insulin also plays a role in lipid metabolism, insulin resistance caused by visceral fat can cause high blood-triglyceride levels and increase the risk of heart disease.

insulin resistance: the body's inability to use insulin efficiently to absorb glucose into cells, which leads to a rise in blood-glucose levels

Pause and Think
Why should teens be concerned about metabolic syndrome?

Determining Healthy Body Size

While the media often presents us with images of "perfect" bodies, there is no ideal weight that suits everyone. Each person is different and their healthy weight is determined by many factors. The genes that you inherit can influence your bone structure, height, body shape, and weight tendencies. Your usual food pattern and exercise habits determine how your genes are expressed. And, as you have seen, diseases have many risk factors, only some of which are related to weight.

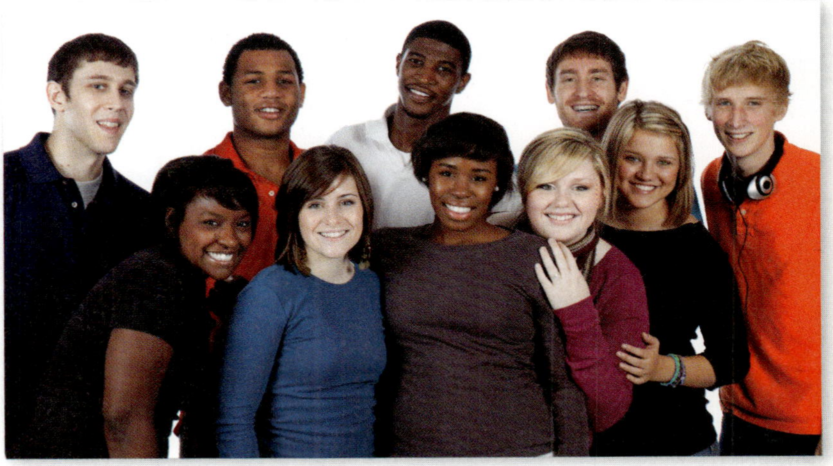

Figure 3.17 Images in the media do not always portray healthy body types. How can this harm individuals trying to maintain good health?

Two people who have the same weight may have very different bodies, and different activity levels. For that reason, medical professionals have developed several ways to measure body size and shape. All of these used together can help them to evaluate health. It is important to remember that none can give an absolute formula for healthy growth and development.

Screening tools commonly used to evaluate healthy growth and development include the following:

Growth charts track children's development by recording weight and measuring height at regular intervals and comparing the data to standard growth charts.

Body Mass Index (BMI) takes height and weight into account to estimate the amount of body fat.

Waist circumference can be used to obtain a rough estimate of the fat stored in the abdomen (fat around the belly), called *visceral adipose tissue (VAT)*.

Waist-to-hip ratio (WHR) is used to more accurately estimate the amount of VAT.

Growth Charts

In 2006, the World Health Organization (WHO) released new child growth standards, which Canada has since adapted. The WHO growth charts show typical heights and weights for children of every age, and are the best tool available for tracking a child's growth. A variety of cultures and ethnic backgrounds were used to develop the WHO Child Growth Standards, which also reflects Canada's multiculturalism. However, some unintentional bias may still be present in the current standards, as many children from certain ethnic groups who seem to be growing in healthy ways do not follow the charts' pattern of typical growth rates. Health professionals take this into consideration when using the new standards. As with any scientific research, the standards may be revised again as further research is conducted. Despite the few exceptions, the WHO research shows that children of all ethnic backgrounds have similar potential for growth when raised in environmental conditions favourable to growth: particularly smoke-free households, access to health care, and adequate nutrition.

FIGURE 3.18 While children develop at their own rates, the heights and weights of most children of a particular age tend to fall within a certain range.

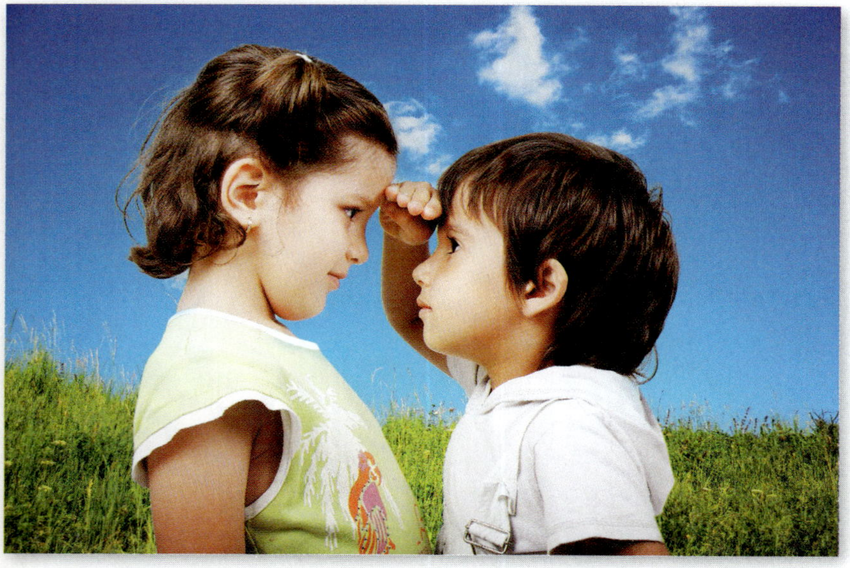

These key messages are important to keep in mind when using growth charts:

- Measurements are one health screening tool among many.
- Growth is one of the signs of general health.
- Growth may reflect family growth patterns.
- Different individuals may have different healthy growth patterns.
- An individual's growth pattern over time is more important than one single measurement.

LIFE CONNECTION

A Free Lunch?

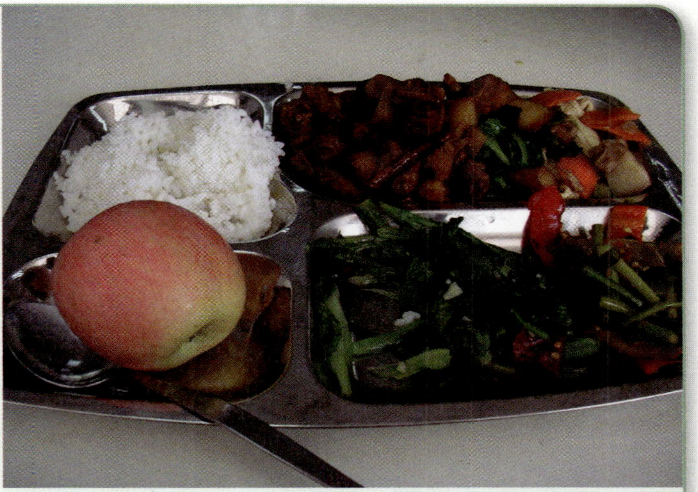

FIGURE 3.19 Providing lunches at school is one way to ensure that children around the world are eating at least one healthy meal a day.

In Canada's past, hot lunches were sometimes provided at school for students, but that practice was gradually abandoned in most schools. As you learned in Chapter 2, many provinces do have guidelines for healthy food options that are provided in schools. However, unlike many other countries, Canada does not have a national school lunch program. Countries that do have national school lunch programs organize them in many different ways. Decisions about what to serve can be made nationally or in local areas. Children can be offered a small number of choices or may choose food from a buffet. Funding for the program can come from the federal government or from regional governments. Students who are able to pay for lunch can be asked to pay (with other students being subsidized), or lunch can be free for all students. In some areas, students themselves get involved in preparing, serving, and cleaning up after the lunches.

Questions:

1. What might be the benefits of a national school lunch program in Canada?
2. What might be the drawbacks to a national school lunch program in Canada?
3. How might a school lunch program help children and adolescents balance their energy needs?
4. Given the different ways countries implement national school lunch programs, what features would you propose the ideal school lunch program in Canada should have?

Body Mass Index

Body Mass Index (BMI) is another tool that can be used to assess healthy body size. BMI is a comparison of weight to height. Because BMI does not distinguish between weight that is adipose tissue and weight that is muscle or other tissue, it is not a precise tool, and should not be used alone for diagnosis. In particular, it may not accurately assess health risks in athletes, pregnant or lactating women, or older adults.

Waist Circumference

Because visceral adipose tissue (VAT) is linked to several serious health risks and because VAT surrounds vital organs in the abdomen, a large belly can be a sign of increased health risks. In fact, waist circumference is one of the factors directly linked to risk of metabolic syndrome. However, waist sizes also vary as a result of a wide variety of other factors, such as height, lifestyle, health, ethnicity, and genetics.

Waist-to-Hip Ratio (WHR)

The waist-to-hip ratio measures the difference between the narrowest part of a person's waist and the widest part of the person's hip. By comparing these two measurements, waist-to-hip ratio attempts to provide a standard reference that can be used to assess health in people of a variety of heights and body types. However, healthy waist-to-hip ratios still vary for children of different ages, and for people of different body types.

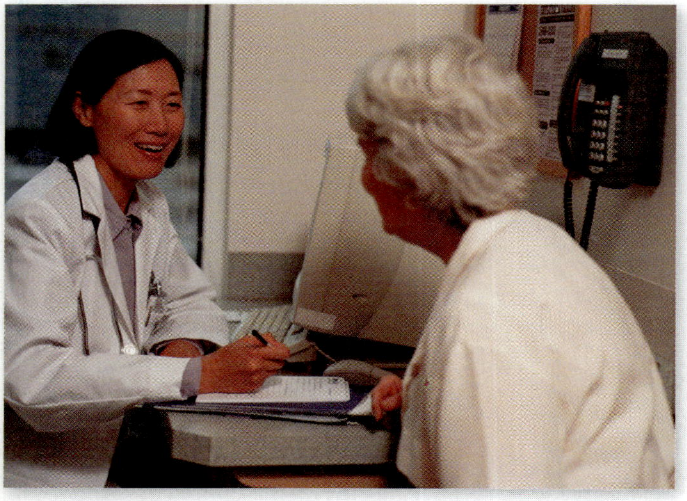

FIGURE 3.20 Health professionals have many tools at their disposal to assess a person's health. Those described on this page are three of many that are sometimes used to predict risks.

THINK CRITICALLY

1. Each of the tools above is an imperfect way to determine health. Explain why some health professionals use them.
2. Create a table to summarize the benefits and limitations of using each of the four tools above for assessing health risks.
3. What factors other than body size can affect a person's risk of developing diseases?

POINT/COUNTERPOINT

"Measuring" Health

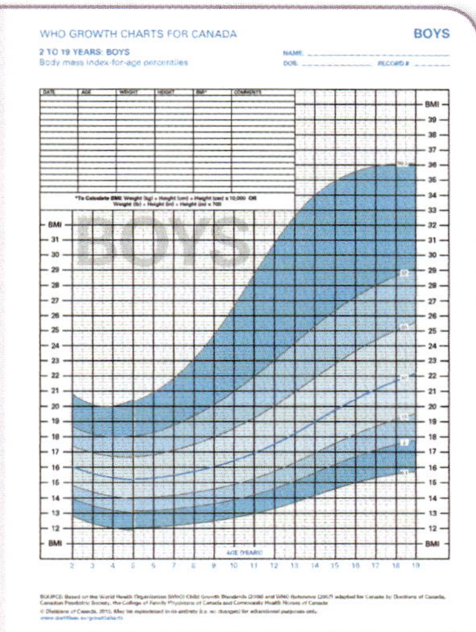

FIGURE 3.21 As concern about the possible health effects of obesity grew, graphs were developed to compare an individual's BMI to those of the general population. Ranges of values classified as underweight, normal, overweight, and obese were established somewhat arbitrarily.

The tools discussed in this section are all imperfect. Should they still be used?

BMI was developed by Adolphe Quetelet in the early 1800s as one of several tools to describe characteristics of the common man. After measuring many men to establish norms, researchers had a way to describe what the average was. Many years later, health professionals became concerned with the health effects of obesity. They began using BMI as an estimate of percent body fat, and established cut-off BMI values that they defined as overweight, underweight, and obese.

BMI was not developed for this purpose. As scientists now know, the cut-off values imposed on the BMI range to indicate underweight, overweight, and obese are somewhat arbitrary and do not apply equally to men and women, to people of different ethnicities, or to people with different body compositions. An athlete with a lot of muscle will have a higher BMI than someone of the same height and less muscle. People may be diagnosed as overweight when they actually have a healthy weight, or as healthy when they have weight-related health risks. Other, more precise ways to assess health exist, including measuring body fat with callipers. While some of these are complicated to use, others—such as measuring waist circumference—are not much more difficult to use than BMI. None of these tools provides a complete assessment of health risks. As you have learned, healthy bodies come in all shapes and sizes. It is not possible to determine the degree of risk for any individual from BMI or any other single measurement.

Those who support the use of BMI to assess health risks point out its advantages. The measurements needed to calculate BMI are easy to take, and BMI is easy to calculate. The cut-off values associated with health risks are round numbers and are reasonably valid for certain parts of the population. This makes BMI an easy tool for health professionals to use. Other simple tools such as waist circumference do not have universally applied cut-off values. As in other areas of life, people are more likely to use a tool that is easy for them to use. Imperfect as it is, the fact that BMI can be easily calculated has resulted in people having discussions with their health care providers about possible health risks and lifestyle changes. A better tool that is not used would not result in these discussions. While most agree that BMI is not an effective tool to diagnose health problems, some believe that when BMI is used as a screening tool—identifying those who should undergo further testing—it can play a valid role in health care.

Questions:

1. What guidelines would you recommend to someone who wanted to use BMI to assess health risks?
2. What lifestyle factors could potentially be used to assess risks to health?
3. How do you think health professionals' use of BMI may change in the coming years? Explain your prediction.

> "What we are really talking about is changing the message from 'Eat Less, Move More' to 'Move More, Eat Smarter.'"
> – James Hill

Maintaining a Healthy Weight

To maintain a healthy balance, health professionals advise people to choose healthy foods and to take part in regular physical activity. When food intake and physical activity are balanced, energy levels are improved and health risks are decreased. A healthy weight can be achieved and maintained throughout your life.

The first step in achieving a healthy balance is becoming aware of what you eat, and why you eat it:

- Listen to your body. When are you hungry? Learn to eat when you are hungry and stop when you are no longer hungry. During a growth spurt or a period of increased activity, you may be more hungry than you usually are because your body needs more energy.
- Learn what one portion of food in *Eating Well with Canada's Food Guide* looks like and watch your portion sizes. Beware of **portion distortion**. Small changes such as ordering smaller size meal deals or sharing a treat with a friend can help maintain a balance.
- Enjoy your occasional indulgences. What you eat on a regular daily basis makes up your diet. Make your diet a healthy plan most of the time, and enjoy a treat occasionally.

portion distortion: large serving sizes that are more than one portion of food, but seem normal due to the size and type of packaging, dinnerware, and serving utensils

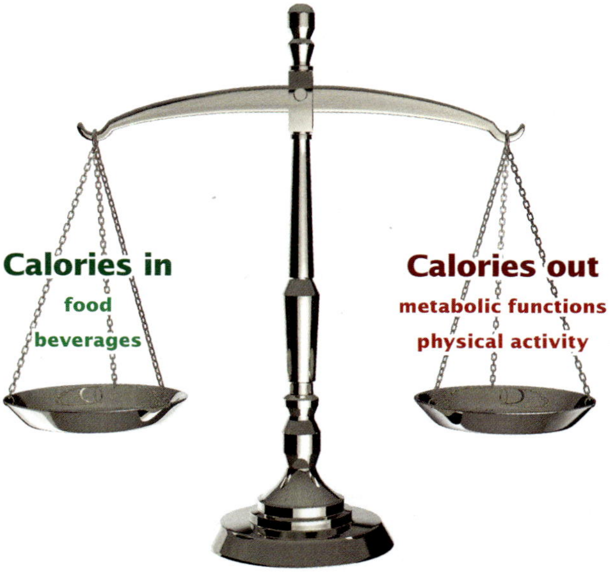

FIGURE 3.22 Maintaining a healthy weight requires balancing the energy you take in and the energy you use. What lifestyle choices can tip the balance scale in one direction or the other?

The next step is to make healthy choices. Remember, as well as energy, food provides you with important vitamins, minerals, and other nutrients. The Dietitians of Canada (2011) recommend that teens follow five strategies to maintain a healthy weight.

1. **Follow the recommendations in *Eating Well with Canada's Food Guide*.**

   In Chapter 2, you learned how to incorporate the recommendations of *Eating Well with Canada's Food Guide* into your diet and how to make the healthiest choices. Make a conscious effort to eat a variety of foods from all four food groups every day, with an emphasis on foods containing iron and calcium. Also make an effort to limit trans and saturated fats, and to eat whole fruits and vegetables more often than juice.

2. **Plan ahead for lunch.**

   Make your lunch with healthy foods that you enjoy from all four food groups. If you get hungry partway through the day, pack a healthy snack for yourself. Having healthy foods available will mean you aren't as tempted by unhealthy ones that you may come across. If you make your own lunch, try to pack it the night before when you have time to select nutritious foods. You read about the benefits of healthy school lunches in *Life Connection* on page 81.

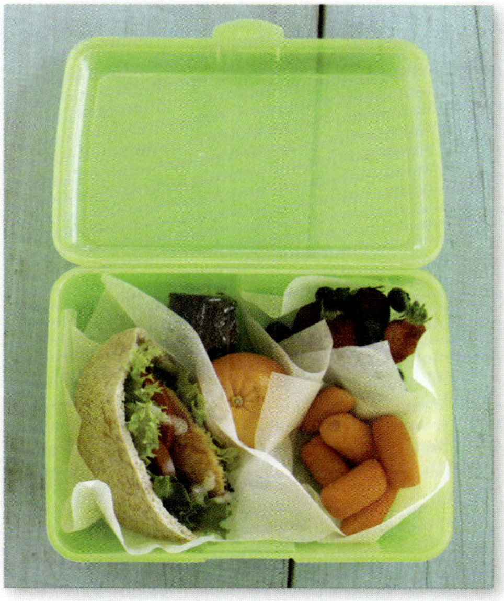

FIGURE 3.23 Lunches you make at home can be nutritious and include your favourite foods. By planning ahead, you can make a lunch for the next day in just a few minutes.

3. **Make smart choices when you eat out.**

   If you choose to eat at a restaurant, use what you know about food groups and serving sizes to choose a healthy option and an appropriate portion size. Apply the principles of *Eating Well with Canada's Food Guide*. If you are not sure what is in a dish or a sauce, the serving staff should be able to help you.

4. **Choose healthy snacks.**

   Choose nutrient-dense foods to make your snacks healthy. Try to combine a fruit and/or vegetable with a healthy choice from another food group, for example cut veggies with a small amount of hummus to dip them in, or yogurt with added fruit. Because protein takes longer to digest than carbohydrates, include some protein in your snack to keep you feeling satisfied for longer.

5. **Be active!**

   Aim for 60 minutes of activity every day. Any activity that lasts for longer than 10 minutes can count toward this total. Regular physical activity helps to keep you healthy, uses energy, and builds muscle. You can see some tips for being active in *Life Connection* on page 76.

TIP for Healthy Living

Limit the amount of sugary drinks such as pop, fruit drinks, and sports drinks to no more than 250 mL (1 cup) per day. They provide little or no nutrition except for extra Calories—one can of pop has as many as 160 Calories—and can cause dental cavities.

Pause and Think

What are some possible obstacles that you might encounter in trying to follow these strategies? What might help you overcome the obstacles?

Case Study

Eating Like an Athlete

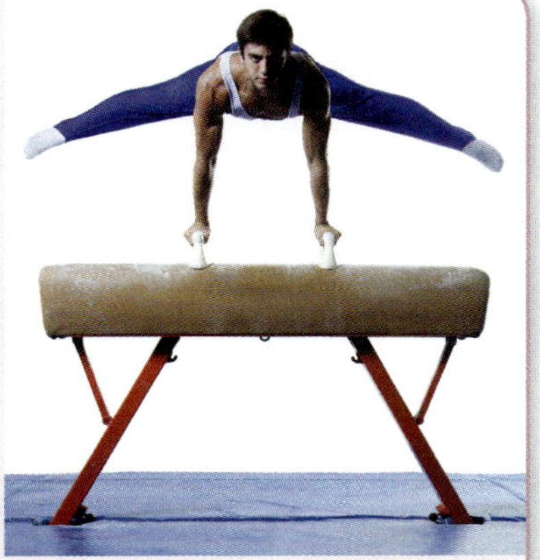

Figure 3.24 The training athletes undergo can place huge demands on their bodies.

Depending on their sport and their physique, athletes' nutritional needs can vary greatly. While an average 20-year-old may use 1900 to 3000 Calories of energy per day, depending on gender, body composition, and activity level, some athletes use 5000 or even 12 000 Calories every day! This energy must all be replenished by eating. In addition, athletes' highly developed muscles and intense activity levels mean that they also have greater needs for protein and many vitamins and minerals that play important roles in cell functioning. For these reasons, although athletes consume thousands of Calories every day, they are still careful to choose nutrient-dense foods to meet their needs. While sports drinks and supplements sometimes form a small part of an athlete's diet, most Canadian Olympic athletes rely on simple nutrient-dense foods for almost all of their needs.

Canada's Olympic athletes work with dietitians to ensure that the food they eat meets all of their needs. Athletes in power sports, such as gymnastics and boxing, need to focus on building and maintaining muscles. They choose foods to maximize high-quality proteins. Athletes involved in endurance sports, like marathon running or cycling, tend to eat larger amounts of carbohydrates to replenish glycogen stores. Dietary needs can also vary as training routines change, or even throughout the day. For example, if athletes ease off training in preparation for a competition, they often work with their dietitian to drastically reduce the number of Calories they consume to maintain the balance. In addition to these requirements, athletes may have religious dietary restrictions, allergies, or sensitivities, or preferences for vegetarian or even vegan foods. Dietitians can help ensure that they adopt a meal plan that meets their needs and is sustainable through the course of their training.

Kelly Anne Erdman, Canadian Olympic Team Performance Dietitian, offers this advice for aspiring athletes:

- Athletes need more carbohydrates, protein, and fluids than inactive people do.
- Get protein at every meal—not just at dinner.
- Iron is critical to support the growth and maintenance of tissues in developing athletes.

Julia Alleyne, Chief Medical Officer of the Canadian Olympic Team, adds a reminder that it is normal to gain weight as you get fitter, because muscle is denser than fat. Athletes often weigh more than their non-active peers.

> "Food is such a huge part of [succeeding in sport] so you can't just open your gob and stuff anything inside ... Even in high school I knew that when I ate good food I felt better."
>
> – Simon Whitfield, Olympic gold medalist (triathlon)

Questions:

1. What factors do athletes consider when planning their meals and snacks?
2. Describe some ways in which one person's nutritional needs can be different from another's.

Maintaining Healthy Habits

Adopting new habits can be challenging. The Dietitians of Canada recommend these strategies to help you maintain healthy eating habits throughout your life:

Develop supportive environments that make healthy choices easier.

Find a network of people and/or groups who can give you reliable food and nutrition information. Encourage your friends and family to join you in your goals. Eat with friends who have also adopted healthy habits. Join online blogs, discussion groups, and cooking classes to keep you motivated and generate new ideas and skills. For more specialized help, find a dietitian that you can talk to and who will support you in your decision to eat smart.

Make breakfast a regular habit.

Eating breakfast helps jumpstart your metabolism after a long period without food and is linked with having a healthy weight. Skipping breakfast may lead to snacking and unhealthy food intake later in the day. Great breakfast choices include fruit, whole-grain cereals, bannock, pita, toast, milk, soy beverage, tofu, eggs, peanut butter, or a carton of yogurt topped with a handful of cereal and dried fruit.

Don't rely on fast food.

Limit your intake of empty-Calorie foods such as chips and fries, and beverages high in Calories, fat, and sugar. Make at least one meal a day a home-prepared meal. If you can, cook together, eat together, and talk together. Family meals help promote healthy eating.

Trends and Change

The United States passed a menu labelling law in 2010 requiring all chain restaurants with 20 or more outlets to provide Calorie counts next to each food item on menus and menu boards. Some states also require sodium, saturated fat, and carbohydrates on printed menus. This allows people to see the energy content of the food available, and order accordingly.

Questions:

1. Would printed Calorie counts on fast-food menu boards influence the foods you ordered? If so, how?
2. Do you think this is a useful policy? Why or why not?

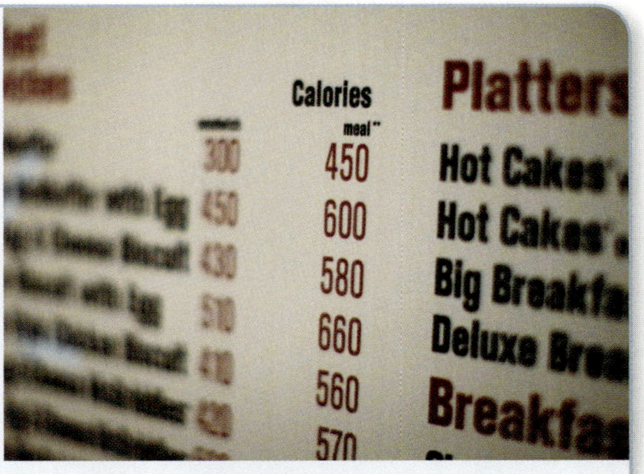

Figure 3.25 Will Calorie labelling influence consumers' behaviour? Will it encourage food companies to make their foods healthier?

starvation mode: a state in which the body perceives a threat of starvation, and conserves Calories and slows metabolism in order to survive

Eat regular meals and a small snack if you are hungry.

Eating more frequently keeps the body from moving into **starvation mode**, which lowers metabolism and activates fat-storing enzymes to conserve energy. By skipping meals, you may also develop an uncontrollable appetite by the next mealtime, often leading to a binge.

"We need some basic food literacy. The entry point to that cultural shift is through a school nutrition program."
– Evan Fraser, professor and author (Leeder, 2011)

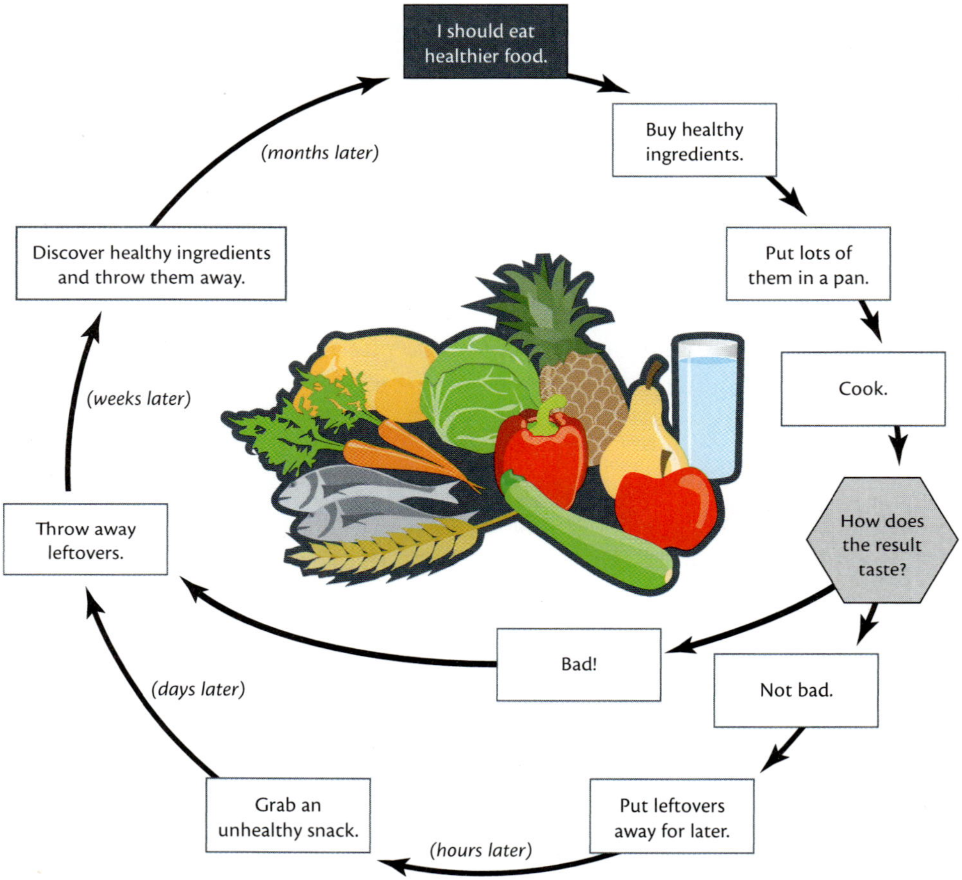

FIGURE 3.26 An unsuccessful attempt to adopt and maintain healthy food habits.

THINK CRITICALLY

1. The flowchart in **Figure 3.26** describes the behaviour of someone who has tried unsuccessfully to eat healthier food. Draw a similar flowchart to show the behaviour of someone who was successful in their efforts to develop healthy food habits.
2. What steps did you include in your flowchart that were helpful to the person?

Active Learning

Make a Healthy Breakfast

The protein and fibre in a burrito will help keep you satisfied until lunchtime. If you keep the ingredients on hand, it can be very quick to prepare.

Microwave Breakfast Burrito

Yield: 1 burrito

Customize this recipe by using vegetables that you enjoy, or by sautéing them first.

Ingredients

1 medium whole-grain tortilla

1 egg

45 mL (3 tbsp) refried beans (canned or homemade)

30 mL (2 tbsp) shredded cheddar cheese

30 mL (2 tbsp) salsa

lettuce, diced tomato, or vegetables of your choice

Method

1. Crack egg into a small microwave-safe cup or bowl. Beat well with a fork.
2. Cover and cook in microwave until done (approximately 1 min). (Alternatively, cook beaten egg in a non-stick pan over medium-low heat until set.)
3. Place egg along diameter of tortilla, add other ingredients, and wrap up your burrito.

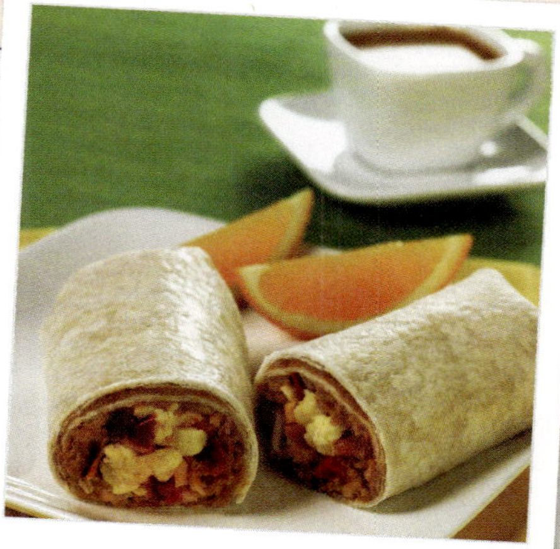

Figure 3.27 By cooking the egg in a microwave oven, a breakfast burrito can be assembled and ready to eat in less than five minutes.

Questions:

1. List the characteristics that make this breakfast healthy.
2. Develop an alternative version of a breakfast burrito using different ingredients. Explain how your version provides the same nutritional benefits as the original.
3. How can a nutritious breakfast such as this one help you maintain healthy eating habits throughout the day?

Strategies to Gain Weight

A healthy weight doesn't necessarily mean a low weight. People may need to gain or regain weight for a variety of reasons. Sometimes people need to gain weight because

- they have had a serious illness resulting in lost weight
- they are very thin and want to look and feel better
- they are athletes who want to build strength and muscle to perform better
- they are older adults who have unintentionally lost weight due to reduced muscle mass, decreased appetite, or other causes

These strategies can help a person gain weight, while remaining healthy (Beck, 2012):

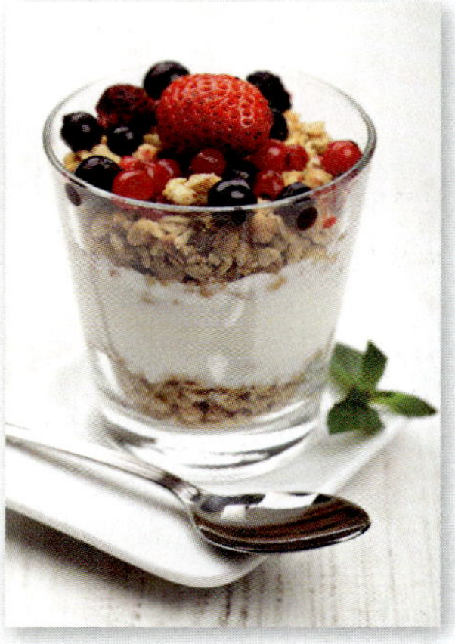

Figure 3.28 Energy-dense snacks such as yogurt and granola provide additional Calories, as well as nutrients to maintain good health.

1. **Eating more frequently.** People trying to gain weight could try to eat three meals a day plus a morning snack, an afternoon snack, and an evening snack, if possible. Snacks should be nutrient-dense foods such as dried or fresh fruit, yogurt, unsweetened fruit juice, low-fat muffins, energy bars, toast, peanut butter, eggs, a bowl of granola, a glass of milk, or a homemade smoothie with nuts. While any high-Calorie foods can result in weight gain, these nutrient-dense foods will help to maintain good health while adding Calories to the daily diet.
2. **Adding extra Calories to foods.** For example, drink juice or milk instead of water, use peanut butter on toast or on bananas, add dried fruit and nuts to breakfast cereals and salads. These nutrient-dense additions to foods will add Calories, but help maintain a balanced diet.
3. **Choosing energy-dense foods.** People working to gain weight can choose an energy-dense juice such as cranberry, cranapple, pomegranate, grape, pineapple, and apricot instead of less energy-dense juices such as apple, orange, and grapefruit. They should work to control their daily sugar consumption, though. They can choose low-fat granola, muesli, and oatmeal instead of lighter cereals; choose hearty lentil, bean, barley, or minestrone soups instead of thinner soups; and choose sweeter, more energy-dense vegetables such as peas, corn, winter squash, and carrots from time to time instead of leafy green vegetables.
4. **Including regular exercise.** Exercise—especially strength training—promotes muscle growth and helps keep the body healthy.

Pause and Think

Describe two pieces of nutritional advice that are given both to people trying to lose weight and to people trying to gain weight. Why is this advice appropriate for both groups?

In Focus

Evaluating Weight-Loss Programs

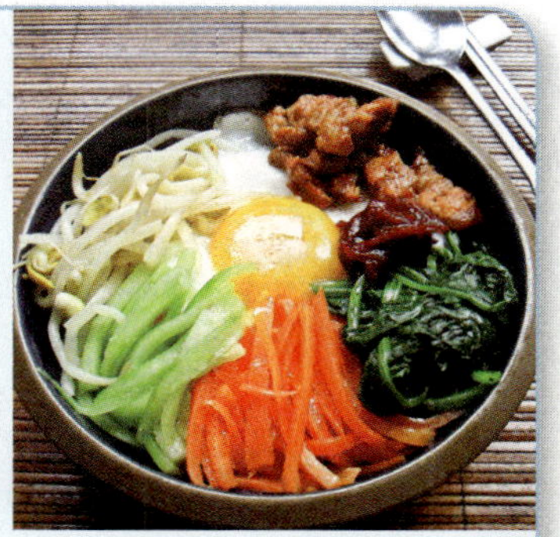

Figure 3.29 A healthy weight-loss program should be based on the principles of healthy eating, and follow the guidelines of *Eating Well with Canada's Food Guide.*

While a healthy balanced diet, combined with appropriate physical activity, is considered to be the best way to balance energy needs, some people do choose to follow a specific program or diet to help them lose weight. Anyone considering a weight-loss program should consult with a health care professional or dietitian before committing to the program. Many weight-loss programs are not effective, and some can be dangerous. The following strategies to help identify safe and effective long-term weight-loss programs are based on guidelines developed by the Dietitians of Canada (2010):

1. Ask questions to make sure the weight-loss program follows *Eating Well with Canada's Food Guide* and sound scientific principles.
    - Does it include all four food groups and at least 800 Calories per day?
    - Does it include a plan for regular physical activity and tips on how to get started?
    - Does it include a maintenance stage to develop a healthy lifestyle over the long term?
    - Does the program rely on unproven or false weight-loss aids, such as starch blockers or fat burners?
    - Is scientific evidence provided that the program can result in safe, successful weight loss?
2. Ask questions to make sure goals and assumptions are realistic.
    - Are details provided about costs, risks, and amounts of time needed to reach goals?
    - Does the program set a weight-loss goal of no more than one kilogram (two pounds) per week?
    - Does the program include flexibility for likes and dislikes, allergies, cultural restrictions, and so on?
3. Ask questions to determine how the owners of the program benefit from clients' participation.
    - Does the program make clients dependent on foods or supplements sold by the program's owners?
    - Are clients required to sign an expensive, long-term contract or to sign up quickly?
4. Decide if the weight-loss program is a good lifestyle fit.
    - Are the diet and physical activity appropriate for the client's current health status?
    - Are any changes to lifestyle manageable by the client and his or her family?

Questions:

1. Why might someone choose to follow a weight-loss plan instead of adopting a healthy lifestyle?
2. What are the disadvantages of following a weight-loss plan instead of adopting a healthy lifestyle?
3. What can people who choose to use a weight-loss plan do to ensure that they maintain the new healthy weight once they achieve it?

CHAPTER 3 REVIEW

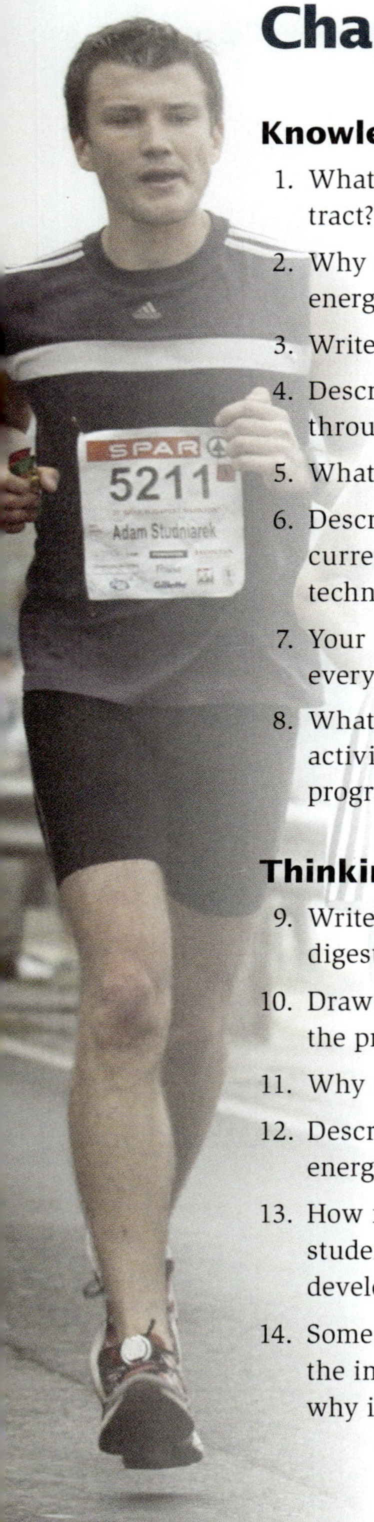

Chapter Review

Knowledge and Understanding/Thinking

1. What important role is played by the cellular membranes that line the digestive tract?
2. Why does your body need to consume protein regularly even if it is getting enough energy from other sources?
3. Write an equation to illustrate the factors involved in maintaining energy balance.
4. Describe three factors that help explain why a person's energy needs change throughout their lifespan.
5. What is meant by the phrase *a healthy weight*?
6. Describe the various techniques that can be used to assess whether a person's current weight is healthy. What are the advantages and disadvantages of each technique?
7. Your friend decides to decrease his energy consumption by skipping breakfast every day. Why is this not a good strategy?
8. What are the advantages of adopting a healthy diet and engaging in physical activity to achieve and maintain a healthy weight, instead of using a weight-loss program advertised online?

Thinking/Communication

9. Write a one-paragraph explanation of what happens to food that you eat during digestion.
10. Draw a diagram to show the steps carbohydrates, proteins, and lipids go through in the process of digestion. Include all steps from ingestion to absorption or excretion.
11. Why can't healthy weight ranges be provided for children and teenagers?
12. Describe two reasons why athletes need to consume more energy to maintain energy balance than unfit, sedentary people do.
13. How might a national school lunch program, in which hot meals were provided to students, impact nutrition in teens? What factors might need to be considered in developing such a program?
14. Some busy people regularly eat fast food instead of home-prepared meals. Describe the impacts this can have on their energy balance and nutritional status. Explain why it can have these impacts.

Communication/Application

15. While your friend is talking to you and eating lunch, he suddenly breaks into a coughing fit. Between gasps, he says, "Sorry, my food went down the wrong tube." What was happening inside his digestive tract?
16. Develop a slide show or a comic strip to show how your body obtains nutrients from foods. Use a real food, such as macaroni and cheese, that is high in carbohydrates, fat, and protein, as an example.
17. Describe concrete steps that a typical Canadian could take to improve their nutrient status. Use the information on page 73 and what you have learned about nutrients and energy balance.
18. Work in a small group to develop an ad campaign that encourages students to practise a healthy energy-balanced lifestyle. Your campaign may include components that use print, video, audio, and/or other media.
19. Describe a breakfast, lunch, and snack that you could prepare for yourself. Explain how each helps you meet your energy and nutrient needs through the day.
20. Your family has agreed to share cooking responsibilities and you need to prepare one dinner per week. Plan three different menus and analyze the degree to which they meet family members' needs for nutrients and energy.

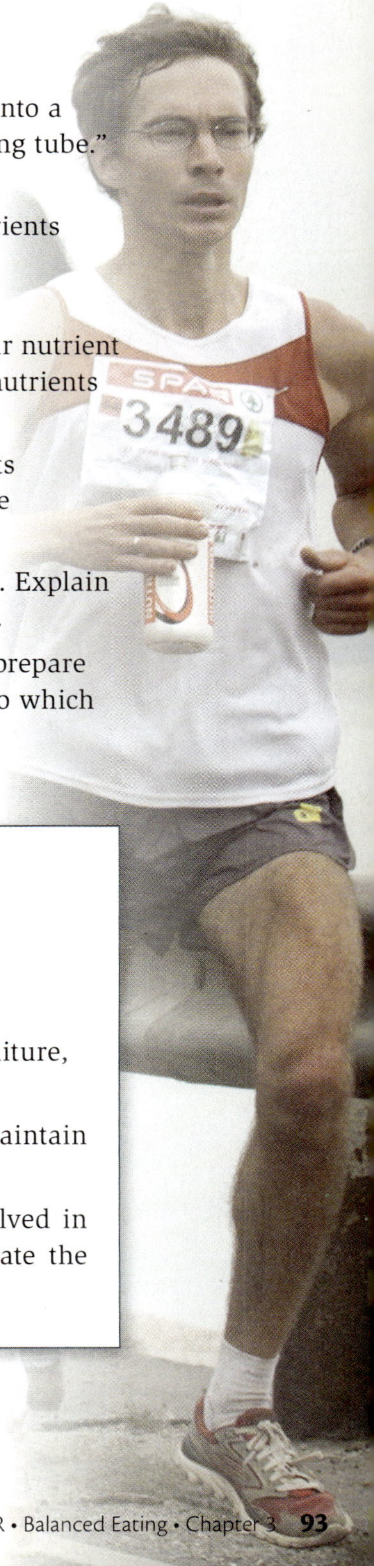

Putting It All Together

In this chapter, you have

- described the process of digestion, absorption, and metabolism of food
- examined the relationship between macronutrient intake, energy expenditure, and energy balance
- investigated various ways of regulating energy balance to achieve and maintain healthy body weight

Create a graphic organizer of your choice to summarize the factors involved in overall energy balance and how energy balance can be maintained. Relate the information to what you have learned in previous chapters.

Unit 2 Lifespan Nutrition

Chapter 4 **Nutritional Needs Through Life**

Chapter 5 **Nutrition and Disease**

Chapter 6 **Emerging Trends in Food and Nutrition**

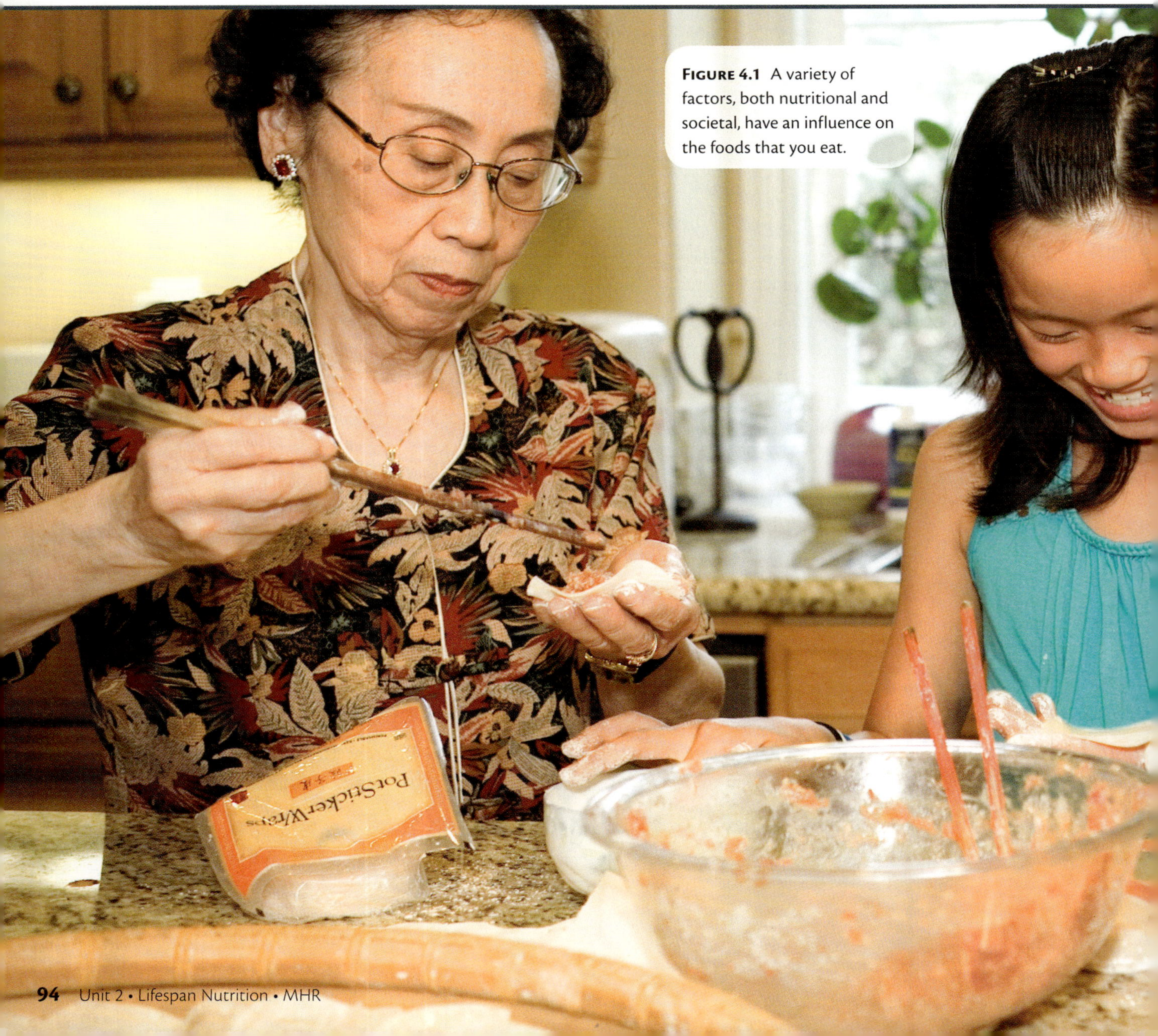

Figure 4.1 A variety of factors, both nutritional and societal, have an influence on the foods that you eat.

the BIG idea **How do our individual nutritional needs and food choices affect our daily lives?**

- Think about the foods you have eaten today. Why did you choose those foods?
- How were the foods you ate as a young child different from those you eat now? Why?
- How do the diets of people with various diseases or health conditions differ from your diet? Why?

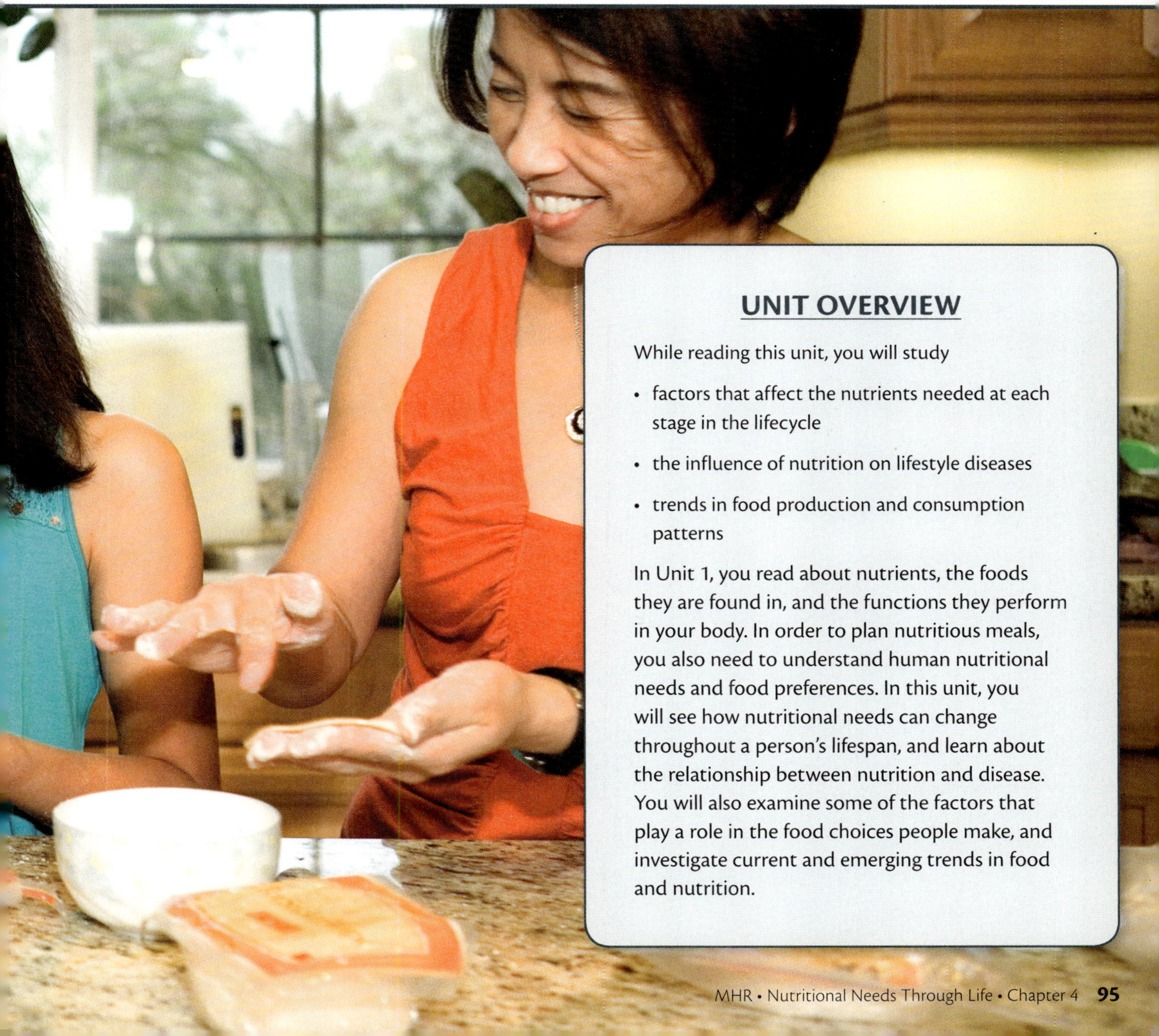

UNIT OVERVIEW

While reading this unit, you will study

- factors that affect the nutrients needed at each stage in the lifecycle
- the influence of nutrition on lifestyle diseases
- trends in food production and consumption patterns

In Unit 1, you read about nutrients, the foods they are found in, and the functions they perform in your body. In order to plan nutritious meals, you also need to understand human nutritional needs and food preferences. In this unit, you will see how nutritional needs can change throughout a person's lifespan, and learn about the relationship between nutrition and disease. You will also examine some of the factors that play a role in the food choices people make, and investigate current and emerging trends in food and nutrition.

Chapter 4

Nutritional Needs Through Life

Key Terms

caries
colostrum
food neophobia
foremilk
hindmilk
neural tube
obesogenic
teratogenic

Research and Inquiry Skills

- Use nutrition and health terminology and concepts correctly

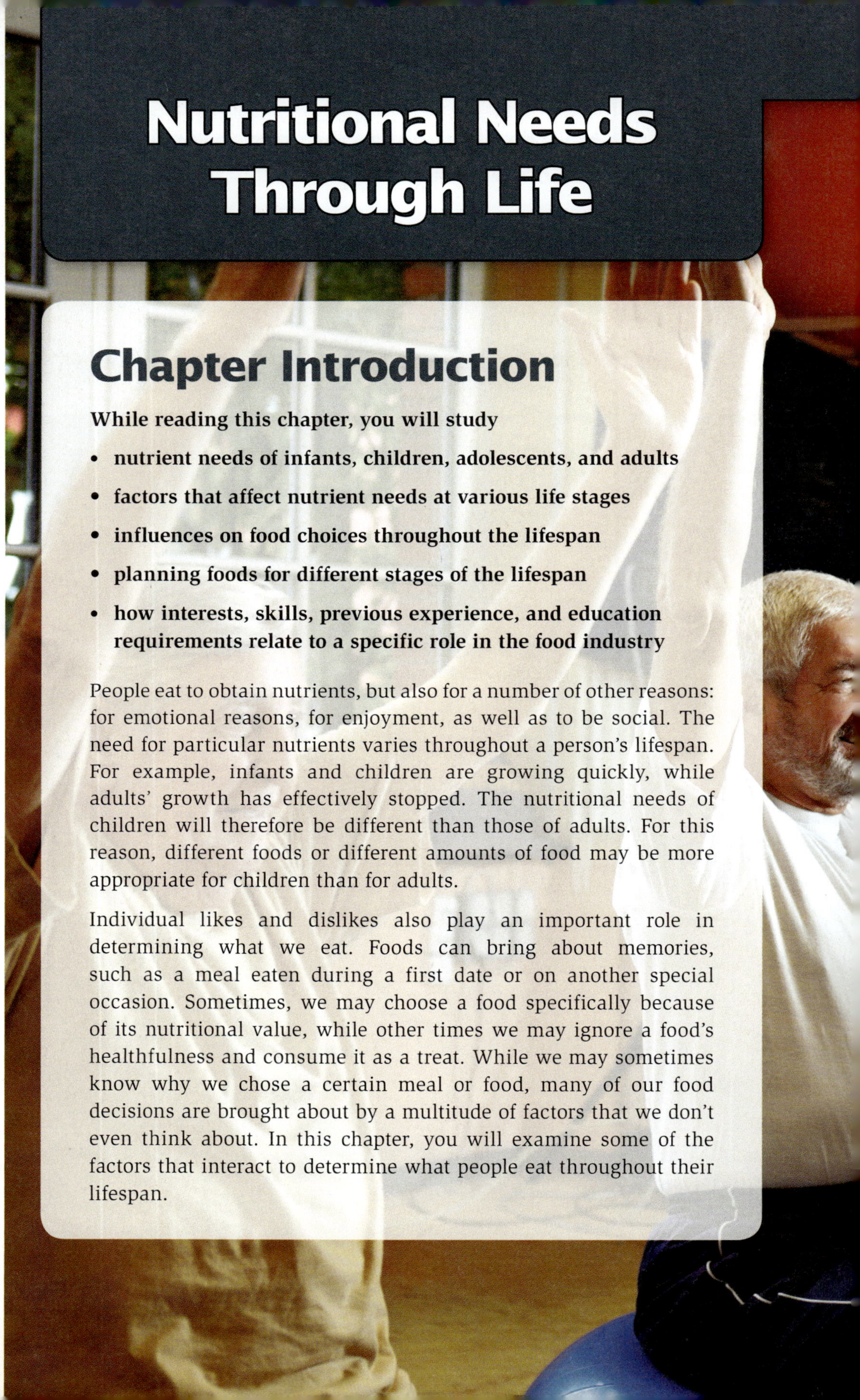

Figure 4.2 Differing needs throughout our lives have an effect on what we eat. How might the needs for older adults be different from your own? How might they be similar?

Chapter Introduction

While reading this chapter, you will study

- **nutrient needs of infants, children, adolescents, and adults**
- **factors that affect nutrient needs at various life stages**
- **influences on food choices throughout the lifespan**
- **planning foods for different stages of the lifespan**
- **how interests, skills, previous experience, and education requirements relate to a specific role in the food industry**

People eat to obtain nutrients, but also for a number of other reasons: for emotional reasons, for enjoyment, as well as to be social. The need for particular nutrients varies throughout a person's lifespan. For example, infants and children are growing quickly, while adults' growth has effectively stopped. The nutritional needs of children will therefore be different than those of adults. For this reason, different foods or different amounts of food may be more appropriate for children than for adults.

Individual likes and dislikes also play an important role in determining what we eat. Foods can bring about memories, such as a meal eaten during a first date or on another special occasion. Sometimes, we may choose a food specifically because of its nutritional value, while other times we may ignore a food's healthfulness and consume it as a treat. While we may sometimes know why we chose a certain meal or food, many of our food decisions are brought about by a multitude of factors that we don't even think about. In this chapter, you will examine some of the factors that interact to determine what people eat throughout their lifespan.

Spotlight On...

Can Food Preferences Begin in Utero?

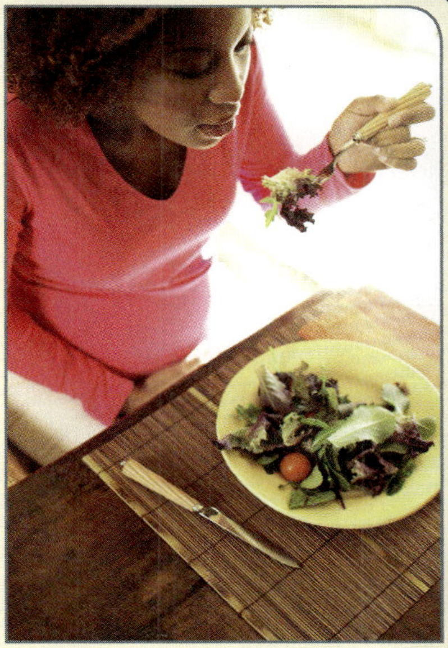

FIGURE 4.3 Are our preferences for certain flavours developed before we're born?

While we may use the terms interchangeably, flavour and taste are different. Taste is one of the senses. We detect five tastes: sweet, sour, salty, bitter, and umami, a savoury taste found in foods like meat, mushrooms, and dashi (Lindemann, Ogiwara, & Ninomiya, 2002). Flavour involves several senses, including taste and smell. Food preferences—our like or dislike for certain flavours and foods—are both innate and learned. Some, like our preference for sweet tastes and high-Calorie foods, are shared among humans (Saad, 2010). Others, like a preference for spicy food or a strong dislike for a particular flavour, differ from one person to another. Our preference for certain foods also depends upon our environment—early exposure to a food or the availability of a food in our environment can affect our preference for it.

Studies have shown that flavours and odours from a food that is consumed by a woman during pregnancy can be transferred via amniotic fluid, and absorbed by her developing fetus. Flavours in a mother's food can also be transferred to the infant via breast milk (Mennella, Jagnow, & Beauchamp, 2001). To what extent do the food choices of a mother during pregnancy and breastfeeding play a role in the food preferences of her baby? Can a baby develop preferences in utero?

To test this, researchers studied mothers in their last trimester of pregnancy (Menella et al., 2001). The mothers were separated into groups. One group of mothers drank carrot juice at a specific time of day for the duration of their pregnancy. The other group drank water at the same time. While a control group drank water both prenatally and postnatally, the group that drank carrot juice during pregnancy drank water during breastfeeding and the mothers who drank water during pregnancy drank carrot juice during breastfeeding. All the mothers refrained from eating carrots during this time.

When the infants were being weaned to solid foods, they were given infant cereal prepared with water, and cereal prepared with carrot juice. Those infants whose mothers drank the carrot juice prenatally and postnatally consumed more carrot-flavoured cereal than those whose mothers drank only water. They also exhibited fewer negative facial responses in response to being fed the carrot cereal.

Questions:

1. How do you believe the results of the study might have differed if the infants were not breastfed?
2. How might this study help describe cultural and ethnic differences in food choices?
3. How could the results of this study potentially be used to increase the consumption of vegetables and fruit by children?
4. Explain why a varied diet is important for pregnant and lactating women.

Research and Inquiry Skills

Use Nutrition and Health Terminology and Concepts Correctly

Being able to use terms and concepts appropriately is an important skill in research. Doing so demonstrates an understanding of the topic you are investigating, and helps you understand any research that you may be reading. There may be subtle or significant differences among terms. Therefore, researchers need to be aware of the differences and ensure that they are using the correct terminology as part of their research. For example, when designing their research and when publishing the results, the scientists studying infants' prenatal and postnatal acquisition of flavour preferences used scientific terms carefully to describe exactly how their study was set up and what they observed. Having a common understanding helps other social scientists understand, review, and critique their colleagues' work. It also allows scientists to articulate very specific questions for their research, allowing them to study a topic in more detail. For example, being able to describe the role of one particular nutrient in the body allows researchers to study the influence of a second nutrient on the functioning of the first. Whenever you write about nutrition and health issues, check that you are using terminology correctly.

When undertaking research, social scientists need to ensure that they use unambiguous terminology. Using incorrect terms or not applying terms properly may lead to inaccurate or misleading results. For example, if a questionnaire includes unclear questions, research subjects may have difficulty interpreting what the researcher is trying to ask and responses may not answer the question the researcher intended. Incorrectly describing or applying a concept could lead to design errors in a study or research in which incorrect questions were examined, both leading to meaningless results. Whenever you design a questionnaire or another research tool, check that all terms are clear and precise. That way, your results have a better chance of being clear and precise as well.

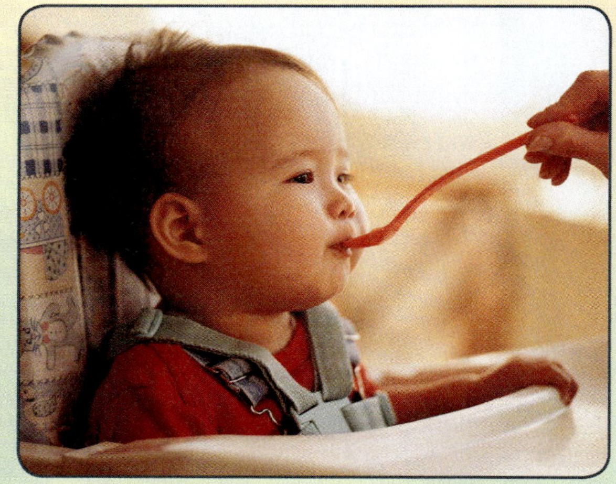

FIGURE 4.4 What errors could be introduced into a study of infant taste preferences if the research design used imprecise terms?

In addition, understanding and using appropriate terms and concepts will help deepen your grasp of what researchers may have been trying to determine, or the results of their study. Therefore, a good understanding of those terms and concepts may allow you to make sense of what you have learned, as well as be better able to explain it to others. When reading results of studies as reported in the media, knowing and understanding the language that was used in the study can allow you to go beyond the headline in order to determine the researcher's intent and discuss their findings. It can also help you detect inaccuracies and potential bias that may have been introduced by the inadvertent or deliberate misuse of scientific terms. Whenever you read about nutrition and health issues, check that terms are used consistently and correctly. Look up the meanings of any terms you are unsure of.

Activities:

1. Below are health and nutrition statements. What terminology would you need to understand in order to accurately assess whether each statement is true?
   a) Obese and overweight mean different things.
   b) Processing foods destroys their nutritional benefits.
   c) Milk products build and strengthen bones.
   d) People can lead sedentary lives, provided they work out a few times a week.
   e) A Calorie and kilocalorie refer to the same thing.
   f) A food product with a high glycemic index means that it is high in sugar.
   g) Quinoa is the only grain that contains eight essential amino acids.
   h) A "light" product is lower in Calories than a regular version of the same product.
   i) Sports drinks and energy gels help the body replace fluids and electrolytes lost during a workout.
2. Where could you find information to help you understand the terms in the statements in Activity 1? Describe the advantages and disadvantages of each source of information.
3. Reread *Spotlight On...* on page 97. List five nutrition or health terms that you need to understand in order to draw accurate conclusions from the study about infants' taste preferences.
4. What nutritional claims have you seen on the front of food packages? Find out which claims are regulated and can only be used if the food satisfies certain criteria. Which claims are not regulated?

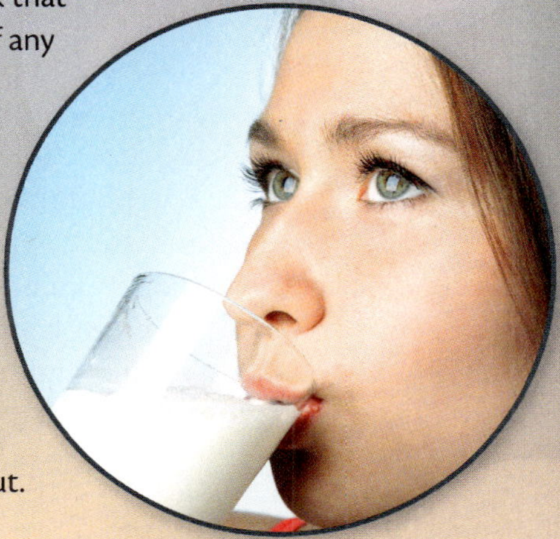

FIGURE 4.5 Some foods are referred to as *processed foods*, but what does that mean? Is pasteurized milk a processed food?

Pregnancy

The nutritional choices that pregnant women make can have a direct bearing on their developing babies. Physicians will often recommend that if a woman is planning on becoming pregnant, she begin making lifestyle changes in advance, as crucial development of the fetus occurs even before a woman may realize that she is pregnant.

Nutrient Needs For Pregnant and Lactating Women

neural tube:
in a developing fetus, the neural tube eventually becomes the central nervous system, including the brain and spinal cord

Folic acid (vitamin B_9) is critical for a baby's development. A lack of this vitamin raises the risk of the baby developing a **neural tube** defect, in which the neural tube fails to close properly during development. Complications arising from this neural tube defect include abnormalities of the brain, spine, and skull. These complications can result in stillbirth or lifelong disabilities such as spina bifida. Neural tube development occurs very early in pregnancy, within the first four weeks after conception. Therefore, health professionals recommend that all women who may become pregnant take a folic acid supplement beginning three months before they plan on conceiving until at least three months into their pregnancy.

Iron is important to support the increased numbers of red blood cells during pregnancy. These blood cells help deliver oxygen to the placenta and the fetus. In the final trimester, the fetus builds its own blood-cell stores from the mother's blood-cell stores, in order to support itself during the first few months of life. Low blood-iron levels can result in babies with low birth weight and premature delivery. Health professionals recommend that pregnant women take a multivitamin containing iron, and consume foods that are rich in iron.

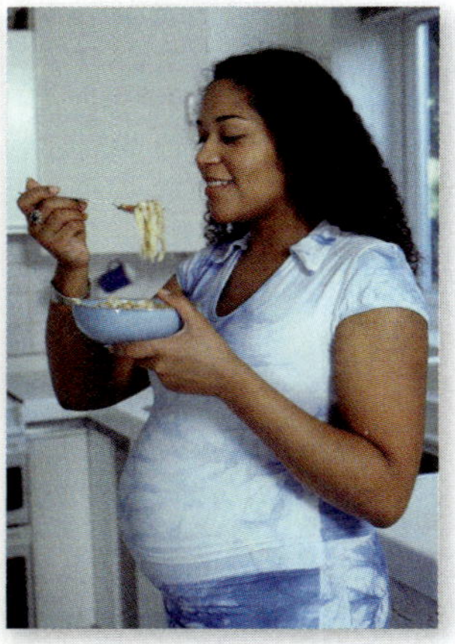

FIGURE 4.6 What stories have you heard about pregnant women and their eating habits? Why do you believe these stories have come about?

Energy needs are higher during pregnancy to support the growth and development of the baby, but the increase in calories required is not as great as many believe. If too much weight is gained, not only will the mother have increased difficulty losing the weight post-partum, but there is an increased risk of complications for both her and the baby during birth. Conversely, gaining too little weight can cause the baby to be born with a low birth weight, which can increase the possibility of various disabilities and health problems as the child ages. Pregnant women are encouraged to follow their health professional's recommendations, follow the guidelines in *Eating Well with Canada's Food Guide*, and continue to be physically active, unless advised otherwise by their physician.

Pause and Think
What factors or influences may cause a woman to gain too little weight during her pregnancy?

Food Safety and Sanitation Concerns

Pregnant women and their developing babies have a higher risk of foodborne illness. A pregnant woman's immune system is weakened, making her more vulnerable to infections. The baby's immune system is not yet developed, so infections can cross the placenta and infect the baby. Foodborne illnesses can cause miscarriage, stillbirth, and increased risk of other complications for the baby. In addition to standard food safety precautions, health professionals caution that pregnant women should refrain from consuming the following foods:

- hot dogs straight from the package without further heating
- non-dried deli meats such as bologna, roast beef and turkey breast
- raw or lightly cooked eggs or egg products, including salad dressings, cookie dough or cake batter, and drinks such as homemade eggnog
- raw or undercooked meat or poultry such as steak tartare
- raw seafood such as sushi, ceviche, raw oysters, clams, and mussels
- raw or unpasteurized dairy products, including soft and semi-soft cheeses such as Brie, Camembert and blue-veined cheese
- raw sprouts such as alfalfa, clover, radish, and mung beans
- refrigerated pâtés and meat spreads
- unpasteurized fruit juice and cider (Health Canada, 2010)

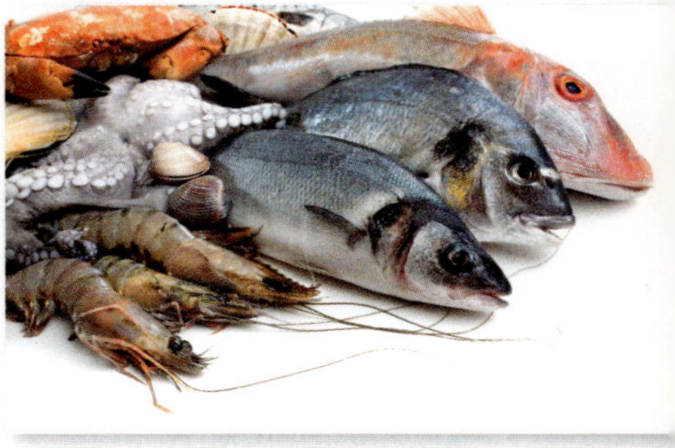

FIGURE 4.7 Why do larger fish usually have higher concentrations of mercury than smaller fish do?

Pregnant women are encouraged to consume fish, as it provides much needed Omega-3 fatty acids in addition to other nutrients. These fatty acids are crucial to the development of the fetus. While *Eating Well with Canada's Food Guide* recommends that adults consume two servings of fish per week, some pregnant women are reluctant to follow this advice due to fear of the mercury content of some fish. Health Canada recommends consuming no more than 0.5 ppm to 1 ppm of mercury as it can have a **teratogenic** effect on the development of the baby's brain. Some fish, such as tuna, shark, and swordfish, does have a higher risk of containing increased levels of mercury. Other fish contain lower levels of mercury and are considered safer.

teratogenic: describing a genetic or environmental factor that can cause abnormal fetal development and lead to birth defects

THINK CRITICALLY

1. Why would the nutrient needs of pregnant women be different than when they are lactating?
2. Review the list of foods above. What characteristics do they share that might place pregnant women at a greater risk of contracting a foodborne illness?

Infancy

In their first year of life, infants are growing and developing rapidly, so not only is their Calorie intake high relative to their size, but the food that they consume can have a noticeable effect. New parents receive a lot of advice from family and friends about whether to breastfeed or bottle feed, when to introduce solid foods, even what foods to give their child. Sorting through the advice to determine the best choice for their child can be difficult.

Breastfeeding

Health professionals agree that breast milk should be the primary source of food for infants. Breastfeeding promotes good health and mother-child bonding. **Colostrum** is full of antibodies and white blood cells, so breastfed children are less likely to develop infections and allergies. Colostrum is easy for infants to digest, and acts as a laxative, making it easier for infants to pass their first stool. Because of this, the World Health Organization (WHO) recommends that babies be fed colostrum within the first hour of birth; exclusively breastfed for the first six months of their lives; and breastfed, supplemented with solid foods, up to age two (2012).

colostrum:
the thick, yellow breastmilk that is produced immediately after birth, continuing through the early days of breastfeeding

Colostrum changes to mature milk within a few days after birth. **Foremilk** quenches infants' thirst. It changes to **hindmilk** as feeding progresses. Hindmilk relaxes the baby, allows the baby to feel full, and encourages weight gain.

foremilk:
the watery milk produced early in a breastfeeding session

hindmilk:
the thicker, almost cream-like milk produced later in feeding that is high in fat

Especially for those infants who may not have consistent access to other food, perhaps due to poverty, breast milk ensures the consistent nutrition that an infant needs to grow and thrive. In addition, breast milk might give some protection from sudden infant death syndrome (Health Canada, 2007). WHO encourages low birth-weight babies to drink breast milk.

Barriers to Breastfeeding

A small percentage of mothers experience physical difficulties breastfeeding. Lactation consultants are available in many communities to help these women. Kaufman, Deenadayalan, and Karpati (2009) noted that the number of women breastfeeding has increased in recent years. However, they found that some mothers believed that their breast milk was not as nutritious as formula, some were uncomfortable breastfeeding around others, and some stopped breastfeeding to return to work.

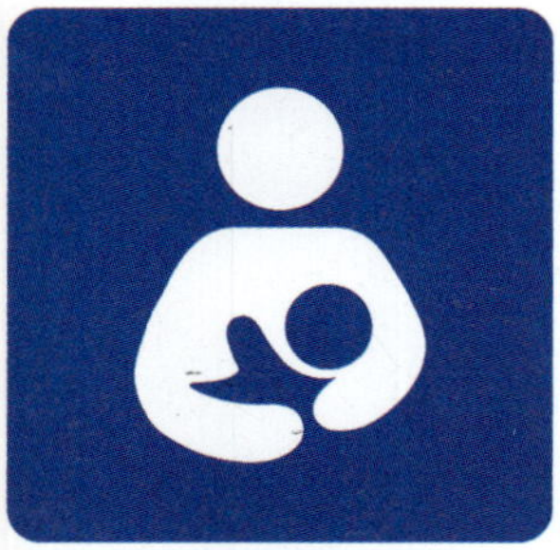

FIGURE 4.8 The International Breastfeeding Symbol. How could the barriers to breastfeeding in public be addressed?

Indeed, society has not always made it easy for women to breastfeed. Breastfeeding women have been banned from public spaces. Women may find it difficult to express and store milk while at work. These reasons may account for the reduction in women who continue to breastfeed three to six months after their baby's birth (Chalmers, Levitt, Heaman, O'Brien, Sauve, & Kaczorowski, 2009).

Life Connection

Donor Milk Banks

Both WHO and the Canadian Paediatric Society recommend the use of human breast milk for sick or low birth-weight babies, as well as for those infants whose mothers are unable to breastfeed. In the 1970s, there were over 20 breast-milk banks in Canada. Due to the increased use of formula, as well as fears about the transmission of diseases through breast milk, the number of milk banks sharply declined. There are currently two, located in British Columbia and Alberta. The banks are stocked by volunteer donations, with deposits made by mothers who have been screened and tested by health care providers. Women who are interested in donating must not be taking certain medications, including herbal supplements. The milk is pasteurized, and made available to mothers on a prescription-only basis.

Question:

Milk banks are currently run on a donation basis. Do you believe that milk banks would become more popular if mothers were paid a fee to provide their milk?

Solid Foods

Starting at around six months of age, solid foods are gradually introduced to children. These should still be combined with breast milk or formula. A primary concern when introducing solid foods is allergies or intolerances to food. Health professionals recommend that foods be introduced one at a time, so that if an infant is sensitive to one particular food, it can be correctly identified. To assess whether a food is an allergen, parents are advised to introduce single foods first, and wait two to three days between introducing new foods to a baby's diet. As the child ages, they may begin to have combination foods (for example, a stew). Babies who have a parent or sibling with a food allergy are at greater risk of developing an allergy themselves. Many parents wait to give certain foods to their child until the child is one year of age, believing it will lessen the chance that their child will develop an allergy to that food. However, the American Academy of Pediatrics states that for those infants who are at a lesser risk of developing an allergy, there is not enough research to recommend delaying potentially allergenic food (Greer, Sicherer, & Burks, 2008).

Feeding also introduces infants to differences in textures and encourages them to develop the ability to chew and swallow. However, choking hazards are a concern. To reduce the risk of choking, foods should be served in small portions (for example, cutting grapes or berries into pieces). Foods should also be soft and moist, as dry foods are more of a choking hazard. Some foods can pose an illness risk in young children. For example, honey can cause serious foodborne illness if served to children under the age of one.

TIP for Healthy Living

As infants should not be exposed directly to sunlight until the age of one, Health Canada recommends that breastfed infants receive a vitamin D supplement until they reach one year of age. Infant formula has been fortified, so a supplement is not required for formula-fed infants.

Unlike older populations, infants under the age of two should drink full-fat dairy products. Fat is necessary for brain development and growth. Letting a child go to sleep with a bottle of milk or juice carries with it an increased risk of the infant developing early childhood **caries**. This tooth decay is most often seen with those infants who drink milk, juice, or formula over extended periods, due to prolonged contact between the sugar in these products and the infants' tooth enamel. To reduce the risk of early tooth decay, the Canadian Dental Association (2012) recommends giving infants water, especially if it is to remain in their bottle overnight.

caries: cavities in teeth, caused by decay of tooth enamel

Pause and Think
Why would infants need more fat than older children?

Familial Influences on Food Choices

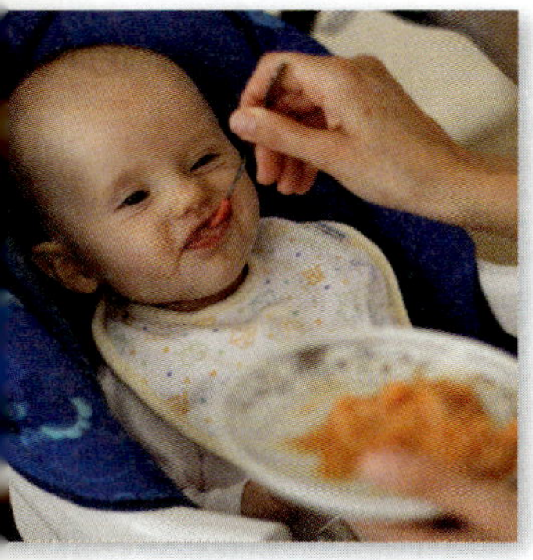

FIGURE 4.9 Solid foods introduce children to a variety of flavours and textures. Why are parents encouraged to introduce one food at a time?

Our families have a significant influence on the foods we eat. Individual family differences help determine the foods we choose to eat, as well as how we eat. Since younger children have their meals prepared for them, adults have an extremely important role in ensuring that good food choices are made during meals and snacks. Feeding infants nutritious diets not only improves their growth and development, but can also set the stage for the food choices those children make as they age and are able to choose what foods they are eating. Our willingness to try new foods is also, in large part, a result of familial influence (Benton, 2004). For example, children whose parents are unwilling to eat vegetables are less likely to eat vegetables themselves. While this specific influence lessens with age, it has laid a foundation for the foods people choose to eat.

In addition to our willingness to try foods, families influence how we perceive certain foods or dishes. Families may hold traditions about special foods that are served during holidays and celebrations, or even on certain days of the week. We may have a well-loved dish that is frequently prepared by a certain family member. Families also influence how we consume food. It is often through our families that we receive information about the timing of meals and about etiquette in a variety of settings.

NUTRITION LITERACY

Homemade baby food is not only less expensive than buying commercially prepared food, but also gives caregivers full control over the ingredients in the food. It is simple to prepare, often involving cooking vegetables or fruit until soft, then puréeing.

THINK CRITICALLY

1. Once children are introduced to solid food, why is it recommended that they continue to consume breast milk or formula?
2. Explain how parental modelling could help a child to make healthy food choices.

Childhood

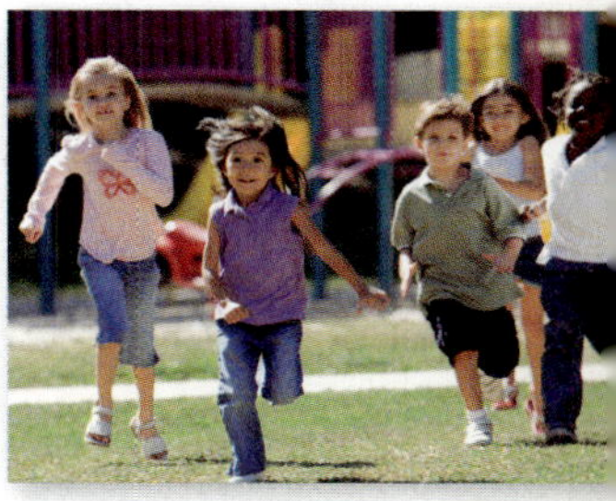

FIGURE 4.10 How can physical activity improve concentration and learning?

Promoting healthy food choices and physical activity for children has a variety of benefits. In addition to encouraging proper growth and development, good nutrition and physical activity also lead to improved concentration and learning. Those who make nutritious food choices during their youth are likely to continue with those choices as they age, lessening their risk of becoming overweight or obese and developing related health problems. Childhood obesity has become a concern in Canada: approximately 17 percent of children are overweight and nine percent are obese (Statistics Canada, 2010). The obesity rate of Canadian children has increased markedly in the past 20 years and fitness levels have decreased (Statistics Canada, 2010). Although the origin of excessive weight in children is complex and relates to both genetics and environmental factors, the issue ultimately results from a high energy intake (diet) related to energy expenditure (physical activity).

General dietary recommendations for children include

- increasing consumption of vegetables, fruits, legumes, and whole grains
- limiting consumption of fats, added sugars, and salt
- participating in at least 60 minutes of physical activity every day (Canadian Society for Exercise Physiology, 2012)

Nutritional Needs in Children

While children need the same nutrients as adults, the amounts they require relative to their body mass differ. For example, children's energy and protein needs are higher than adults', due to children's greater growth patterns. While they are not growing at the rate that they were during infancy, children are still growing; therefore, care needs to be taken that they receive adequate amounts of nutrients such as protein to help sustain their growth. Feeding children a wide variety of foods helps to ensure not only that they are exposed to a variety of flavours, but also that they receive a variety of nutrients.

Poor nutrition in children is related to health concerns such as constipation, iron-deficiency anemia, and vitamin D deficiency. Vitamin D is produced through exposure to the sun, but the amount of sunlight that children are receiving has reduced due to increased indoor play, increased use of sunscreen because of concerns of skin cancer, and wearing clothing that covers much of the skin. Darker-skinned individuals are more at risk of being deficient in vitamin D because the pigment melanin reduces the ability of UV light to penetrate their skin. In addition to exposure to sunlight, vitamin D is available in some food products. Milk (but not milk products) has been fortified with vitamin D, as well as soy, almond, and rice beverages. Egg yolks and fatty fish are other sources of the vitamin.

Children's Food Choices

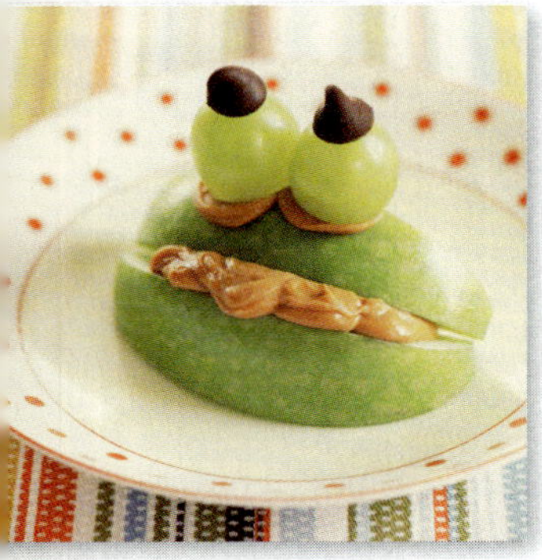

FIGURE 4.11 Describe a healthy snack that you believe is appropriate for a school-age child.

As children age, they have more access to a variety of foods and it becomes important that their choices be healthy whenever possible. Nutrient dense foods should be chosen more often and those high in salt, sugar, and fat should be limited. As you have learned in Chapter 2, beverages can be high in Calories, so juices and sugary drinks should be limited as well. In reality, the majority of many children's fruit intake is in the form of juice (Lorson, Melgar-Quinonez, & Taylor, 2009).

Child Control of Food Choices

Most children will go through a time when they are considered picky eaters, refusing to eat all but certain foods. This can be frustrating for parents and caregivers, especially as it can turn mealtimes into what seem like battles. Children do not necessarily dislike healthy food. Instead, they learn from watching how others around them react to food. Modelling appropriate food choices tends to result in children consuming a wider variety of foods (Wardle, Carnell, & Cooke, 2005). Conversely, pressuring children to finish their food tends to result in children having a negative reaction to that food, and consuming less food (Galloway, Fiorito, Francis, & Birch, 2006). Some children may not like the taste or texture of certain foods. Children have more taste buds than adults do, so they find many flavours stronger than adults will. Researchers also find that girls recognize more tastes than boys. Boys, on the other hand, are better at recognizing the taste of sweet and sour (University of Copenhagen, 2008).

food neophobia: fear of and unwillingness to try new foods

Children may experience **food neophobia** and need to be introduced to new foods several times before they will try it. Allowing children to try smaller amounts of a new food may make them more likely to try it. Presenting the food in a novel way, such as cutting it into shapes may also help. Many nutritionists, cookbooks, and parents extol the virtue of hiding less favoured foods, such as vegetable purées, inside other foods, such as a spaghetti sauce or a baked good. While this practice does ensure that the child gets much-needed nutrition, others worry that ultimately, it will dissuade children from becoming familiar with, and eating those foods separately.

Social Influences on Food Choices

Eating is often a social event. When people get together in social situations, food is often served. In fact, the *Nunavut Food Guide* specifically includes images of people eating together to highlight the importance of social eating, as well as the importance of learning from elders about food and food preparation methods.

As we age, the role of our social circle in helping determine what we eat becomes more important. Seeing what their family, friends, and classmates consume can have a strong influence on children's food choices. When we eat with others, we may eat more food, as we are not as conscious of how much we are actually putting in our mouths (Wansink & Park, 2001). Think about the last time that you ate a meal or snacks with friends. Were you aware of how much food you were consuming? When people are with others, whether it be one friend or a group, they may be less likely to decline food, as it may appear to be rude. This may be an unconscious, rather than conscious decision, but in an attempt to get along with others and mirror what they are doing, we often match what and how much others are eating (Exline, Zell, Bratslavsky, Hamilton, & Swenson, 2012). While this phenomenon may lead us to ingest more Calories, it can also lead us to eat foods that we may not otherwise try.

NUTRITION LITERACY

While the Percent Daily Values listed on a nutrition label are meant for the general population, they may not always be relevant for children, especially if a child's daily needs for a particular nutrient are markedly below that of adolescents or adults (Baylor College of Medicine, 2004).

THINK CRITICALLY

1. Many children like foods from one food group much more than they like foods from another food group. What strategies could be employed to encourage children to eat a variety of foods from all food groups?
2. How can caregivers model and encourage physical activity?

TRENDS AND CHANGE

Fruit and Vegetable Programs

Programs have been developed across the country, as well as in the United States and the United Kingdom, to increase children's consumption of vegetables and fruit. Often created in conjunction with ministries or departments of health, local health units, and other organizations, the programs deliver vegetables and fruit to be served as snacks to school children. The British Columbia School Fruit and Vegetable Nutritional Program delivers produce every other week to school children in the province to eat as an in-school snack, while in Northern Ontario, the Northern Fruit and Vegetable Project aims to deliver produce to elementary school children in the north of the province who may not always have access to fresh produce throughout the year. In Manitoba, the Canadian Cancer Society has created programs for students and their families promoting the use of vegetables and fruit and has trained peer leaders to teach about the importance of consuming vegetables and fruit.

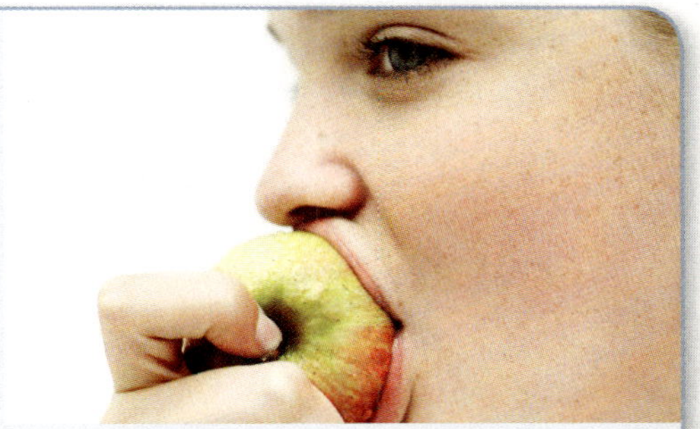

FIGURE 4.12 Fruit and vegetable programs allow students to try potentially unfamiliar produce and emphasize the importance of healthy snacking options.

Question:

How might a researcher determine the influence of fruit and vegetable programs on children's eating habits?

Preadolescence and Early Adolescence

"You should know what's being cooked in the kitchen otherwise you might eat a forbidden food."
– African proverb

Puberty is one of the most important developmental changes to occur during this stage. Both girls and boys are likely to go through puberty between the ages of 10 to 17. However, girls are much more likely than boys to go through puberty earlier, with many more girls experiencing puberty by age 13 (Arim, Shapka, Dahinten, & Willms, 2007). Puberty brings heightened growth, including growth spurts, so nutrient intake, including energy intake, often increases.

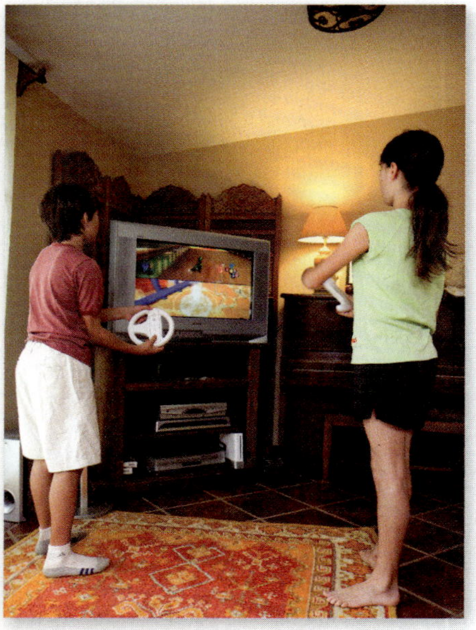

FIGURE 4.13 Video game producers have introduced game systems that involve the player becoming the controller. How effective are these as alternatives to other physical activity?

Effects of Nutrition on Puberty

The age at which children, especially girls, begin to experience puberty has lowered over the decades (Olesen, Jeune, & Boldsen, 2000; Anderson, 2005). While genetic factors play a role, with girls whose mothers went through puberty early being more likely to go through it early themselves, it is only one factor in the lowered age of puberty. Researchers have studied and proposed a variety of reasons for earlier puberty, including the increasing weight and nutritional intake of both males and females (Cheng, Buyken, Shi, Karaolis-Danckert, Kroke, Wudy, Degen, & Remer, 2012). Mumby, Elks, Li, Sharp, Khaw, Luben, Wareham, Loos, et al. (2011) found that girls with a higher BMI (usually those with a higher percentage of body fat) were more likely to have experienced early puberty. Researchers have theorized that increased levels of body fat may trigger the release of hormones that begin the process of puberty (Cheng et al., 2012).

Researchers have also investigated the effect that food choices play in early puberty. Cheng, Gerlach, Libuda, Kranz, Günther, Karaolis-Danckert, Kroke, and Buyken (2010) found that children with poor diets are more likely to go through puberty earlier. Children with diets that are higher in vegetable protein tend to go through puberty approximately seven months later than average, while those with diets higher in animal protein go through puberty approximately seven months earlier (Cheng et al., 2012). Soy products, which are rich in isoflavones—compounds that are similar to the hormone estrogen—have been linked to later puberty in girls, but had no effect on boys (Cheng et al., 2012). Because isoflavones are also found in whole-grain products and both animal and vegetable protein sources, it is difficult for researchers to determine conclusively the effect that this single substance has on the timing of puberty.

Role of Media in Food Choices

While the voluntary guidelines from the Children's Advertising Initiative set limits for the advertising of foods, they are directed only at children's programming. As they age, children and youth have increased access to media and programming that do not fall under the guidelines set out by the Advertising Initiative. Some estimate that children are exposed to as many as 40 000 advertisements per year (Kaiser Family Foundation, 2004). We do know that children who have high levels of media usage are more likely to consume foods that are less nutrient dense and more energy dense (Scully, Wakefield, Niven, Chapman, Crawford, Pratt, Baur, Flood, & Morley, 2012).

In addition, children and youth who were exposed to more food advertising tended to have a higher BMI than those who were not (Halford, Boyland, Hughes, Oliveira, & Dovey, 2007). Scientists theorize that the use of media itself may be an issue, with increased use of media (for example, television and computers) reducing the time that youth spend participating in physical activity. However, while there are correlations between media use and obesity rates, that is, while populations with high rates of media use also tend to have high rates of obesity, a causal link between media usage and weight gain has not been proved (Kaiser Family Foundation, 2004).

OPEN FOR DEBATE

Debate with your class the following: Advertising of fast food or "junk" food should be banned in any programming that youth are likely to watch.

THINK CRITICALLY

1. In what ways can children's eating habits affect their health as early adolescents?
2. Research has shown a correlation between media use and obesity. Why do you think research has not shown a causal link?

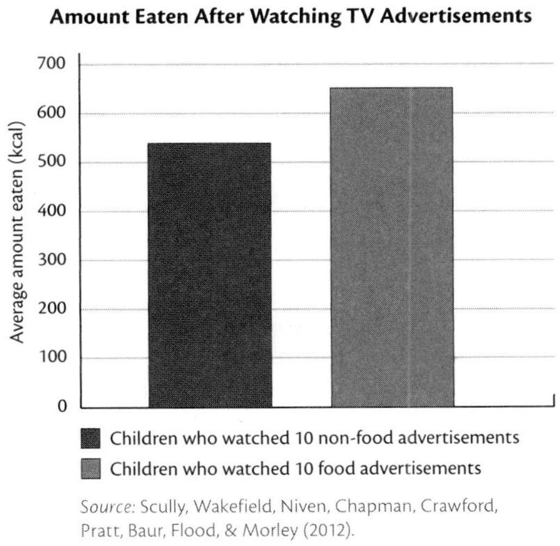

FIGURE 4.14 Normal-weight children who watched advertisements for food increased their consumption of energy dense foods.

ACTIVE LEARNING

Make Your own Healthy Snack

Granola and granola bars are often touted as a healthy food, though with large amounts of fat and sugar, they are not always the best choice. Making your own version means that you have control over the ingredients that go into the recipe.

Granola Bars

Yield: 12 servings

You can vary the fruits, nuts, and seeds in these granola bars to suit your own taste.

Ingredients

250 mL (1 c) old fashioned or quick cooking rolled oats

250 mL (1 c) shredded wheat cereal

250 mL (1 c) walnuts or almonds (optional)

60 mL (¼ c) sesame or sunflower seeds (optional)

125 mL (½ c) coconut

375 mL (1 ½ c) dried fruit (e.g., raisins, cranberries, dates, prunes, apricots)

5 mL (1 tsp) cinnamon

2 mL (½ tsp) salt

2 eggs

60 mL (¼ c) honey

5 mL (1 tsp) vanilla

30 mL (2 tbsp) chocolate chips (optional)

Method

1. Preheat the oven to 180 °C (350 °F). Lightly grease a 20 cm (8 in.) square baking pan.
2. Place the oats, shredded wheat, walnuts, seeds (if using), dried fruit, cinnamon, and salt in the bowl of a food processor. Pulse until the mixture is finely chopped.
3. In a large bowl, blend the eggs, honey, and vanilla. Stir in the oat mixture and chocolate chips (if using). Mix well.
4. Spread the mixture evenly in the prepared pan. Flatten gently with the back of a spoon.
5. Bake about 20 minutes, or until the edges turn golden brown. Let cool completely in pan, then cut into 12 bars.

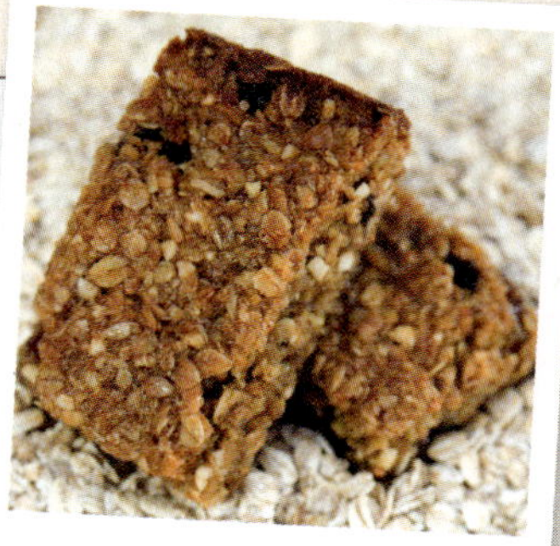

FIGURE 4.15 Homemade granola bars.

Activities:

1. Research to find another recipe for granola bars.
2. Which recipe do you think is healthier? Why?
3. Make both recipes and comment on similarities and differences in the final products.

Adolescence

From a biological, standpoint adolescents are children. They are working their way to adulthood however, and, not surprisingly, many of their nutrition needs fall between recommendations for both groups. Adolescents are increasingly responsible for the foods that they consume, both at school and at home. Unfortunately, not all are making good food choices, but those choices are often related to their level of nutrition knowledge. Greene-Finestone, Campbell, Gutmanis, and Evers (2005) found that the majority of adolescents they studied had inadequate diets. However, those who considered themselves health conscious were more likely to consume nutritionally adequate diets. While energy and fat intakes were close to current recommendations, a substantial number of young women were reported to consume inadequate amounts of nutrients that are especially important during their reproductive years, namely calcium, folate, and iron (Health Canada, 2009).

"Tell me what you eat, and I'll tell you who you are."
– Jean Anthelme Brillat-Savarin

Nutritional Needs in Adolescence

While iron-deficiency anemia can affect both males and females, due to rapid growth at this stage, it is more of a concern among adolescent girls. Girls lose iron when they menstruate, and are therefore at a higher risk of being deficient in iron. For this reason, girls' recommended intake of iron is higher than that of boys. While poor nutrition can also lead to iron deficiency, so can poor bioavailability of the iron source. Iron from animal sources is generally easily absorbed from the gastrointestinal tract and used by the body. Calcium and substances in plants called *phytates* can reduce the bioavailability of iron from vegetable sources making it more difficult for the body to use (Derbyshire, 2012). However, other foods can increase iron's bioavailability. Vitamin C helps to increase nutrient absorption, so including foods high in the vitamin, such as citrus fruits, kiwi, tomatoes, and broccoli will help.

FIGURE 4.16 Which foods pictured here are good sources of iron? Which foods are good sources of protein?

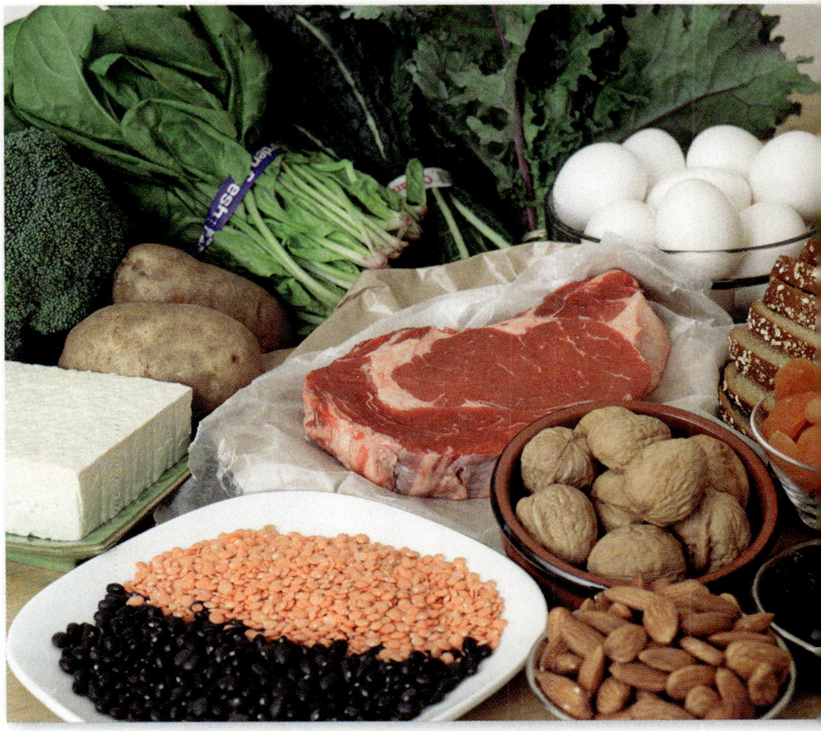

While vegetarian eating patterns exist around the world, often due to cultural, religious, and economic reasons, Canadian teenagers are increasingly turning away from meat sources and towards more vegetarian choices. Approximately 20 percent of teenage girls report not consuming meat products, with another 35 percent consuming fewer than the recommended number of daily servings (Jacobs Starkey, Johnson-Down, & Gray-Donald, 2001). While vegetarian diets can be nutritionally sound, some vegetarians, especially those who are new to vegetarianism, may not ensure that they consume foods high in protein, iron, and calcium, as well as vitamin B_{12}. With appropriate education, vegetarians can have healthy diets.

Protein needs continue to be as important for adolescents as they are for children, due to the rapid growth that happens at this time. Since almost all vegetable protein is incomplete—it does not contain a full complement of amino acids—vegetarians may need to consume more protein than the stated RDI (Kniskern & Johnston, 2011). Those who consume meat products also need to be mindful of their protein choices. While meats may provide complete proteins, they may also be high in fat, especially saturated fat.

Psychological and Emotional Influences on Food Choices

We associate food with both positive and negative experiences. Comfort foods are often foods we associate with home and a sense of belonging (Troisi & Gabriel, 2011). These can be foods that remind us of our childhood, such as consuming chicken soup when sick, or a favourite meal at a special event such as a birthday.

Our psychological state can also determine how much we eat and what types of foods we choose. For example, researchers find that people who are well rested will make better food choices than people who are sleep deprived (Wells & Cruess, 2006). Certain emotions make us more likely to eat, including anger, confusion, and loneliness (Nguyen-Rodriguez, Unger, & Spruijt-Metz, 2009). A concern with emotional eating is that the overconsumption of food can lead to weight gain and may be a factor in rising obesity levels in society, especially as the foods consumed in stressful situations tend to be energy dense or even empty-Calorie foods. Because emotional eating is a learned response, people can be taught to deal with negative emotions in other ways, to avoid emotional overeating.

THINK CRITICALLY

1. Why do some vegetarians need to take a vitamin B_{12} supplement?
2. Describe your comfort foods. Why do they hold positive feelings for you?

POINT/COUNTERPOINT

Protein and Sports Supplements

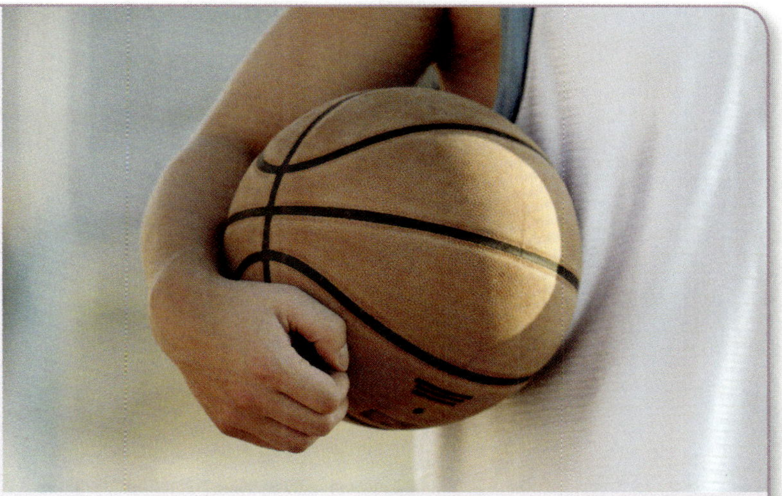

FIGURE 4.17 Many athletes use supplements, as they believe it will help them grow muscles and give them an edge over their competition. Are these supplements safe and effective?

Protein or sports supplements are increasingly used by bodybuilders, athletes, and the general public in the belief that they will help them build and increase their muscle mass. Those who market supplements maintain they are a way to build muscle mass and help with recovery after a workout, often citing research to back their claims. A wide variety of supplements exist, including drinks, meal replacement bars, pills and tablets, protein powders, and vitamin-enhanced waters. In Canada, drinks, bars, and powders are classified as foods, while tablets and vitamin-enhanced waters are classified as supplements and regulated accordingly. It is often difficult to determine if certain products should be classified as a food or a supplement, as they display characteristics of both. A product classified as a supplement should not be thought of as stronger or better.

However, are these products necessary? While athletes may need increased protein levels, the amount required varies by age, gender, body size, and diet (Nutrition Working Group of the IOC, 2003). For most athletes, many nutritionists state that a healthy, nutrient-rich diet will meet their daily protein requirements. Not all ingredients in supplements may be regulated, and as a result, their effectiveness and safety are not always known. How, then, could a person determine whether protein and sports supplements have any value?

Activities:

1. Choose a protein or sports supplement or ingredient (examples include creatine, amino acids, glucosamine, whey protein, caffeine, vitamin-enhanced waters, bee pollen, DHEA, geranium oil, yohimbine). Using reliable computer-based sources, find an article supporting the use of your chosen supplement, and one article opposing its use.
2. List the source of each article you chose and explain why you chose that article, site, or link. What criteria did you use to determine the reliability of the authors?
3. Summarize the content of each article.
4. Based on what you have read, come to a conclusion about the effectiveness of your chosen supplement. Would you recommend its use? Justify your answer.

Adulthood

Studies on Canadian adults' food intake show that younger adult males are most likely to meet the recommendations of *Eating Well with Canada's Food Guide* (Jacobs Starkey, Johnson-Down, & Gray-Donald, 2001). People of both sexes were unlikely to consume the daily recommendations for vegetables and fruit, and received 25 percent of their daily energy needs from foods high in sugar, salt, and fat.

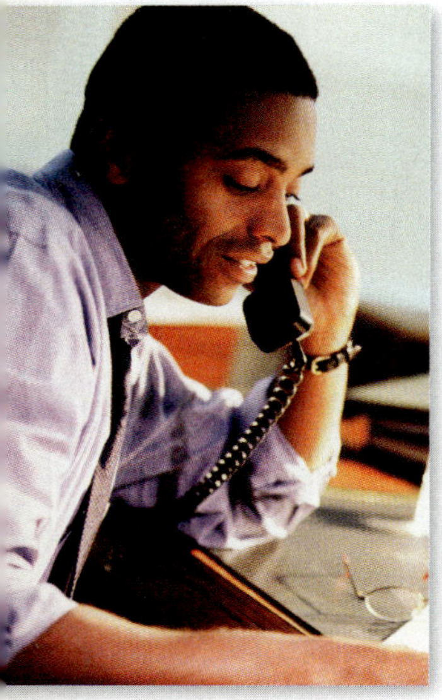

FIGURE 4.18 What are some activities or exercises that a person with a sedentary job could fit into their daily work routine?

Many adults find that their metabolism gradually slows down, which means that it can be easier to gain weight, and harder to lose weight. Adults who had no difficulty maintaining a healthy weight as adolescents may suddenly find that they gain weight every year. While a weight gain of five pounds in a year may not seem like much, if that gain is consistent every year, in a decade a person could be 50 pounds heavier. Once adults enter the workforce, many find that their activity level drops from when they were students. At the same time, they may have fewer opportunities for physical activity than they previously did.

As with all other age groups, daily physical activity is important for adults. Some adults find it difficult to find time in their schedules to be active, as they take on work responsibilities, enter into relationships, and have children. While some were involved in sports or other activities on a regular basis in their youth, they may no longer participate in those activities, and find it inconvenient to substitute another activity.

Nutrient Needs of Adults

As adults are no longer growing, their nutrient needs will be different from when they were younger. For example, Calorie needs may be reduced, as the metabolism slows down as part of the aging process. In addition, the nutrient needs of a younger adult may be different than those of an older adult. For example, iron and folic acid are important nutrients for women in their childbearing years, while calcium and vitamin D are increasingly important for older men and women.

A nutritional concern among all age groups in North America, but particularly among adults, is the overconsumption of macronutrients (chiefly, fat, protein, and sugar), coupled with the underconsumption of micronutrients and fibre (Physicians Committee for Responsible Medicine, 2008). One of the consequences of this imbalance is obesity, but it can be related to other health issues as well. For example, researchers are finding a relationship between poor diet, obesity, and fertility for both sexes (Attaman, Toth, Furtado, Campos, Hauser, & Chavarro, 2012; Nichols, Curtis, Rayman, & Taylor, 2008).

Economic Influences on Food Choice

How Canadians spend their food money has changed significantly over the past 20 years. They now spend more of their food dollars at restaurants, and less to purchase foods at grocery stores (Canadian Council of Food and Nutrition, 2008). Several factors have influenced this change. An increased availability of restaurants and other food-service establishments has created more choice in dining options. Eating out has become a more common leisure activity. For some Canadians, the cost of spending money on restaurant food is worth more than the time to make the food themselves. Whatever the reasons, we're spending less money on food to prepare at home, and more on food that has been prepared for us.

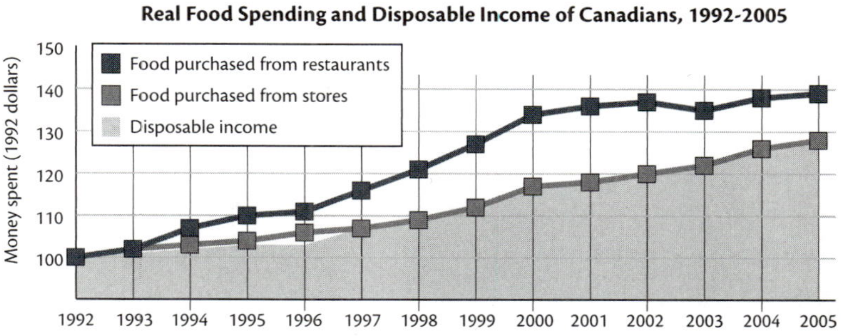

FIGURE 4.19 Using the data in the graph, describe the relationship between income and food expenditures.

As adults move away from their family home, they are introduced to daily tasks with which they may have had limited experiences. Preparing meals is one of those tasks. Some young adults developed food preparation skills by cooking for themselves or their families on a regular basis. For others, it is entirely new. In addition to learning how to prepare nutritious, flavourful meals, adults need to learn how to budget for groceries, shop, and safely store food. While it can be tempting to simply eat out or use pre-prepared meals, being able to prepare foods is important. When you prepare a meal, more control can be placed over the ingredients in a dish. Ingredients and cooking methods can be altered to increase the nutritional value, or to suit personal tastes. Also, portion size can be controlled.

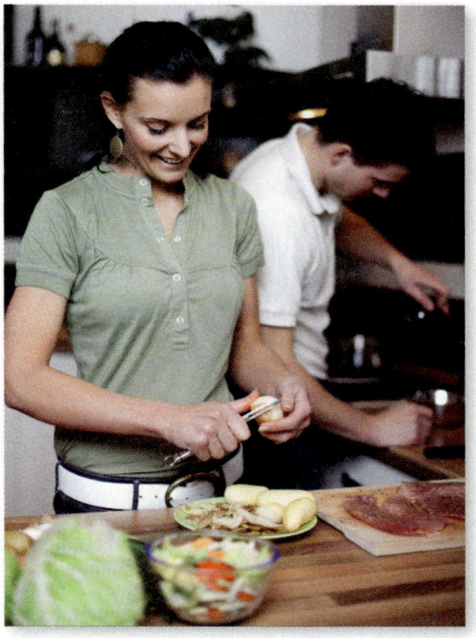

FIGURE 4.20 Being able to plan and prepare meals is a skill many adults use all their lives. What are some benefits of being able to cook for yourself?

FINANCIAL LITERACY

Using online or other resources, create a meal for four people that costs no more than $10. The meal must follow recommendations from *Eating Well with Canada's Food Guide* or another food guideline. Calculate the price of each ingredient in your meal to determine the total price of the meal.

THINK CRITICALLY

1. Why is the recommended daily intake of nutrients often higher for adults than it is for adolescents, even though adults have stopped growing?
2. What aspects of preparation might cause foods to lose nutritional value?

Older Adults

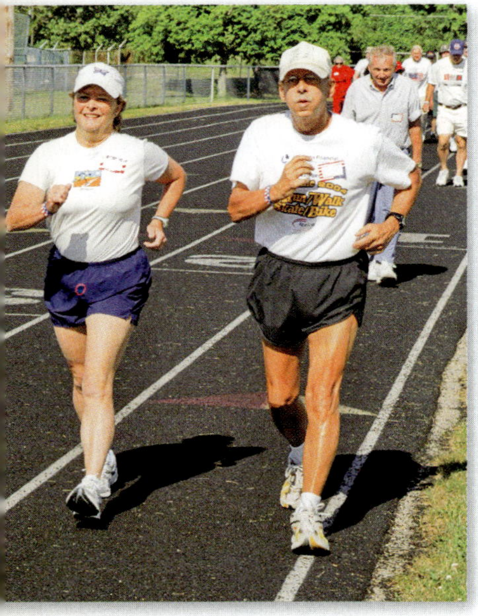

FIGURE 4.21 Increased levels of physical activity reduce obesity levels and the risk of falls. What are ways to encourage physical activity among seniors?

As we age, our metabolism slows down. Energy needs diminish, but nutrient needs generally remain the same as they are for younger adults. Therefore, seniors need to ensure that they consume foods that are high in nutrients, but lower in Calories. For some, this means that portion sizes of foods need to be adjusted. Nutrient dense foods, such as vegetables, fruits, and whole grains can help ensure that nutritional needs are met while consuming fewer calories. Some seniors may find that their appetite has become smaller. Energy dense foods may be beneficial for these people, because they provide needed Calories and other nutrients in smaller portions.

Physical activity can reduce the risk of chronic illness and obesity, and improve cognition. Retaining muscle strength in the elderly is also very important, as it has a bearing on daily functions such as the ability to pick up items, walking speed, and endurance (Nied & Franklin, 2002). It also plays a role in maintaining bone mass (Guadalupe-Grau, Fuentes, Guerra, & Calbet, 2009).

A variety of factors may impair an older adult's ability to acquire and prepare food, such as lack of transportation, poverty, and physical disabilities. The result may be a very limited diet, with few or no fresh foods. Community programs such as Meals on Wheels, as well as for-profit companies, will deliver prepared meals once a day to the elderly and others with chronic health conditions or recovering from surgeries. Some grocery stores also have ordering and delivery options, thus making it possible for people with reduced mobility to receive fresh groceries on a regular basis.

Pause and Think
In addition to food, what other benefits could seniors gain from food delivery programs such as Meals on Wheels?

Nutrient Needs of Older Adults

"Man is what he eats."
– Ludwig Andreas Feuerbach

Food moves through an older adult's digestive system more slowly, which means that constipation may be more of a concern than it is in younger adults. Therefore, eating a diet high in fibre, such as whole grains, fruits, vegetables, nuts, and seeds, and consuming an adequate amount of water are important. Since older adults are less likely to experience thirst, dehydration can be a concern, especially during the warmer months.

Vitamin D deficiency can result in osteomalacia, the softening of bones, when it occurs in adulthood. Researchers have also found that adequate vitamin D and calcium levels among older adults help to reduce the number of falls people experience (Bischoff-Ferrari, Dawson-Hughes, Staehelin, Orav, Stuck, Theiler, Wong, Egli, Kiel, & Henschkowski, 2009). Because aging skin synthesizes vitamin D less efficiently from the sun, Health Canada recommends that adults over the age of 50 take a vitamin D supplement.

Prescription and over-the-counter medications can affect the absorption of some nutrients into the bloodstream. As well, some nutrients, such as grapefruit juice, may reduce the effectiveness of a medication. All medications, including supplements, should be discussed with health professionals, to help determine if any unwanted interactions may occur.

CAREER CONNECTION

Seniors' Meals Volunteer

Volunteering allows people to connect to their community, and helps them develop important skills. For adolescents with little job experience, volunteer work can build skills, demonstrate experience to potential employers, and help identify strengths. Volunteering can also allow people to determine whether they are interested in a particular career area.

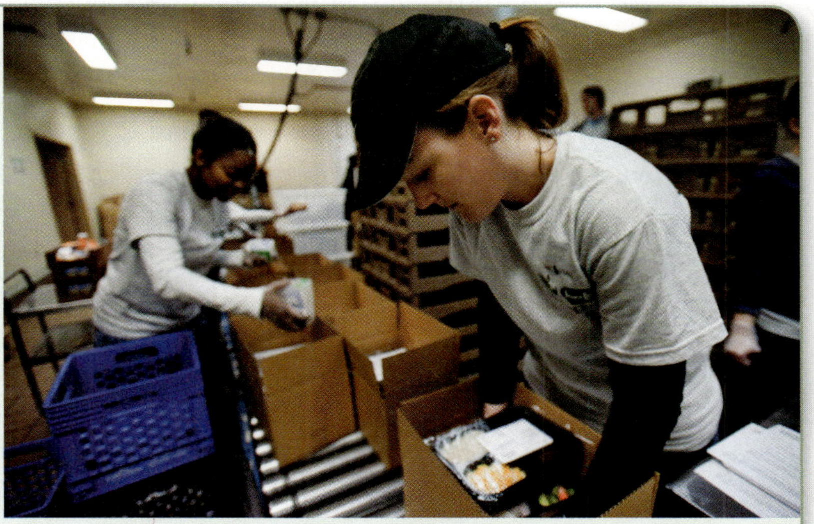

FIGURE 4.22 How might your school get involved in a seniors' meal program?

Seniors' meals services aim to address the issue of hunger as it affects the elderly. They may take the form of meals served at a seniors' centre or place of worship. Delivering meals can help those who find it difficult to leave their homes. Both types of programs often rely on the work of volunteers.

Volunteers who deliver meals often also check on the safety of their clients and provide some social interaction, as their delivery schedule may incorporate time to visit. While it is preferable to have access to a vehicle, some organizations that run delivery programs make use of car-sharing services, and have begun bike delivery programs. Other volunteer opportunities exist for individuals and groups, from helping to prepare and package meals and cleaning up, to coordinating schedules and loading and unloading delivery vehicles.

Questions:

1. What characteristics would make someone a good volunteer for a meal delivery service?
2. Why might it be beneficial for adolescents to volunteer with seniors' meals programs?

Cultural Influences on Food Choice

obesogenic: describes environmental factors and influences that encourage or promote obesity

Our society is increasingly **obesogenic**, which makes it increasingly difficult for people to maintain a healthy weight. While rising rates of obesity have been linked to our environment since the 1990s, scientists have not yet reached consensus as to what constitutes an obesogenic environment (Kirk, Penney, & McHugh, 2010). By examining a variety of possible influences, researchers hope to create more effective strategies to address obesity.

These influences include the widespread availability of inexpensive, energy-dense foods. There are also many opportunities to consume food throughout the day, not only from food-service establishments, but also from vending machines, food delivery options, and increasing numbers of ready-to-eat foods available to us. Elements of the food industry have promoted the sale of increased portion sizes of some foods for a small increase in price.

TIP for Healthy Living

Research shows that families who eat at home together are more likely to be healthier than those who don't eat together. In addition to eating more vegetables and other nutrient-rich foods, families who eat together are more likely to interact positively with one another.

In addition, our daily lives present us with fewer opportunities for physical activity, from neighbourhoods that discourage walking or biking while encouraging the use of cars, to an increase in the number of sedentary jobs. However, just as our society has created conditions that have promoted obesity, it can also promote healthy eating and physical activity. For example, a coalition of regional health authorities, urban planners, and other organizations have created Healthy Canada by Design, which is examining how communities can be designed to improve aspects of health. For example, creating bike lanes and walking or running paths can encourage people to rely less on cars as a form of transportation.

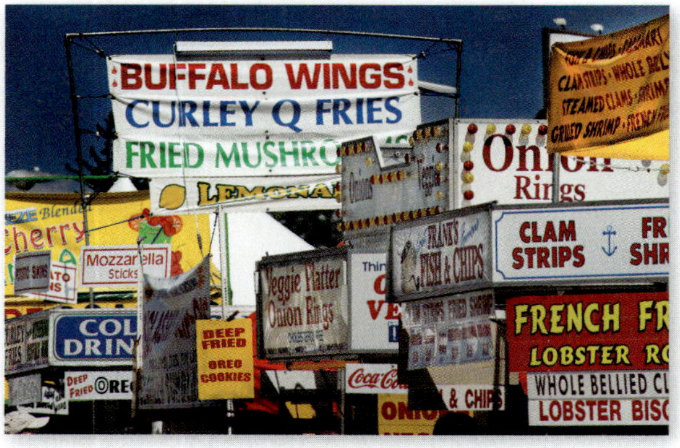

FIGURE 4.23 What aspects of your neighbourhood are obesogenic? What aspects encourage a healthy lifestyle?

THINK CRITICALLY

1. Delivery services bring one meal per day. How could older adults ensure they are making good food choices for the remainder of the day?
2. Propose other approaches that communities could take to increase physical activity. Explain your choices.

Case Study

Meal Planning for a Multigenerational Household

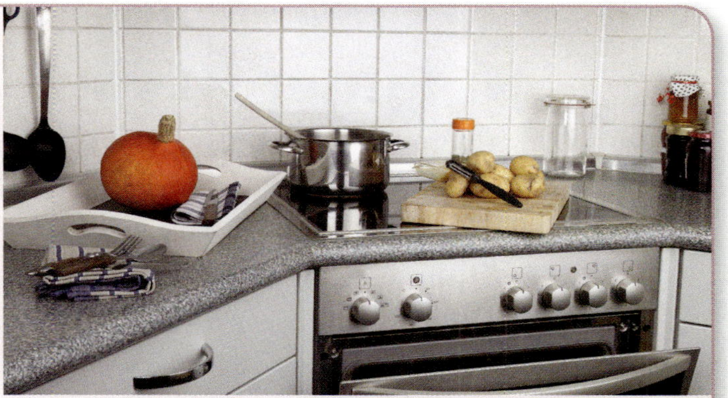

Figure 4.24 Research shows that eating together is beneficial to families. Do you believe these same results would be true for a family eating meals at a restaurant, rather than at home?

The Lees live in a single-family home on the outskirts of a city. There are seven people in the Lee household.

The parents are both 43 years old. They have a wide variety of interests. While they would like to be more active, they find that family activities often interfere. One of the parents has been advised by a physician to control fat and sodium intake, due to a family history of heart disease. As a result, the couple has resolved to participate in a physical activity at least three times per week.

The Lees have three children, a one-year-old baby, and 10-year-old twins. One of the twins is quite involved in martial arts. The other twin plays soccer. With twice weekly soccer practices, and a weekly soccer game, plus occasional tournaments and special training sessions, life is quite busy. Both twins are also involved in dance classes, taking hip-hop lessons once a week. While they are twins, they have very different food preferences. One twin loves spicy food, while the other doesn't. One twin loves vegetables, while the other prefers meat. They also have different appetites, with one eating almost twice the amount of food as the other.

The baby has been growing quickly, and is enjoying the ability to self-feed.

The children's 17-year-old cousin has also been living with them while attending high school. In addition to being a vegetarian the cousin is also on the school's track and field team. As an ovo-lacto vegetarian, the cousin eats eggs and milk products but not meats, fish, or poultry.

In addition, a 67-year-old grandparent is also a part of the household. The grandparent participates in local, provincial, and national track and field competitions. As an athlete, any healthy food is appreciated, though the grandparent will admit to a serious sweet tooth.

Activities:

1. Using the information provided, plan meals for a week for the family that follow the recommendations of *Eating Well with Canada's Food Guide*. Plan one meal to celebrate the cousin's graduation from high school.
2. Describe the factors that you needed to take into account when determining what dishes to serve.
3. Using a variety of sources, create a list of recipes that you believe would be appropriate, explaining why you have chosen each recipe.
4. As an extension, you may choose to make one or more of the recipes in class or at home.

CHAPTER 4 REVIEW

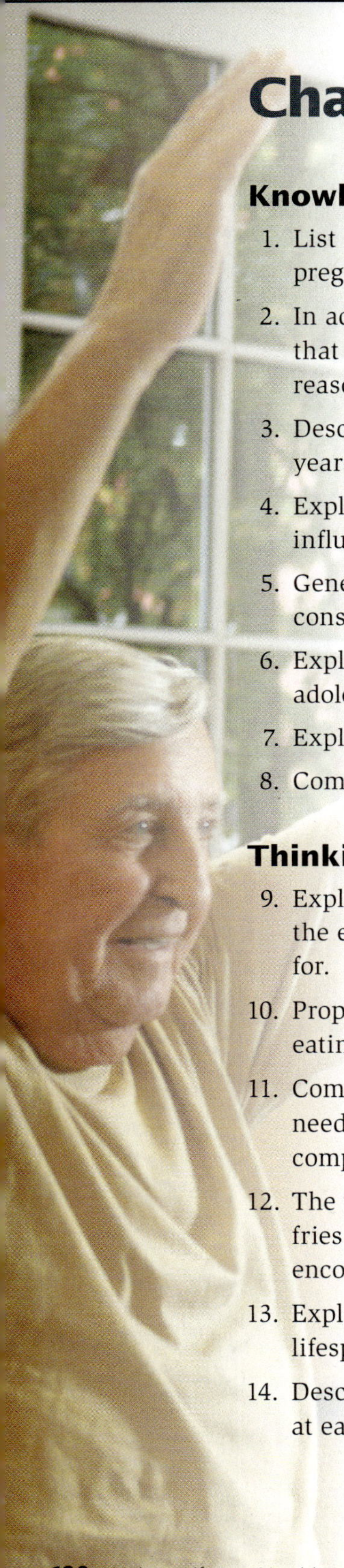

Chapter Review

Knowledge and Understanding/Thinking

1. List sources of foods that are high in Omega-3 fatty acids and are appropriate for a pregnant woman who is a vegetarian.
2. In addition to taking a folic acid supplement, describe other nutritional safeguards that a woman might need to take if she is planning on becoming pregnant. Provide reasoning behind your response.
3. Describe how the nutrient needs of an infant are different than those of a seven-year-old child.
4. Explain how fruit and vegetable programs in schools can make use of social influences on our food choices.
5. Generate a list of protein-rich foods that would be appropriate for athletes to consume.
6. Explain why different nutrient amounts are recommended for male and female adolescents and adults, but not for children and preadolescents.
7. Explain why a 21-year-old woman requires more iron than an 11-year-old girl.
8. Compare and contrast the nutrient needs of adolescents with those of the elderly.

Thinking/Communication

9. Explain the job skills a person could develop working at a meal delivery service for the elderly. Then describe a job that each of the skills you listed might be useful for.
10. Propose reasons to explain why there is a positive correlation between families eating meals together and measures of health.
11. Compare and contrast nutrient needs across the lifespan. What nutrients are needed in increased amounts at each stage? You may use a table to present your comparison.
12. The vegetable most commonly eaten by children is potatoes in the form of French fries (Wardle, Carnell, & Cooke, 2005). What strategies could be employed to encourage children to increase their consumption of other vegetables and fruits?
13. Explain how familial influences would affect food choices at various stages of the lifespan.
14. Describe what you think would be the three main factors influencing food choices at each life stage. Explain your reasoning.

Communication/Application

15. Create an advertisement targeted to children to promote fruit and vegetable consumption.
16. Develop a poster or a computer presentation highlighting strategies to reduce the risk of foodborne illness for pregnant women.
17. Design a fact sheet with tips for adults to plan, shop for, and prepare meals for one person.
18. Investigate which meal delivery services are available to the elderly in your community. Compare the options using price, nutritional value of meals, variety of foods offered, and convenience. Explain which program you believe is the most effective, based on your results.

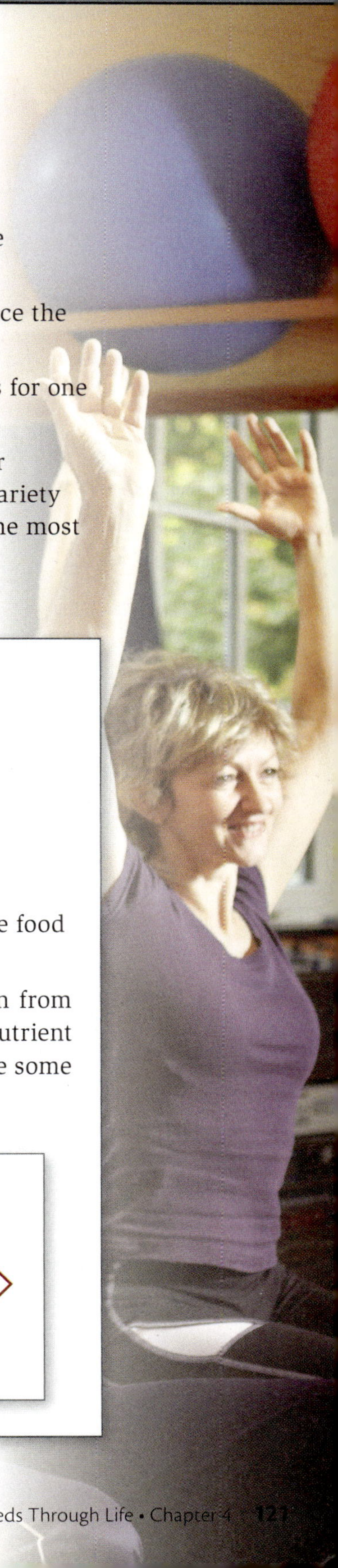

Putting It All Together

In this chapter, you have

- compared nutrient needs of various life stages
- identified influences on nutrient needs throughout the lifespan
- described various influences on food choices
- used nutrient needs throughout the lifespan and food preferences to make food and meal choices

On a long sheet of paper, create a time line to represent a person's lifespan from infant to older adult. On one side of the time line, indicate important nutrient requirements of each stage of life. On the other side of the time line, describe some of the factors that may influence food preferences at each stage.

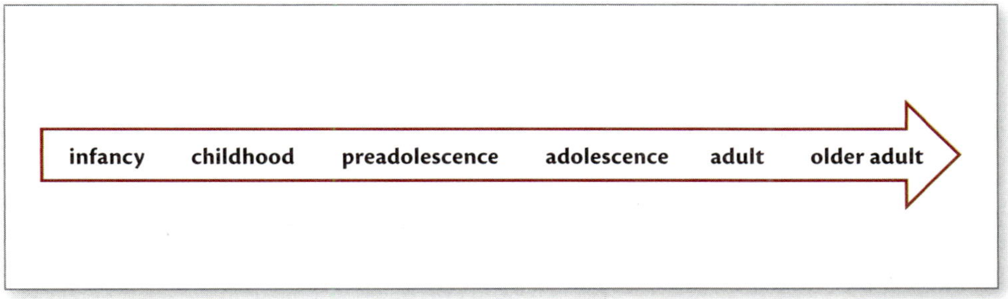

Chapter
5

Nutrition and Disease

KEY TERMS

allergen
anaphylaxis
histamine
hyperglycemia
insulin
neuropathy
stress

RESEARCH AND INQUIRY SKILLS

- Analyzing research information

Chapter Introduction

While reading this chapter, you will study

- **conditions that can contribute to the development of illness and disease**
- **the effects of eating habits on the prevention and management of health conditions**
- **the incidence of specific nutrition-related illnesses and concerns among population groups**
- **nutrient needs and dietary requirements of people with specific illnesses or diseases**

Canadians are living longer because of advances in science and technology. However, not all are living well. Chronic diseases such as cancer, diabetes, cardiovascular disease, and osteoporosis can have a drastic effect on a person's well-being. Many of these conditions start developing several years before they become an issue. To prevent them, specific risk factors need to be addressed early in life.

Although causes of chronic diseases are complex and not fully understood, eating a healthy diet and engaging in regular physical activity are two important strategies to reduce the risk of many diseases. A healthy diet can also reduce symptoms, prevent complications, and increase quality of life for someone who has a disease.

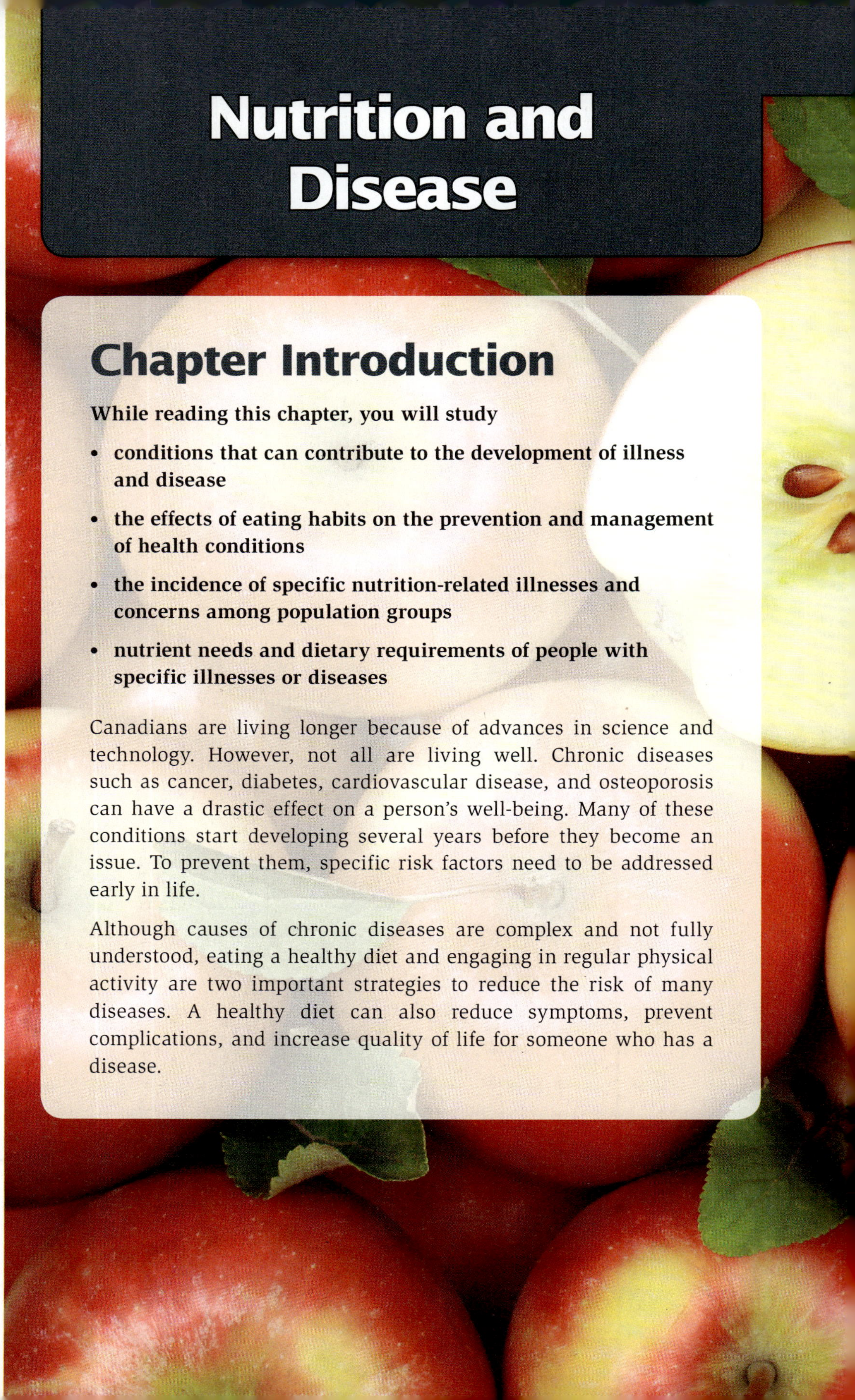

FIGURE 5.1 It takes more than an apple a day to keep you healthy but it's a good start. What other practices can help prevent disease?

Spotlight On...

Misconceptions about Nutrition and Disease

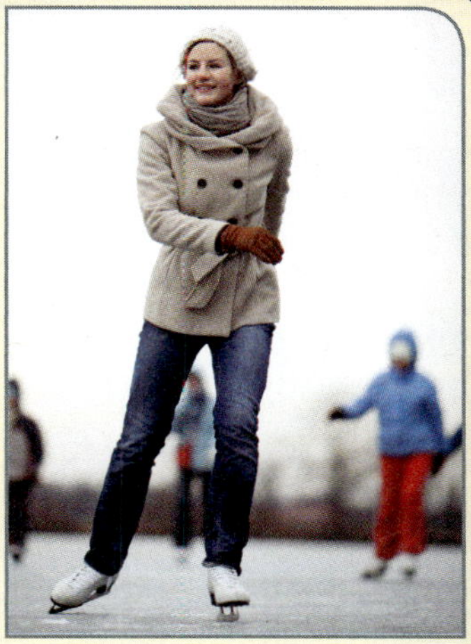

FIGURE 5.2 What can this young woman do today to help keep her healthy throughout her lifespan? What can you do to stay healthy?

Many misunderstandings have contributed to the prevalence of diseases such as cancer, heart disease, and type 2 diabetes. Young people sometimes think that they do not need to be concerned about these diseases. In reality, habits adopted as a child or teenager can influence health throughout the lifespan and poor health habits can be very difficult to change as you age.

Misconception 1: We're all going to get cancer anyway.
The reality is that many causes of cancer and other chronic diseases can often be avoided. If three major risk factors—an unhealthy diet, a sedentary lifestyle, and tobacco use—are eliminated, over 40 percent of cancer, and 80 percent of heart disease, stroke, and type 2 diabetes can be prevented (WHO, 2012).

Misconception 2: If your lifestyle is unhealthy, you are to blame for developing type 2 diabetes.
Although unhealthy lifestyles play a role in developing many chronic diseases such as type 2 diabetes, family history, social inequalities, and other factors also play a role. Type 2 diabetes may be related to overconsumption of Calorie-dense, nutrient-poor foods, but it is also linked to heredity.

Poverty, food insecurity, and other social factors can all interfere with people's abilities to make choices about their lifestyle. Vulnerable groups such as children cannot choose the environment in which they live, and have limited choices about the food they eat. Reports of type 2 diabetes in children and adolescents—previously unheard of—have increased worldwide.

Misconception 3: Chronic diseases affect only old people.
Worldwide, almost half of all deaths from chronic disease occur in people under 70 years of age. In 2005, one-quarter of all deaths from chronic disease occurred in people 30 to 60 years of age (WHO, 2012).

Misconception 4: People who eat more organic than conventional fruits and vegetables are healthier.
While organic fruits and vegetables generally include fewer synthetic pesticide and fertilizer residues than other fruits and vegetables, the amounts in all fruits and vegetables sold in Canada are within a safe range. There is no hard evidence that eating organic fruits and vegetables is healthier than eating conventionally grown fruits and vegetables (National Collaborating Centre for Environmental Health, 2010). It is more important for your health to eat seven to eight servings of fruits and vegetables a day than it is to worry about whether those fruits and vegetables are organic or not.

Activities:

1. Why is it important for teenagers to understand these misconceptions?
2. Describe some of the factors that cause chronic disease.
3. Besides eating more vegetables and fruits, what do you think are the most important food choices you could make to help prevent chronic disease?

Research and Inquiry Skills

Analyzing Research Information

Reputable scientific studies are based on large amounts of data. These large pools of data help ensure that results and conclusions are valid and reproducible.

To analyze large amounts of data, researchers look for patterns by using statistical, graphical, and analytical techniques. Similarly, when you gather data from research, the same techniques can help you analyze the data you gather.

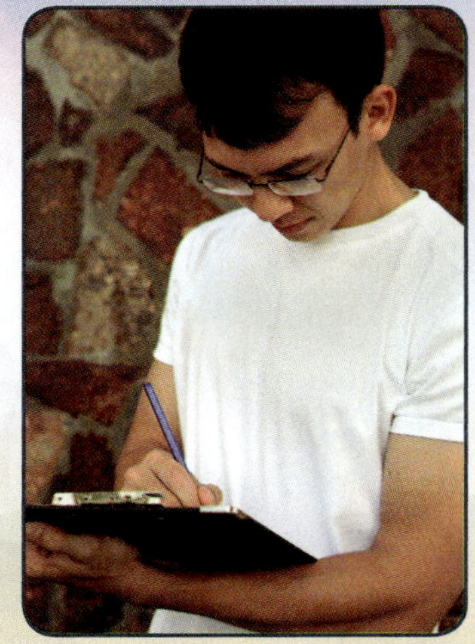

FIGURE 5.3 Write questions for questionnaires carefully so that the answers will be as easy as possible to analyze.

The following strategies will help you analyze information you gather during any research process:

1. Before you start collecting data, develop a research question. Once you have gathered some information, use your research question to help organize the information and focus your analysis. For example, if you are conducting research to determine what foods can help prevent heart disease, you can organize information by whether it helps answer that question or not. Once you have done that, you can organize the information further, perhaps grouping it into information about foods that protect the blood vessels and foods that help reduce stress on the heart.
2. Organizing your data should also help you decide whether you have enough data to fully answer your research question, or whether you need to gather more data to answer parts of the question.
3. Organize qualitative data (comments and opinions) into categories. For example, you might categorize the results of a series of interviews about careers in the food industry into *education, skills, experiences on the job,* and *benefits of the career.* Then examine the categories and try to identify patterns, trends, or causes and their effects.
4. Organize quantitative data (numbers and statistics) into tables or columns. Once the data is organized, you can calculate statistical measures such as mean, median, and range. You can graph the data to see trends or to compare two sets of data. For example, if a survey question asked people to rank three recipes on a scale of how filling they found them, you could construct a bar graph to compare the rankings.

Different types of graphs can help you see different kinds of trends.

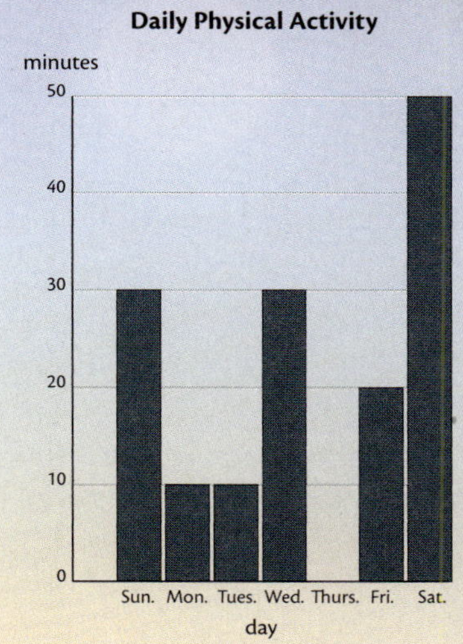

Figure 5.4 Bar graphs can help you compare two or more sets of quantitative data.

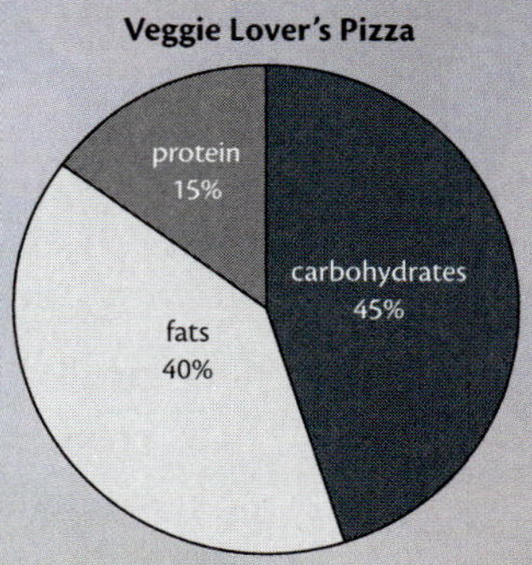

Figure 5.5 Circle graphs can help you compare parts of a whole.

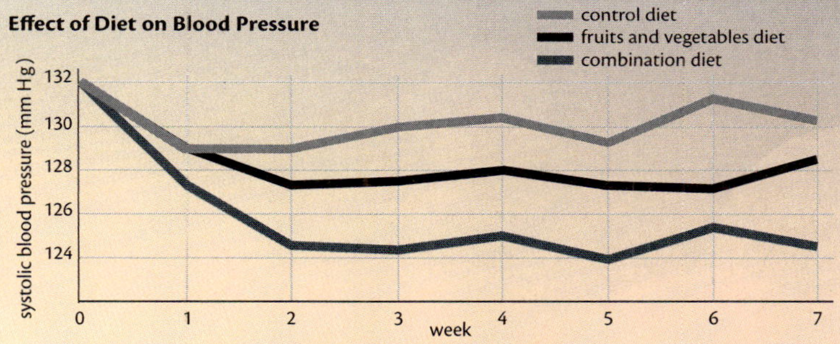

Figure 5.6 Line graphs can help you analyze how something changed over time, and can also help analyze cause-and-effect relationships.

Questions:

1. By writing questions for questionnaires and interviews carefully, you can ensure that the answers you obtain will be as easy as possible to analyze. Rewrite each question to result in a set of answers that you will be able to analyze more easily.
   a) How much cooking experience do you have?
   b) What is your favourite snack?
   c) How large a lunch do you usually eat?
2. Analyze the data shown in one of the graphs above. Explain how the graph helps you to see relationships.
3. Write a research question about one of the misconceptions in *Spotlight On...* (page 123) and describe the type of data you would try to gather to answer your question. Then explain how you might analyze the information you gathered to help you answer your question.

What Makes You Healthy?

What determines the state of your health? Is it your weight? your diet? your lifestyle? the genes you inherited from your parents? Actually, your health is determined by a combination of all of these factors and more. Sometimes, people assume that by making one change to your life you can avoid disease. According to the Public Health Agency of Canada, it's not that easy. Their research has led them to the view that our health status is determined by a complex combination of factors. Physical factors such as genetics and age play a central role, but health is also influenced by individual lifestyle factors, such as diet and exercise. Interactions with family, friends, and others can affect health, as can the supports available in society, such as access to employment and health care. Finally, environmental and social factors such as air quality or poverty can influence health. While some of these factors are beyond our control, by making changes to those we can control, we can improve our chances of being healthy.

The Main Determinants of Health

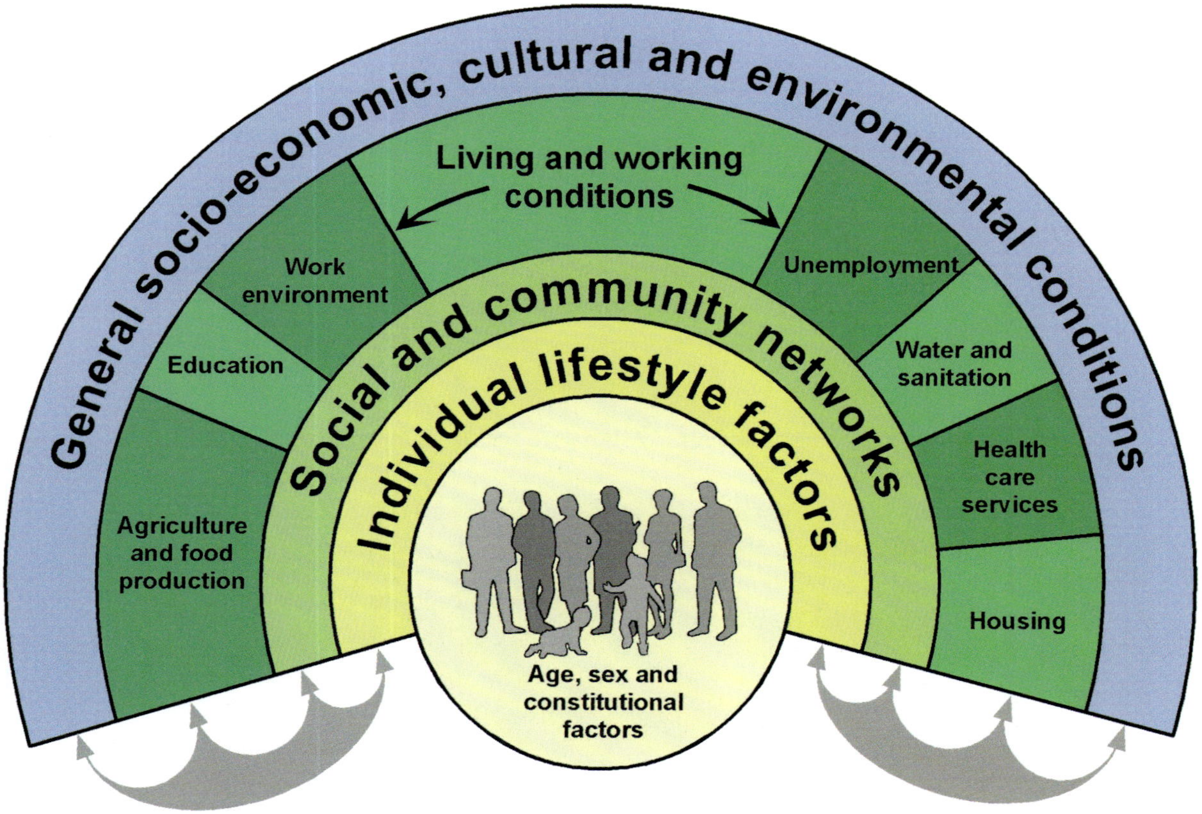

Source: Dahlgren and Whitehead (1993).

FIGURE 5.7 Our health is affected by many factors. What determinants of health do you know of that could be placed within each ring of this diagram?

To help learn about and influence determinants of health, researchers often group them into categories.

Income and social status	The more financially secure people are, the longer their life expectancy and the better their overall state of health.
Education and literacy	Education develops knowledge and skills that help with effective problem solving, and helps people cope with life's difficulties.
Employment and working conditions	People with a higher degree of control over their work conditions and less job-related stress are healthier and have a longer life expectancy.
Social environments	The type of social supports—for example, groups to belong to, financial assistance, help with learning new skills—available in the community influence health.
Physical environments	Health can be compromised as a result of contaminants in the natural environment: the air, water, food, and soil. Our built environment, including the way our homes and communities are designed and the materials used, also affects our health.
Biology and genetics	A person's genetic make-up may make them more likely to develop particular diseases or health problems, such as heart disease.
Healthy child development	Early childhood experiences and development set the foundation for future well-being or ill health.
Gender	Men and women have different life expectancies: men generally die earlier than women, but women tend to suffer more from depression, arthritis, and injuries from family violence.
Culture	Attitudes towards medical professionals, language skills, cultural beliefs, and stigma can influence people's ability to address health issues.
Health services	Health is benefited by access to services that prevent disease, as well as access to those that maintain and promote health.

Source: Public Health Agency of Canada (2012).

FIGURE 5.8 Some of these determinants of health are under our control, and some are not. Which do you have the most control over?

THINK CRITICALLY

1. Which of the determinants of health in **Figure 5.8** do you think play a greater role in Canada? Which might play a greater role in another part of the world? Explain.
2. Choose two of the determinants of health in **Figure 5.8**. Conduct research to find one or more examples of specific ways each factor can impact health.
3. Identify two determinants of health in **Figure 5.8** that people have some control over. Describe changes someone could make to those two factors to improve their chances of being healthy.

POINT OF VIEW

A Little Health from Your Friends

According to researcher Elizabeth Svoboda (2012), the more social connections you have, the greater your ability to fight infection—people with active social lives are 50 percent less likely to die of any cause than their nonsocial counterparts are. In contrast, low levels of social interaction have the same negative effects as smoking 15 cigarettes a day—and even worse effects than being obese or not exercising. But it's not just how many relationships you have that's important—the type of relationship seems to play a role in health. Close friendships may have protective effects on our cardiovascular systems, especially in times of anxiety. Researchers speculate that the stress associated with low social support sets off a cascade of damaging reactions within the body, including cardiovascular dysfunction and weakened immune resistance (Svoboda, 2012).

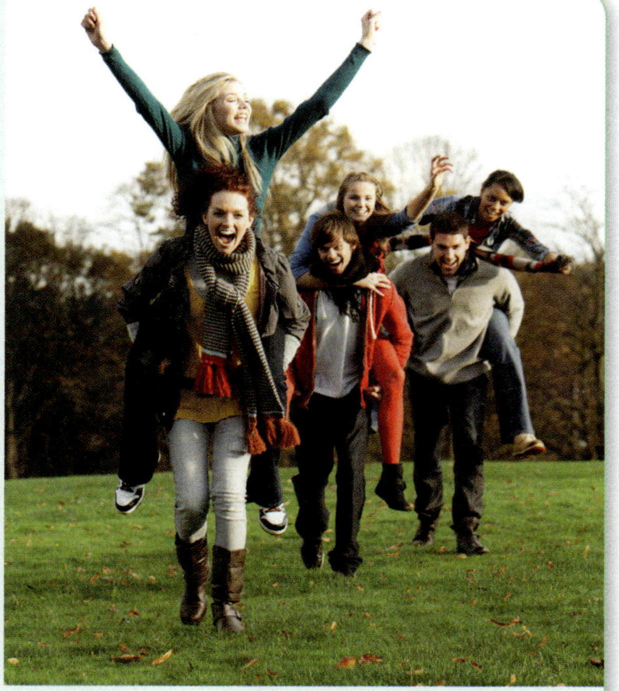

FIGURE 5.9 How can friends help you stay healthy?

Questions:

1. In your experience, is there one ideal number of close friendships to have, or does the optimal number vary from one individual to another? Explain.
2. In what ways might close real-life relationships affect a person's health differently than online relationships?

Stress

Stress can relate to any of the determinants of health. People experience stress related to their workplace, their family life, their education status, and their culture. If you have experienced diarrhea or indigestion right before a major exam, or a headache when you receive bad news, you have experienced the effects of **stress**. Stress is challenging to pinpoint because the signs and symptoms vary from person to person and because it can be caused by many different issues.

stress: excessive pressure that causes a physical or emotional response

Stress can be short-term, chronic, or traumatic. Some stress is good. Mild stress before an exam motivates you to study. However, the immune system may not work as effectively under severe stress, increasing the susceptibility to, or severity of, certain diseases—particularly those closely associated with immune function, such as infection, cancer, allergies, and autoimmune diseases. Stress can also cause inflammation—an underlying cause of many chronic diseases such as heart disease and diabetes—and exacerbate conditions such as irritable bowel syndrome (IBS) (Kline, 2008). The body has built-in systems to recover from many forms of stress but with prolonged stress, illness and disease can develop.

The good news is that stress can be controlled. Learn to recognize your own symptoms of stress. Then learn techniques for controlling them. Many people manage stress through activities such as exercise, yoga, meditation, and support groups. Ultimately, determining the cause of the stress and making changes to your environment or lifestyle to minimize those causes, if possible, will help the stress from becoming chronic.

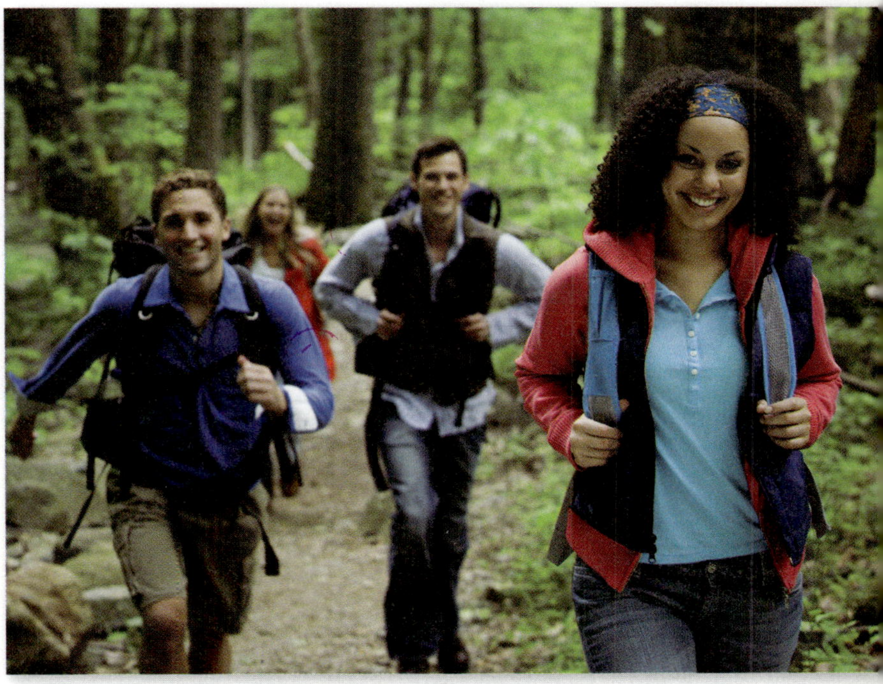

FIGURE 5.10 What potential stress relievers might work together when you engage in physical activity outdoors?

Choosing and Preparing Foods to Prevent Disease

"Approximately 18% to 25% of deaths are caused by diet-related risk factors and a small amount [are] due to physical inactivity."
– World Health Organization

The foods we eat are an important determinant of health. They can help us avoid diseases such as nutrient-deficiency diseases and infectious diseases in the short-term, and can help us avoid chronic diseases in the long term. In fact, researchers have determined specific nutrients that play a role in protecting us from various types of chronic disease.

Chronic diseases usually progress slowly, and last for many years—usually throughout a person's lifespan (WHO, 2012). Three common chronic diseases are cardiovascular disease (heart disease, stroke, chronic respiratory diseases), diabetes, and cancer. Although genetic factors and social determinants contribute to the development of these diseases, they also have controllable risk factors, including an unhealthy diet, a sedentary lifestyle, and tobacco use.

Cardiovascular Disease

Cardiovascular diseases (CVDs) are a group of disorders of the heart and blood vessels. They include coronary heart disease, heart attacks and stroke. While coronary heart disease develops over a long period of time, heart attacks and strokes are usually acute (or sudden) events and often caused by a blockage that prevents blood from flowing to the heart or brain. The most common reason for a blockage is a build-up of fatty deposits on the inner walls of the blood vessels. Strokes can also be caused by bleeding from a blood vessel in the brain or from blood clots (WHO, 2012).

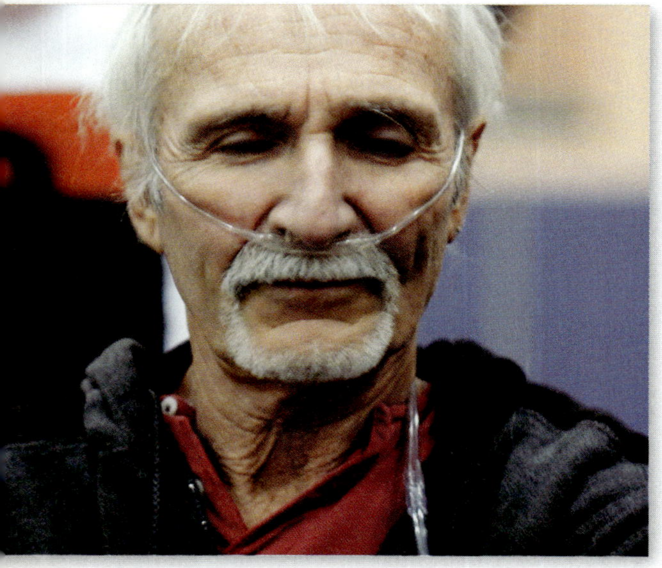

FIGURE 5.11 Some chronic diseases result in low levels of oxygen in the blood, necessitating the use of ongoing oxygen therapy.

The World Health Organization (WHO) recommends four strategies to protect heart health: avoiding tobacco use, engaging in physical activity for at least 30 minutes every day, eating at least five servings of fruits and vegetables every day, and limiting salt intake to less than 5 mL (1 tsp) per day. This salt intake includes salt you may add at the table, and also any salt used in preparing the food. Some convenience foods and fast foods contain large amounts of salt. Limiting consumption of saturated fats can also help to protect heart health.

Pause and Think
Describe one breakfast menu, one lunch menu, and one dinner menu that follows the WHO guidelines for protecting heart health.

LIFE CONNECTION

Apps for Healthy Living

Since you can download apps to help you manage other areas of your life, it's not surprising that there are apps that you can use to adopt and manage a healthy diet.

For example, the Heart and Stroke Foundation has an app designed to provide information and support to people as they work to reduce their risk of heart disease and stroke. People still need to manage their lifestyle themselves, but the app can help by providing information, identifying priorities, and providing motivation. The Dietitians of Canada have an app that provides daily healthy eating tips. Other organizations have produced apps that support exercise programs, provide information about food products based on barcodes, and help ensure a good night's sleep.

For people who prefer to use desktop or laptop computers instead of mobile devices, there are many software programs and online resources that can help with adopting and sticking to a healthy diet.

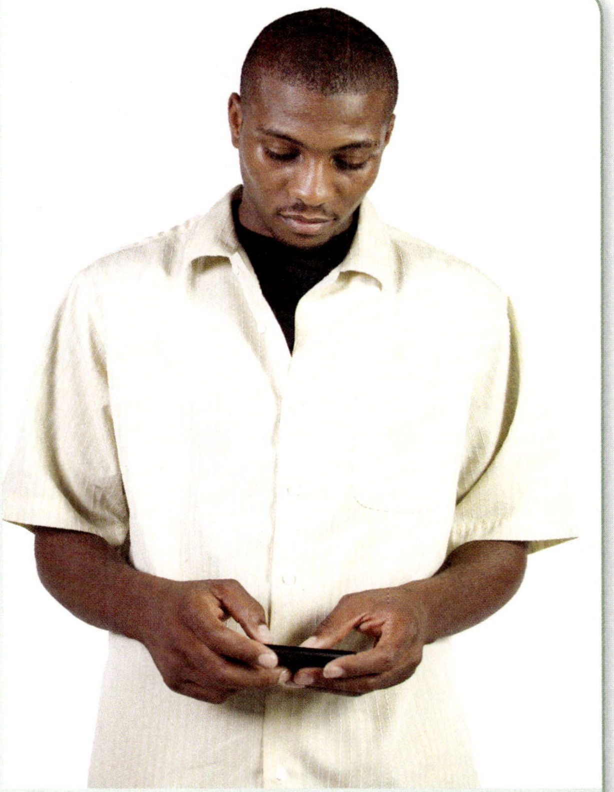

FIGURE 5.12 How could you use a mobile application to help modify your diet and lifestyle?

Questions:

1. What features do you think would be most useful in an app to help manage the risk of cardiovascular disease? Why?
2. Do some research to find other apps that can help people to adopt healthy lifestyles, including adopting diets that can help prevent disease. Describe two apps that you think are among the most useful. Explain why you think each one is useful.
3. What are the advantages of using an app to help you adopt components of a healthy lifestyle? What are the disadvantages?
4. What other tools or techniques can people use to help them organize priorities, find information, and stay motivated as they work to adopt a healthier lifestyle?

Diabetes

insulin: a hormone produced by the pancreas that regulates blood sugar (glucose)

hyperglycemia: abnormally high levels of glucose in the blood

Diabetes occurs when the pancreas does not produce enough **insulin** or when the body cannot effectively use the insulin it produces. Since insulin helps to transport glucose from the blood into the cells of the body, blood-sugar levels rise due to diabetes. If left uncontrolled, **hyperglycemia** can cause serious damage to many of the body's systems, especially nerves and blood vessels.

Type 1 diabetes is characterized by insufficient insulin production and requires daily administration of insulin. Symptoms include excessive excretion of urine (*polyuria*), thirst (*polydipsia*), constant hunger, weight loss, vision changes, and fatigue. The cause of type 1 diabetes is unknown and it is not currently preventable.

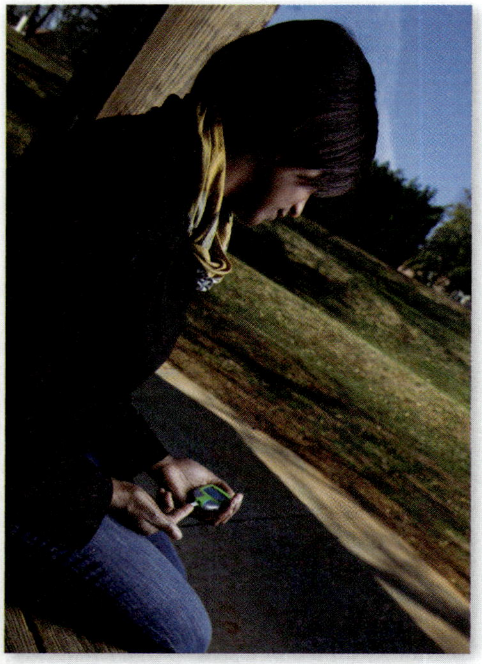

Figure 5.13 People with diabetes must monitor their blood-sugar levels regularly. For many, diet and exercise controls are not sufficient to regulate blood sugar, and injecting insulin is a daily routine.

Type 2 diabetes results from the body's ineffective use of insulin. Symptoms may be similar to those of type 1 diabetes, but are often less marked. As a result, the disease may be diagnosed several years after onset, once complications have already arisen. It is largely caused by excess body weight and physical inactivity and makes up 90 percent of diabetes cases worldwide (WHO, 2012). Until recently, type 2 diabetes was seen only in adults but it is now also occurring in children.

People of Aboriginal, Hispanic, Asian, South Asian, or African descent are at particularly high risk for developing type 2 diabetes (Canadian Diabetes Association, 2012). Type 2 diabetes can be hereditary and researchers believe that certain genes affecting insulin function—which are more prevalent in particular populations—may contribute to the development of type 2 diabetes.

Gestational diabetes is characterized by hyperglycemia with onset during pregnancy. Symptoms of gestational diabetes are similar to type 2 diabetes, and may predict a risk of developing type 2 diabetes in the future. Gestational diabetes is most often diagnosed through prenatal screening, rather than by reported symptoms.

Skills Focus

Describe the types of analysis the researchers might have carried out to form their hypothesis about genes affecting insulin function.

Pause and Think

Type 1 diabetes used to be known as *juvenile diabetes*, or *childhood-onset diabetes*. Type 2 diabetes used to be known as *adult-onset diabetes*. Why do you think this was? Why do you think these terms are no longer used?

Effects of Diabetes

- Diabetes increases the risk of heart disease and stroke.
- Combined with reduced blood flow, **neuropathy** in the feet increases the chance of foot ulcers and eventual limb amputation.
- Blindness can occur as a result of long-term accumulated damage to small blood vessels in the retina.
- Diabetes is among the leading causes of kidney failure.
- People with diabetes have double the risk of dying prematurely, compared to their peers who do not have diabetes (WHO, 2012).

neuropathy: an abnormal and usually degenerative state of the nervous system or nerves

The best diet to help prevent diabetes is the one recommended in *Eating Well with Canada's Food Guide:* a variety of fruits and vegetables and other food groups, low amounts of saturated fat, and energy intake that balances the energy you use every day. Whole grains and fibre tend to stabilize blood sugar and help with weight control. By eating healthy and engaging in regular physical activity, even people who have a genetic predisposition to type 2 diabetes can lessen their chances of developing the disease.

IN FOCUS

Immigrants to Canada

Many people make changes to their diets, but many immigrants to Canada are forced to make radical changes. They may no longer have access to foods they are used to eating, and instead they have access to a variety of other foods. As researchers have learned, these changes can have long-term effects on health.

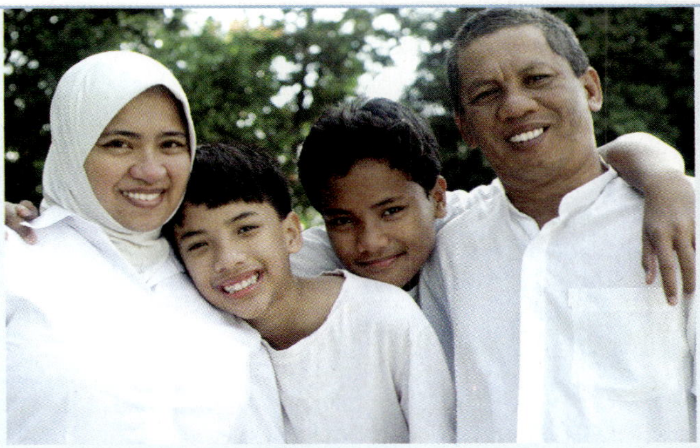

FIGURE 5.14 Many immigrants to North America are healthier than the average North American. What might contribute to this effect?

When immigrants first arrive in North America, they are typically healthier than the general population (Zhao, Xue, & Gilkinson, 2010). This is referred to as the healthy immigrant effect and may have several causes. One explanation is that immigrants may have diets that are healthier than the average North American diet—for example, their diets may include more whole grains and vegetables. Another is that new immigrants must pass rigorous medical screening before being approved so they may represent a healthier-than-average sample of the population in their own country and in North America.

continued on next page

continued from previous page

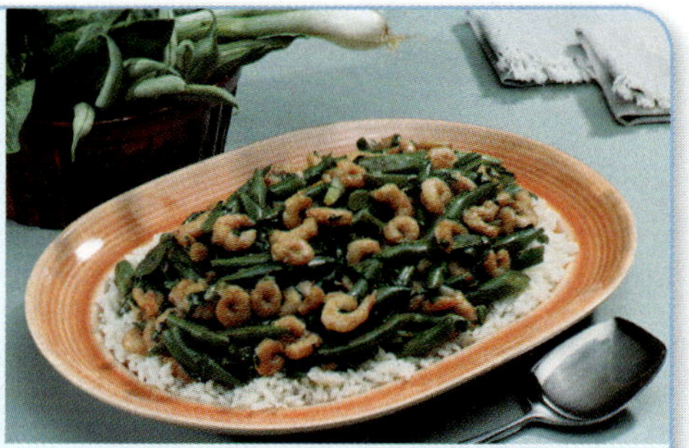

FIGURE 5.15 Which parts of a traditional meal would a person who has recently immigrated to Canada likely find easiest to purchase? Which might be the most difficult to purchase? Why?

Unfortunately, this health effect deteriorates the longer new immigrants live in Canada or the United States. Immigrants living in Canada for over 30 years have the same risk as non-immigrants of developing many chronic illnesses such as cardiovascular disease, type 2 diabetes, and cancer. In comparison, immigrants living in Canada for less than 29 years have a lower risk of chronic illness (Beiser, 2005). In some cases, immigrants' risk of chronic illness becomes greater than that of non-immigrants. After 30 years, immigrants from South Asia, for example, have a higher rate of type 2 diabetes than the general population does (Beiser, 2005).

What could cause this change? Adopting a Western diet, high in fat and sugar and low in nutrients and fibre, is often suggested as a key factor. Eating larger portion sizes, smoking, excessive alcohol consumption, and a sedentary lifestyle could be other factors. Access to affordable, nutritious food can also affect health.

- Several studies show that recent immigrants in Canada and the United States are more likely to lack money for food, eat fewer meals, and eat less nutritious food than people who immigrated earlier or who were born in Canada (Koc & Welsh, 2001).
- Immigrants may start cooking Western meals when they cannot find or afford the ingredients necessary to prepare traditional dishes. Even when familiar foods are available, immigrants have different experiences. For example, many immigrants from Africa, Asia, and South America are used to shopping daily for fresh produce and typically do not use frozen or canned goods. When surveyed, they reported being dissatisfied with the quality of fresh produce they could find in Canadian and American supermarkets (Thomas, 2006; Koc & Welsh, 2001). In these cases, adapting their diets to the foods available often means increasing fat and sodium consumption.
- For some immigrants, the colder climate in Canada and shopping weekly rather than daily can decrease levels of physical activity, and lead to related health problems (Thomas, 2006).

If the changes in diet caused by these factors are affecting the health of immigrants, it is a clear illustration of the long-term effects of dietary habits.

Questions:

1. According to the research cited above, the health of immigrants to Canada only deteriorates significantly after they have been in Canada for at least 30 years. How can changes to diet affect health 30 years later?
2. What changes other than diet could affect the long-term health of immigrants to Canada?
3. Suggest some strategies that could be used to prevent the deterioration of immigrants' health status.
4. Have you or a family member made sudden changes to the foods you eat? How do you believe these changes may affect long-term health?

Cancer

Cancer is a generic term for a large group of diseases that can affect any part of the body. One defining feature of any cancer is the rapid creation of abnormal cells that grow beyond their usual boundaries. In many cancers, these cells can then invade adjoining parts of the body and spread to other organs in a process known as *metastasis*. The cancers that most often lead to death in Canada are lung, breast, and colon cancer (Canadian Cancer Society, 2011). Many cancers have a high chance of cure if detected early and treated appropriately.

Eating to Prevent Cancer

Do artificial sweeteners cause cancer? Is it harmful to microwave plastic containers? These are a few of the many cancer myths and controversies that confound the management of cancer risk. Because carcinogens exist in many parts of the environment, there is no sure way to prevent cancer. However, certain dietary habits can help.

- Fibre and antioxidants from vegetables, fruits, and whole grains can reduce the risk of intestinal cancers (WebMD, 2012).
- Limiting consumption of processed meats and meats cooked at very high temperatures can help reduce the risk of certain types of cancer (Canadian Cancer Society, 2012).
- Limited consumption of saturated fats and sugar can help reduce the risk of developing cancer.
- Maintaining a healthy body weight can reduce the risk of cancer. Excess adipose tissue can release chemicals that may contribute to the development of cancerous cells (Mayi et. al., 2012).
- Most current research shows that sweeteners such as aspartame do not cause cancer in humans.
- While some plastics are safe to use in a microwave oven, glass and ceramic are usually more reliable choices.

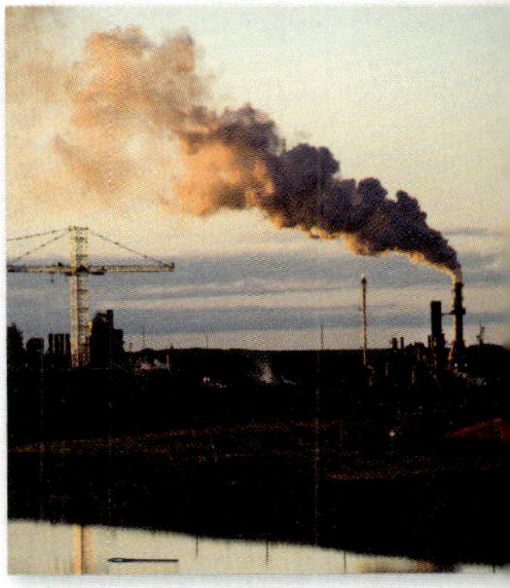

FIGURE 5.16 Exhaust from industry combines with the air we breathe and can affect our health. Environment Canada has developed the Air Quality Health Index to help Canadians make decisions to protect their health.

THINK CRITICALLY

1. Create a Venn diagram with three circles to compare dietary habits that can help prevent heart disease, type 2 diabetes, and cancer. Place habits that help prevent more than one of these diseases in overlapping areas of your diagram. What strategies appear in the centre section of your diagram—that is, in all three circles?
2. Plan a dinner menu that includes choices that can help prevent cancer. How does the menu you planned also protect against heart disease?

Active Learning

Vegetables and Fruits to Prevent Disease

One of the most important changes most people can make to their diet to reduce the risk of developing chronic diseases is to increase vegetable and fruit consumption. Although *Eating Well with Canada's Food Guide* recommends that young people eat between six and eight servings of vegetables and fruits every day, the reality is most teens eat less than one serving a day (Health Canada, 2004). A serving of most vegetables or fruits is 125 mL (½ cup). If you eat two or three servings at every meal, you will meet the daily recommendation. Steam, stir-fry, or roast vegetables to preserve nutrient content.

Vegetables provide a variety of nutrients, including fibre, which helps maintain a healthy digestive tract; potassium, which helps to regulate blood pressure (Haddy et. al., 2005); magnesium, which also helps promote normal blood pressure and helps regulate blood-glucose levels (National Institutes of Health, 2009), and phytochemicals, which perform a variety of disease-fighting roles.

Ratatouille with Sweet Potato

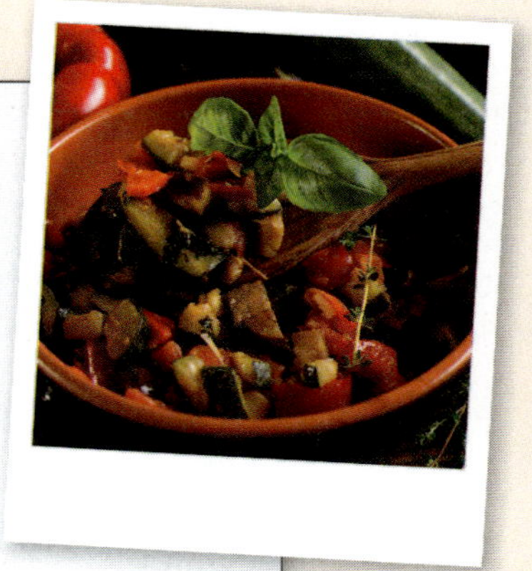

Figure 5.17 Ratatouille with sweet potato includes several vegetables and fruits. What could you serve with it to make a meal that included all four food groups?

Yield: 6 servings

Who said vegetables are boring? The truth is, people who are not eating enough vegetables are missing out on some exciting combinations of flavours as well as missing out on nutrients. Perhaps it all lies in the way vegetables are presented.

Ingredients

3 large sweet potatoes

75 mL (5 tbsp) olive oil

1 medium onion, sliced thinly

2 garlic cloves, minced

½ eggplant, cut into 1–2 cm pieces (about 750 mL or 1 ½ c)

1 small zucchini, scrubbed, quartered lengthwise, and cut into thin slices

300 mL (1 ¼ c) chopped tomatoes, fresh or canned

1 red bell pepper, chopped

1 mL (¼ tsp) dried oregano, crumbled

1 mL (¼ tsp) dried thyme, crumbled

pinch ground coriander

1 mL (¼ tsp) fennel seeds

salt and pepper to taste

125 mL (½ c) shredded fresh basil leaves

Recipe continues on next page.

Ratatouille with Sweet Potato

Method

1. Wash the sweet potatoes well but don't peel them. Prick the skin with a fork in four or five places.
2. Microwave the sweet potatoes on high for 5 minutes. Turn over, and cook another 8–10 minutes until soft. Let them rest.
3. In a large skillet, heat 30 mL (2 tbsp) of the oil over medium-low heat. Add the onion and garlic and cook, stirring occasionally, until the onion is soft.
4. Add the remaining 3 tbsp oil and heat over moderately high heat until it is hot but not smoking. Add the eggplant and cook the mixture, stirring occasionally, for 8 minutes, or until the eggplant is softened.
5. Stir in zucchini, tomatoes, and bell pepper and cook the mixture over moderate heat, stirring occasionally, for 5–7 minutes, until the vegetables are tender.
6. Stir in the oregano, thyme, coriander, and fennel seeds. Add salt and pepper, to taste, and cook, stirring, for 1 minute. Stir in the basil.
7. Slice the sweet potatoes in half and spoon the ratatouille over or beside each potato. Serve.

Questions:

1. How can fibre in vegetables help lower your risk of developing chronic diseases?
2. Propose reasons why many teens do not eat enough vegetables and fruits.
3. Describe how the ratatouille in the recipe above can help
   a) build strong bones
   b) protect your heart
   c) maintain a healthy body weight
   d) prevent diabetes
4. How might you modify the ratatouille if you were preparing it for your friends or family? Why would you make this modification?
5. Describe another vegetable dish that you enjoy eating. In what ways do the ingredients of that dish help to prevent disease? In what ways could the dish be modified to make it even healthier?

Fatty Liver Disease

When a person consumes high levels of fat and Calories for a long period of time, fatty tissue builds up in the liver. This fatty tissue puts the liver at risk of sustaining further damage, known as *fatty liver disease* (Canadian Liver Foundation, 2012). Other factors may contribute to fatty liver disease as well, including protein malnutrition, insulin resistance, high blood pressure, and genetic factors. Fatty liver disease can result in irreversible damage to liver tissue, which can lead to liver failure, and even death.

POINT/COUNTERPOINT

Should Some Foods Have Warning Labels?

All around us, advertising prompts us to purchase tasty foods, including some that may not contribute to a healthy diet. Since a healthy diet can help prevent so many chronic diseases, to what degree should people be discouraged from purchasing empty-Calorie foods? Should the foods be outlawed or taxed at a high rate? Should they carry warning labels as proposed by the Ontario Medical Association? Or should people be trusted to make their own decisions about the foods they eat? Naturally, there are many different opinions.

The proposals and counterarguments in **Figure 5.20** illustrate two opposing viewpoints.

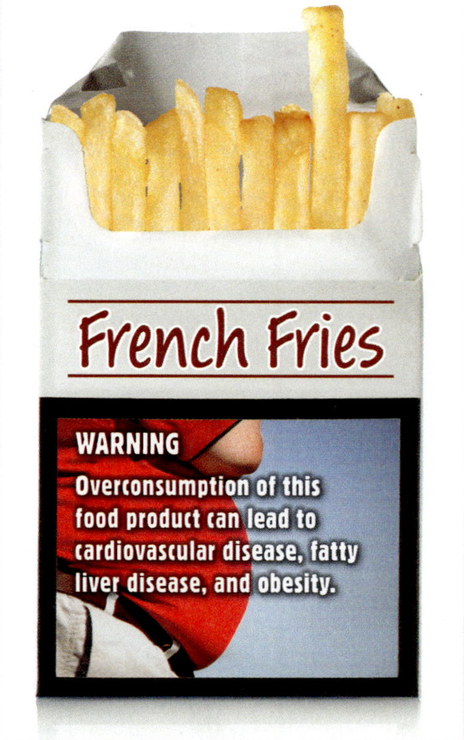

FIGURE 5.18 How would a label like this one influence the foods you choose to buy?

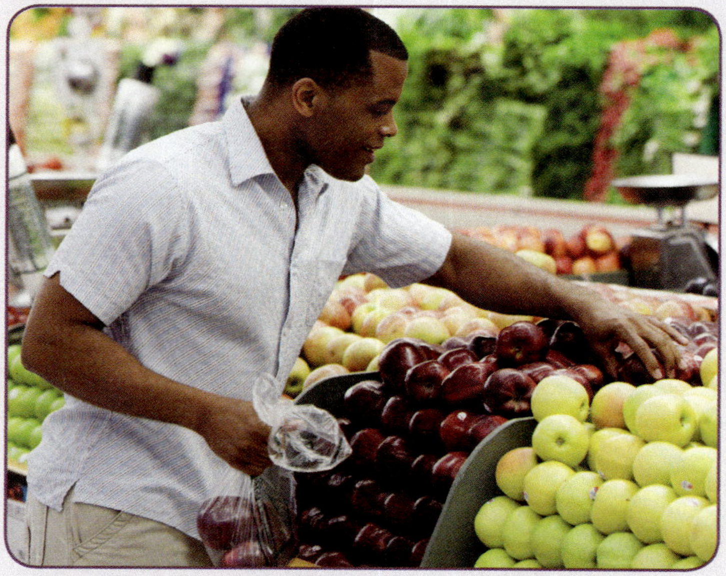

FIGURE 5.19 What strategies do you think would be most effective to encourage you to purchase healthy foods?

As with many other chronic diseases, the best way to prevent fatty liver disease is to lead a healthy lifestyle. Eat a well-balanced diet, low in saturated fats and high in fibre, and engage in regular physical activity. If you are overweight and decide to lose weight, do so gradually by following recommendations in *Eating Well with Canada's Food Guide*.

Yes	No
The Ontario Medical Association (OMA) argues that the following measures could help battle childhood obesity (CBC, 2012): • We should decrease taxes on healthy foods and increase taxes on unhealthy food. • We should restrict marketing of fatty and sugary foods to children. • We should place graphic warning labels on pop, French fries, fruit drinks, and other high-Calorie foods with little to no nutritional value. • We should add retail displays for high-sugar, high-fat foods that prominently advise consumers of the health risks. • We should restrict the availability of sugary, empty-Calorie foods in sports and other recreational facilities frequented by young people.	Food and beverage groups and other experts argue that • Taxing groceries is a simplistic approach to a complex issue. • Warning labels on alcohol products have no significant impact on purchasing decisions (WHO, 2003, as referenced in Therien, 2012). • Taxation does not change behaviour, it hurts middle- and lower-income families and it costs food and beverage manufacturing jobs (Jim Goetz, president of the Canadian Beverage Association, as quoted in CBC, 2012). • The government of Denmark introduced a tax on saturated fat in 2011 and has since dropped the surcharge (Food & Consumer Products of Canada, as quoted in CBC, 2012). • Dramatic government intervention is not the solution to the obesity problem, since poor eating is only one of the factors that cause weight problems (Brett Skinner, health analyst, Canadian Health Policy Institute, as quoted in Blackwell, 2012).

FIGURE 5.20 Viewpoints supporting and opposing taxes and warning labels on foods that could be unhealthy.

Questions:

1. What assumptions might the OMA be making when they propose the above strategies to battle childhood obesity?
2. Which of the OMA's proposals do you think would have the most significant effect? Why?
3. Which of the opposing arguments do you think is the strongest argument? Explain.
4. List possible sources of bias in the arguments on each side of the issue.
5. What steps do you think should be taken to combat childhood obesity? Why do you think the steps you recommend might be the most effective?

Osteoporosis

Osteoporosis is a condition that causes bones to become thin and porous, decreasing bone strength and leading to increased risk of breaking a bone. This, in turn, can lead to disfigurement and loss of mobility. Although osteoporosis reduces the quality of people's lives significantly, there may be no symptoms as bone mass begins to decline. While no single cause of osteoporosis has been identified, adequate calcium and vitamin D intake along with regular weight-bearing physical activity will help build healthy bones. Genetic factors also play a role in osteoporosis.

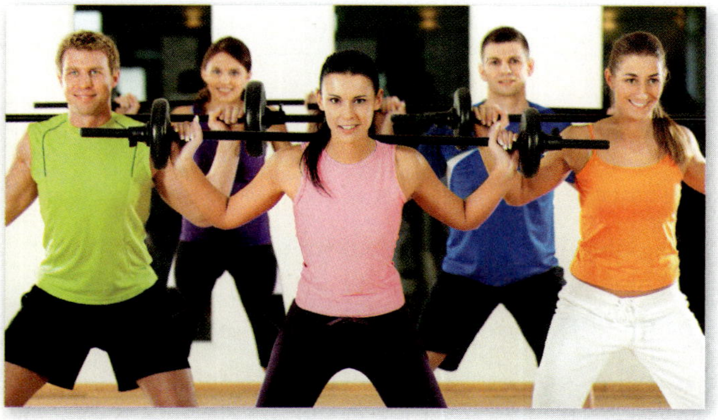

FIGURE 5.21 Regular weight-bearing exercise throughout the lifespan can help strengthen bones, and help prevent osteoporosis.

Peak bone mass is achieved at an early age: at age 16 to 20 in young women and age 20 to 25 in young men. Women and men alike begin to lose bone mass in their mid-30s. Osteoporosis can affect both men and women at any time, but most commonly as an older adult. Osteoporosis has been called a *pediatric* disease with *geriatric* consequences because building strong bones during childhood and adolescence can be the best defence against developing osteoporosis as an older adult.

CASE STUDY

Building Strong Bones

Eighteen-year-old Zara has a busy school schedule but manages to go out dancing once a month. She considers this her way of staying physically active. To make up for her lack of regular exercise, she tries to follow a healthy diet that includes lots of dark, green, leafy vegetables, fortified soy milk with her breakfast cereal, canned salmon with the bones, and vitamin D supplements during the winter. In an effort to learn more about her culture's traditional meals, Zara spends every Sunday helping her grandmother cook. Zara often writes these recipes down and adjusts them later to make them healthier. One Sunday, as Zara's grandmother bent over to pick up a spoon that had fallen while she was cooking, she cried out in pain. As the pain in her grandmother's back was severe and unrelenting, Zara brought her grandmother to the hospital. There, she learned that her grandmother had suffered a spinal fracture. Further testing revealed that Zara's grandmother had osteoporosis.

Questions:

1. What lifestyle choices has Zara made to prevent osteoporosis?
2. What advice would you give to Zara to help her build and maintain strong bones?
3. Would this advice also be useful for Zara's grandmother, father, or mother? Explain.

Managing Disease

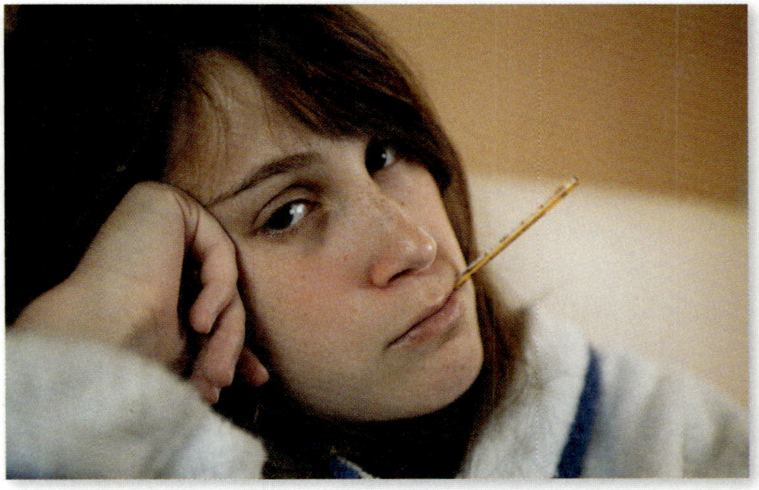

FIGURE 5.22 Nutritious food and relaxation can often help you feel better when sick. What do you normally eat or drink when you are sick?

When you are sick, it is important that you follow your health care professional's recommendations, eat nutrient-dense foods, drink plenty of fluids, and get lots of rest. Even colds or the flu put stress on your body, and appropriate nutrition can help you heal. Many studies have found that malnutrition is a variable associated with poor healing and higher complication rates, as well as higher rates of morbidity and mortality and ultimately increased hospital costs. Studies reveal that up to 55 percent of hospital patients are undernourished or at risk of being so (Dietitians of Canada, 2012).

Despite our best intentions, we cannot completely control our health and people do develop diseases. Choosing appropriate foods and preparing them carefully can help reduce the severity of many disease symptoms and, for some diseases, can speed healing.

Pause and Think
Why do you think so many hospital patients are undernourished?

Cardiovascular Disease

People with cardiovascular disease can reduce their risk of stroke and heart attack by making modifications to their diet. High blood LDL cholesterol levels, low blood HDL cholesterol levels, and high blood-pressure all increase the risk of life-threatening cardiovascular events.

Research suggests that a diet low in saturated fats, and high in potassium, calcium, and magnesium can lower blood pressure (Kromhout, 2001). Unsaturated fatty acids can lower LDL cholesterol levels. In addition, a balanced energy intake, to achieve and/or maintain a healthy weight, reduces the strain on the cardiovascular system and also reduces risk.

Diabetes

People with diabetes cannot adequately regulate their blood-sugar levels. Many administer insulin daily, which can help. Food choices and meal timing can also help regulate blood sugar.

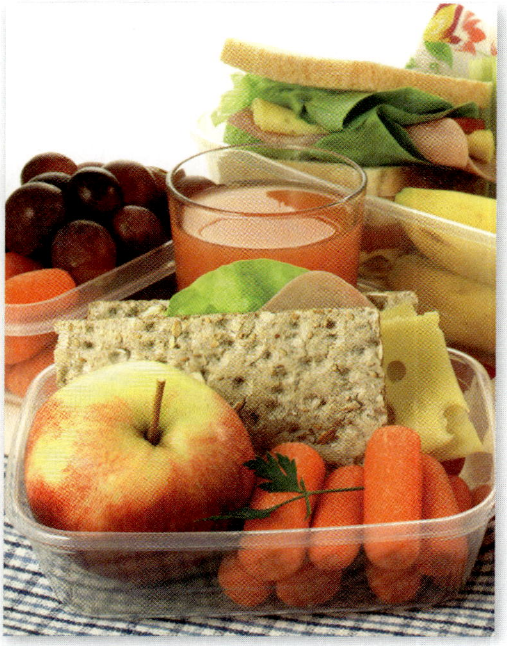

FIGURE 5.23 Which nutrients in these snacks can help a person manage their diabetes?

While simple sugars are absorbed through the intestinal wall quickly, complex carbohydrates take longer to digest, so they are absorbed more gradually. Fibre regulates the digestion process. Because of this, eating foods that contain complex carbohydrates, including fibre, helps to slow the release of sugar into the blood. Eating simple sugars can cause a spike in blood-sugar levels. Foods high in fibre and low in simple sugars, including whole grains, many vegetables, and legumes, are recommended. In general, consumption of sweetened drinks, jams, candies, and honey should be limited.

Eating regular meals and eating healthy snacks when needed can also help to regulate the release of sugar into the blood. Carrying a healthy snack in a purse or pocket can ensure that it is possible to eat when blood-sugar levels drop.

Maintaining a healthy weight can help with blood-glucose control and minimize stress on the heart. Strategies to maintain a healthy weight include limiting consumption of high-fat foods and choosing reasonable portions. Instead of fried food and cookies, which can lead to weight gain and provide few nutrients other than fat, servings of nutrient-dense foods from the four food groups can help control some of the symptoms and complications associated with diabetes (Canadian Diabetes Association, 2012).

TIP for Healthy Living

The Canadian Diabetes Association has created a mobile application that uses nutrient information from Health Canada to keep track of the carbohydrates eaten and build grocery lists for a user's recipes or the Association's healthy recipes.

THINK CRITICALLY

1. How do the strategies for choosing and preparing food to prevent common chronic diseases compare to the strategies for choosing and preparing food to manage the effects of the diseases? Explain similarities and differences that you find.
2. Create a T-chart to compare strategies for managing cardiovascular disease and type 2 diabetes. Highlight strategies that are helpful for both diseases.
3. Describe some portable healthy snacks that would be easy for someone with diabetes to carry in their purse or pocket.
4. Choose a recipe, and adapt it to be suitable for someone who is managing diabetes. Explain why you made the modifications you did.

Cancer and HIV/AIDS

Cancer—especially when undergoing chemotherapy—HIV/AIDS, and some other diseases can lower the body's immune system response, making it easier to contract diseases from bacteria and viruses. For this reason, preventing foodborne illness is extremely important for patients suffering from these diseases. Special care needs to be taken when handling, storing, preparing, and shopping for food (Health Canada, 2012). Cook meats to recommended internal temperatures, store leftovers in the fridge for no longer than 48 hours, and keep hands and anything that comes into contact with food clean. Washing them with soap and water and rinsing with 5 mL of bleach in 1 L of warm water can help disinfect utensils.

Chemotherapy can also alter a person's sense of taste, sometimes making many foods unappealing and diminishing appetite. When preparing foods for cancer patients, it is more important to ensure that they consume a reasonable number of Calories than to worry too much about the degree to which their diet is balanced (Livestrong Foundation, 2009). Nutrient-rich smoothies and the addition of healthy high-Calorie and high-protein foods to fruits and vegetables can help achieve an optimal diet when appetite is reduced.

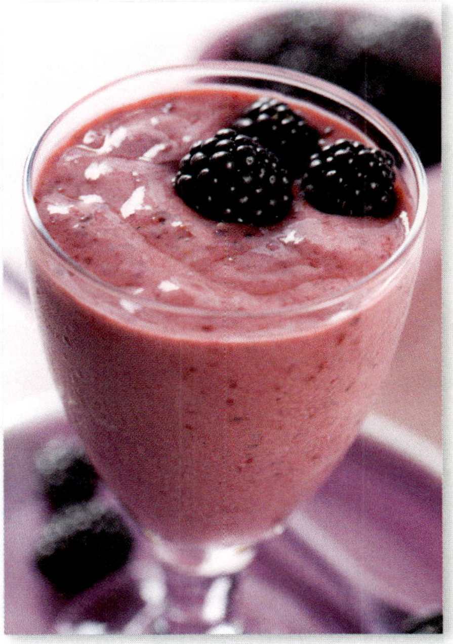

FIGURE 5.24 Fruit smoothies made with yogurt can help a person undergoing chemotherapy obtain key nutrients. What other nutrient-rich foods may help to stimulate appetite?

Kidney Disease

People with kidney disease should follow the recommendations of a health professional. Depending on the extent of kidney disease, their dietary needs can vary. Common considerations in kidney disease include (National Kidney Foundation, 2006)

- controlling the amount of protein in the diet. Everyone needs protein to build and repair tissues, but the byproducts of metabolizing protein are excreted through the kidneys. People with kidney disease can minimize stress on their kidneys by controlling the amount of protein they consume.
- controlling the amount of salt and potassium in the diet to help control blood pressure.
- controlling the amount of phosphorus in the diet. High levels of phosphorus in the blood can cause calcium to be lost from the bones. Diseased kidneys may not remove phosphorus from the blood as efficiently as normal kidneys, so it may be necessary to limit the amount that is consumed. Rice and oat bran; flax, sesame, and pumpkin seeds; and cheese are all high in phosphorus.
- controlling the amount of fluid consumed. In the early stages of kidney disease, this is normally not necessary, but it may be recommended in later-stage kidney disease.

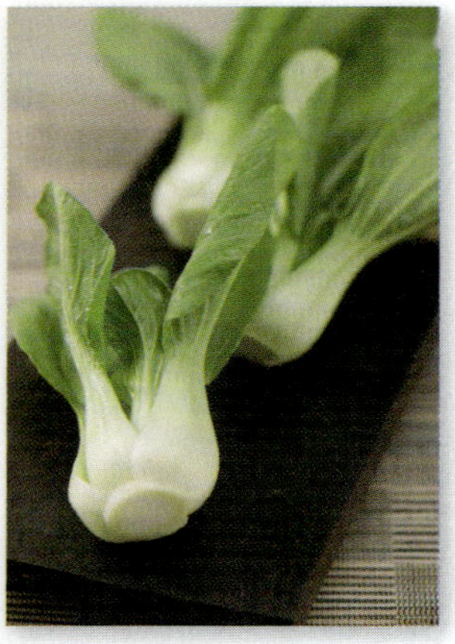

FIGURE 5.25 This bok choy is a good source of folate. What foods do you know of that are suitable for people with celiac disease and good sources of vitamins B_{12}, C, or D?

Celiac Disease

In people with celiac disease, portions of the small intestine lining become damaged as a result of eating foods containing gluten. This damage limits the absorption of key nutrients and causes malnutrition. Other common symptoms of celiac disease include nausea, abdominal pain, decreased appetite, constipation, and diarrhea.

For people with celiac disease, a gluten-free diet is essential to help the intestinal lining heal and restore nutrient absorption. Gluten can be found in foods made with wheat, rye, barley, and oats, including baked goods, pasta, some beverages, and some medications.

Because iron-deficiency anemia is common in people with celiac disease, dietary considerations often include eating iron-rich foods.

Many vitamins and minerals are not absorbed efficiently with celiac disease. It is important to plan nutrient-dense meals, including foods that are rich sources of vitamins B_{12}, C, and D; calcium; and folate.

Symptoms of diarrhea can be reduced by limiting the consumption of simple sugars. Consequences of diarrhea, such as dehydration, can be limited by ensuring an adequate intake of fluids and of electrolytes (salts). Symptoms of constipation can be reduced by ensuring adequate fluid and fibre consumption (Canadian Celiac Association, 2008).

NUTRITION LITERACY

Iron from animal sources is easier for our bodies to use. Iron from plant sources becomes more bioavailable when it is consumed with vitamin C.

Gastroenteritis

Gastroenteritis is an inflammation of the intestinal tract caused by viruses or bacteria. Symptoms resemble those of the stomach flu, and it is caused by contact with infected people, objects, food, or water. Some gastroenteritis can be prevented by following careful kitchen hygiene procedures.

Because diarrhea and vomiting are common in gastroenteritis, it is important to consume fluids and electrolytes. For older children and adults, once some solid food can be kept down, simple grain products and fruits can be added, such as mashed bananas, rice, applesauce, and toast (known as the *BRAT diet*), to add additional nutrients. Once a person with gastroenteritis can tolerate those foods without further vomiting, other bland foods can be introduced, including protein sources. Certain foods should be avoided during and immediately after an episode of gastroenteritis because they may further irritate the intestinal lining. These include citrus fruits, corn, caffeinated drinks and alcohol, dairy foods, oily foods, and spicy foods (HealthHype.com, 2012). It is often recommended that young children with gastroenteritis continue to follow their normal diet, with additional fluids and electrolytes. Follow a health professional's advice.

THINK CRITICALLY

1. Design a card to summarize the most important things to remember when preparing food for someone with

   a) kidney disease b) HIV/AIDS c) celiac disease

2. You are helping to look after a 12-year-old boy with gastroenteritis. Describe some foods suitable for him to eat at different stages of recovery. Explain what stage each food would be suitable for and why.

Food Allergies and Intolerances

Food allergies can be very serious, in some cases leading to death. It is vitally important that a person with a food allergy not consume any of the food they are allergic to. This often means keeping the food out of the home, to avoid cross-contamination, choosing where to eat carefully, and asking detailed questions about the content of meals.

Because food allergies can have such severe consequences, it is important for anyone who suspects an allergy to a particular food to consult with a health professional to help obtain a clear diagnosis.

Sometimes food intolerances are confused with food allergies. Due to the serious consequences of being exposed to an **allergen**, recognizing the difference is essential.

A food allergy is an abnormal response to a particular ingredient (usually a type of protein) triggered by the body's immune system. Symptoms can occur within minutes and can be mild—such as a runny nose or itchy eyes—or severe and life-threatening. The first time an individual is exposed to the allergen, the body's immune system responds by creating antibodies. When the individual is exposed again to the same allergen, antibodies and chemicals such as **histamine** are released. The reaction to the allergen may be identical, or more or less severe. A severe reaction can lead to anaphylaxis.

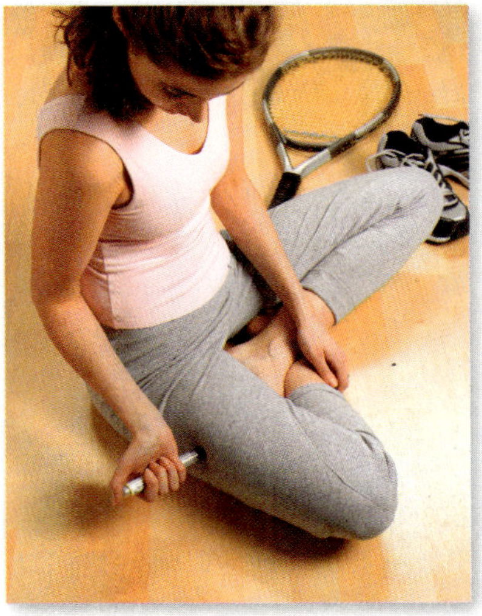

FIGURE 5.26 People with severe allergies often carry an injectable form of adrenaline, to stop an allergic reaction as quickly as possible.

SAFETY AND SANITATION

Mild Allergy Symptoms Can Become More Severe
Initially mild symptoms that occur after ingesting a food allergen can become more serious in a very short amount of time, and could lead to **anaphylaxis** (Health Canada, 2009).

anaphylaxis:
the most serious type of allergic reaction, often including throat swelling and low blood-pressure; it can progress very quickly and can cause death without proper medical attention

allergen:
a substance that causes allergic reactions

histamine:
a powerful chemical produced by the body that can cause an inflammatory reaction in the respiratory system, gastrointestinal tract, skin, or cardiovascular system

A person experiencing an allergic reaction may have any of the following symptoms:

- trouble breathing, speaking, or swallowing
- rapid heart beat
- loss of consciousness
- flushed face, hives, rash, or red and itchy skin
- swelling of the eyes, face, lips, throat, and tongue
- cramps, diarrhea, and/or vomiting (Health Canada, 2012)

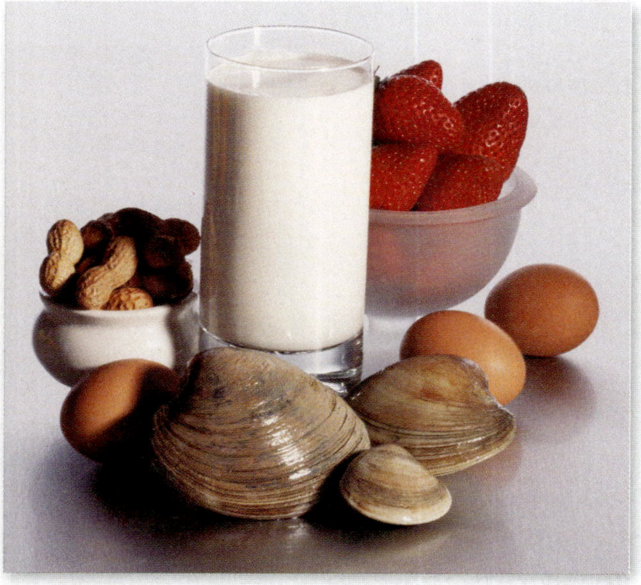

FIGURE 5.27 In what dishes are you likely to find these common allergens? How can the dish be modified so it is safe for people allergic to these ingredients?

Any food can provoke an allergic response. According to Health Canada (2012), the food allergens that cause the most severe allergic reactions are peanuts, tree nuts, sesame seeds, milk, eggs, soy, fish (including shellfish and crustaceans), wheat, and sulphites.

In contrast, a food intolerance occurs when you are unable to digest a certain component of a food because of a lack or insufficient amount of a particular chemical or enzyme in the body. Examples include lactose (milk sugar) intolerance and wheat intolerance. Food-intolerance symptoms occur within hours or days after eating and do not involve the immune system. Symptoms can include headaches, bloating, diarrhea, and a feeling of poor health.

Managing Allergies and Intolerances

People with food allergies or intolerances need to avoid foods that make them sick. If these foods are excluded from the diet, suitable alternatives must be introduced to prevent nutrient deficiencies. A dietitian can help people plan appropriate meals and learn about foods to avoid and ingredients to watch for on labels.

For example, lactose intolerance results from lactose malabsorption and a decreased ability to digest lactose due to a deficiency of the enzyme *lactase*, which breaks down lactose into glucose and galactose. Lactose is normally digested in the small intestine, but when lactase levels are low, lactose is transported intact to the colon where intestinal bacteria ferment the lactose and cause uncomfortable symptoms such as gas, cramps, diarrhea, and bloating. Some people who have lactose intolerance cannot digest any milk products. Others can eat or drink small amounts of milk products or certain types of milk products without problems.

Lactose intolerance is common in adults. It occurs more frequently in First Nations peoples and people of Asian, African, and South American descent than among people of European descent (Health Canada, 2012). Once a doctor confirms that a person has lactose intolerance, the challenge then becomes how to obtain adequate amounts of calcium and vitamin D without consuming milk products. Fortunately, alternatives to milk products exist. Soy milk, canned salmon, and sardines contain calcium and vitamin D. Dark green vegetables such as turnip greens, kale, broccoli, and collards also contain some calcium and some orange juice is fortified with calcium and vitamin D.

CASE STUDY

Nut Allergies

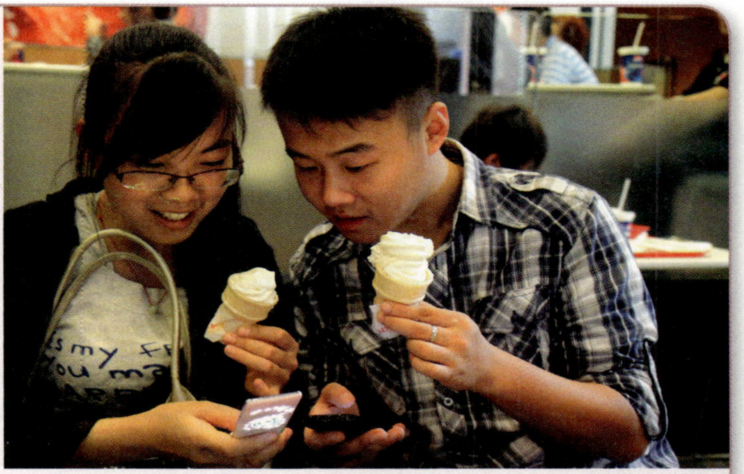

FIGURE 5.28 Can vanilla ice cream cause an allergic reaction in someone with an allergy to nuts?

A 15-year-old boy was on holiday with his parents when he had a taste of vanilla ice cream and began vomiting. His family also noticed that his face had begun to swell and he had trouble breathing, so they took him to a hospital. Paramedics at the hospital injected him with epinephrine (a form of adrenaline) to stop the allergic reaction and with hydrocortisone to prevent it starting again.

Later, doctors learned that when the boy was five years old, he had vomited after eating a chocolate bar containing nuts. At the age of eight, he ate a few peanuts and experienced some facial swelling. Other than these two episodes, he had avoided eating nuts. When his family thought back to the most recent episode, they realized that the ice cream vendor had used a scoop to serve a previous customer a flavour of ice cream that contained nuts, then used the same scoop to serve the boy his vanilla ice cream.

The boy was admitted to the hospital overnight for observation and recovered quickly and uneventfully. Testing showed a severe allergy to peanuts and tree nuts. He was advised to avoid all peanuts and tree nuts, to pay particular attention to hidden nut ingredients in foods, to wear a medical-alert bracelet, and to carry epinephrine in injectable form with him at all times in case of an allergic reaction (Chapel, Haeney, Misbah, & Snowden, 2006).

Questions:

1. In what circumstances could a medical-alert bracelet help the boy?
2. Describe four foods that can have hidden nut ingredients.
3. In what ways is this boy's experience similar to that of someone who has lactose intolerance? In what important ways are the two conditions different?

CHAPTER 5 REVIEW

Chapter Review

Knowledge and Understanding/Thinking

1. Choose a popular type of empty-Calorie food. Create a label that would warn people about the possible health effects of consuming large quantities of the food.
2. The OMA believes warnings on empty-Calorie foods could improve the health status of Canadians. Many food manufacturers disagree. What factors would governments likely consider before they passed legislation requiring this type of labelling?
3. What are the physical, social, and psychological determinants of disease?
4. List three factors that can contribute to the development of chronic diseases. Explain how each factor may influence the likelihood of a person developing a chronic disease.
5. Why is it important for children and teens to eat a healthy diet when most chronic diseases don't develop until later in life?
6. Why is it important for someone who already has heart disease to adopt a healthy diet?
7. What is the difference between a food allergy and a food intolerance?
8. Describe three chronic diseases and describe strategies for preventing each one.
9. Use a T-chart to summarize the major differences between type 1 diabetes and type 2 diabetes.
10. Osteoporosis is often called *the silent thief*. Explain why this is, or is not, a suitable nickname for the disease.

Thinking/Communication

11. Your cousin is undergoing chemotherapy. She is losing weight, but her family eats spicy food and she really has no appetite for it. In an email to you, she says she thinks she'll just drink juice in the weeks when she has chemotherapy, and try to eat more normally in other weeks. Write an email that you could send in response, based on what you have learned in this chapter.
12. Investigate to find logos used on food packages in Canada to indicate foods that are healthy choices. Create a display for the school showing the logos, what they indicate about the food, and on which foods they might be found.

13. Create a graphic organizer to explain the difference between a food intolerance and a food allergy.
14. The first time a child eats eggs, she develops a rash and mild swelling around her eyes, but the reaction soon subsides. Should her parents be concerned? Explain.
15. Write a list of the top 10 eating strategies to maintain good health. Place the one you think is most important first on your list and the one you think is least important last on your list.
16. Write a letter to your local government representative in support of, or opposing, warning labels on empty-Calorie foods. Conduct research and incorporate it into your letter.

Communication/Application

17. Choose a common chronic disease. Design a fridge magnet to remind people of the most important food-related strategies to help prevent the disease you chose.
18. Find and prepare a recipe designed for a person with diabetes, lactose intolerance, or heart disease. Explain why your recipe is suitable for someone with the condition you chose. Rate the food you created for appearance, texture, and flavour.

Putting It All Together

In this chapter, you have

- identified determinants of health
- described nutrition-related diseases
- learned about eating practices that can help prevent and manage diseases and health conditions

Design a poster to encourage adolescents to adopt healthy food habits that will help them prevent chronic diseases. Include text and visuals, key strategies, and details to support each strategy.

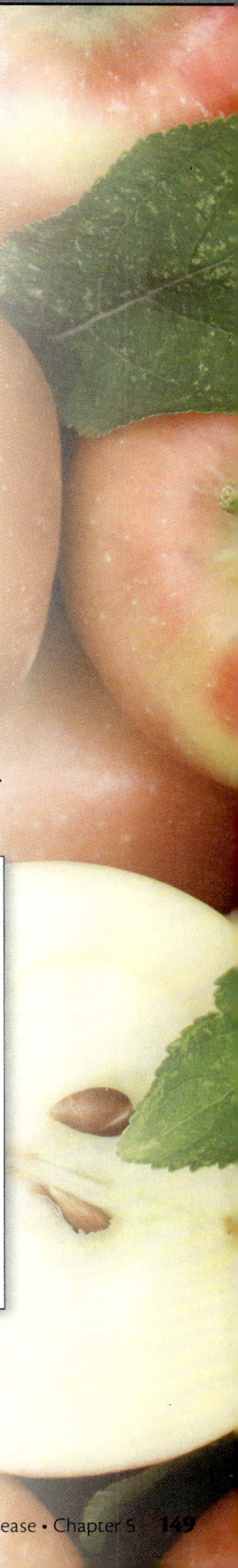

Chapter 6

Emerging Trends in Food and Nutrition

KEY TERMS

bioactive compounds
carotenoids
food additive
functional food
genetically modified/engineered
locavore
nutraceutical
phytochemicals
probiotics
proprietary

RESEARCH AND INQUIRY SKILLS

- Communicate results of research and inquiry effectively

Chapter Introduction

While reading this chapter, you will study

- **trends in nutrition, food production, and consumption patterns**
- **how trends influence food products and services available to the consumer**
- **the use of additives and functional foods in food production**
- **the role of legislation in controlling food products**
- **nutritional health claims**
- **how interests, skills, previous experience, and education requirements relate to specific career opportunities in the food industry**

Like clothing and music, food goes through trends, or fashions. These trends affect the foods that are available to us: what is grown, and what is produced and sold. Some trends describe preferences—a style of food, cooking technique, or flavour that is currently popular. Other trends describe improvements—the addition of key nutrients or an agricultural innovation that increases yield. Every day, we are bombarded with messages that highlight the latest trend. Foods are promoted as nutritious, instant, low-priced, organic, natural, sustainable, and more. How do we make informed, healthy choices?

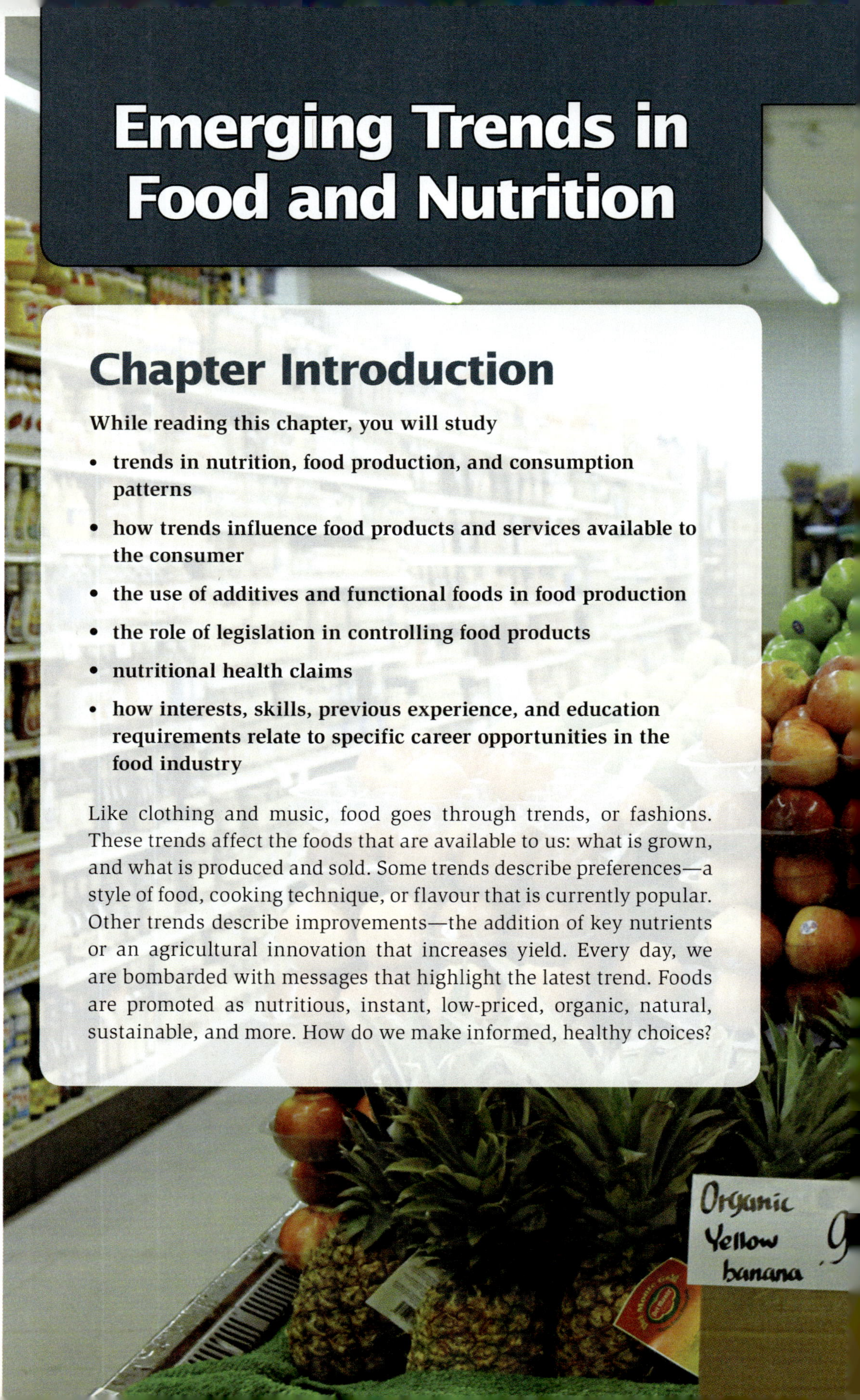

FIGURE 6.1 How can consumers look past food trends in order to make healthy decisions about what they eat?

Spotlight On...

Canadians and What We Eat

Understanding who Canadians are and what they believe about food can help companies to determine what food products are likely to be popular in the Canadian market. To help food producers, Agriculture and Agri-Food Canada (2010) gathered available data and published a summary report. A rich portrait of Canada emerged, showing strong regional variations and some definite trends.

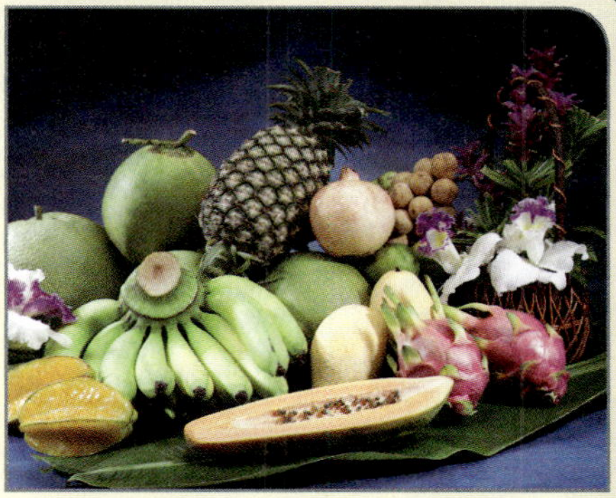

FIGURE 6.2 Canadians are consuming more tropical fruits. Which of these fruits have you tasted?

The population of Canada is aging: by 2050, Canada will probably have twice as many seniors as children. More Canadians are living alone, and there is an increase in lone-parent families and in families with fewer children. While Canada is the second largest country in the world, its population is clustered in the southern part of the country, with almost half of its citizens living near six major cities. Immigration continues to fuel our population growth, with Canadians reporting over 200 ethnic origins on the 2006 Census.

Approximately half of those surveyed report being overweight, and the same number don't get enough physical activity. Cancer and cardiovascular disease are the leading causes of death. Many Canadians consider themselves knowledgeable about nutrition, and look for products that would allow themselves and their families to improve their well-being and live healthier lives.

The Canadian labour market has also undergone changes, with the employment rate for women increasing 17 percent since 1976. Canadians are spending less time preparing food, and are looking for ways to streamline meal preparation. They also consume more meals on the go. Canadians' expenditures on prepared foods at restaurants and stores totals 17 percent of their personal spending.

The percent of household budgets devoted to food and beverage purchases has declined over the past 40 years, to approximately 10 percent. Almost 80 percent of Canadians indicate that value for money is the most important factor in determining how they spend their food dollars. Freshness, nutrition, safety, appearance, and flavour are other important considerations. While value for money is important, there is a smaller but growing demand for foods that are seen as authentic and sustainable.

As a result of these and other changes, the foods that Canadians consume have changed. Canadians now consume more fresh vegetables and fruit, especially tropical fruits such as mangoes and guava. Canadians consume less milk, and are switching to lower-fat options. They consume more yogurt and cheese. Consumption of shellfish has declined, but consumption of freshwater fish and red meats has increased. In general, cereal consumption has declined, however consumption of rice has increased.

Questions:

1. Propose reasons why the percent of household budgets spent on food has declined over the past 40 years.
2. What trend above did you find the most surprising? Explain your answer.
3. How might a company that produces food be able to use this information about Canadians?

Research and Inquiry Skills

Effectively Communicate Results of Research and Inquiry

As with fashion, food goes through trends. While some trends come and go quite quickly, others may last for years and even decades, becoming accepted parts of our food culture. Food companies, retailers, and food-service establishments want to capitalize on current food trends, to create products and services that will appeal to consumers. But how do they know what consumers want?

Market researchers survey consumers' needs, analyze the data to determine societal trends, and report on the results. Food manufacturers, restaurants, and retailers can then use the information to help create and market successful products.

Market research is an area of research that focusses on how decisions may affect customers and allow a food company to increase their share in the marketplace. In trendspotting, market researchers conduct research to discover and name new trends. They may make use of surveys and focus groups to help identify new trends such as increasing health concerns or changes in eating patterns, family relationships, or leisure activities. Researchers will analyze data from their research to determine its significance and help predict upcoming trends. Some researchers make use of trendhunters or coolhunters, people who help spot trends by focussing on those in communities who are more likely to set trends, such as youth, celebrities, and technology users. They may look for immediate, short-term trends, or may attempt to forecast further into the future. The trends that trendspotters and coolhunters predict are used by food manufacturers, retailers, and food-service establishments to create products and services that embody that trend and become popular.

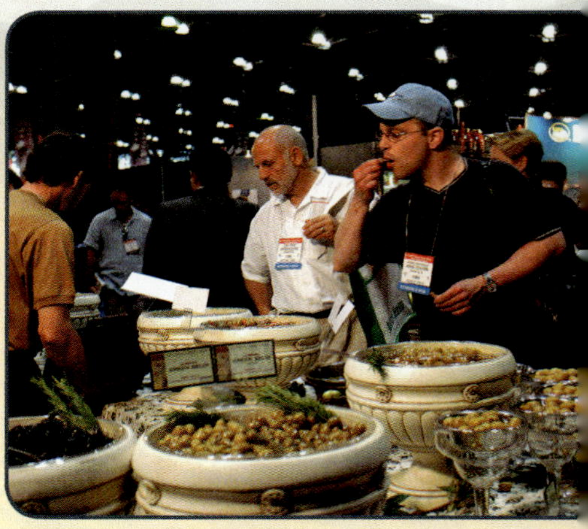

FIGURE 6.3 How might a researcher use a trade show to help identify new trends?

However they gather data, market researchers must present it in a way that will be useful to food companies and others who make decisions based on consumer trends. As with any research, many tools are available to help communicate results:

- Graphs can help summarize statistical information.
- Diagrams can help describe spatial information.
- Lists and bullet points can help readers locate key conclusions or facts.

In addition, an introduction helps readers to know how, when, and where the research was gathered, and a conclusion can summarize overall trends or suggest questions for further research. Clear writing and careful editing make the report informative and easy to read.

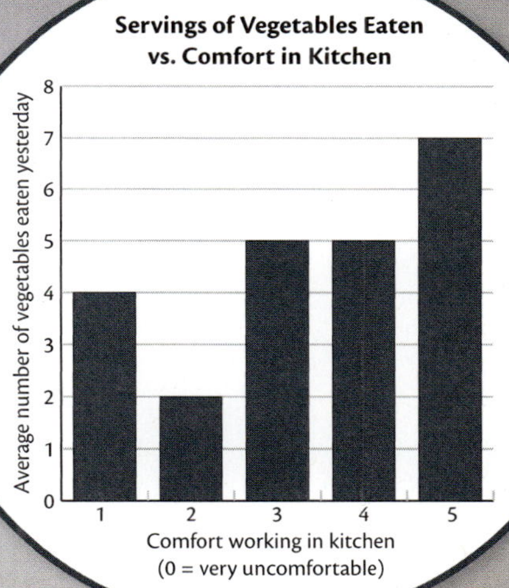

Figure 6.4 What information can you learn from this graph? In what ways are trends in the data more obvious than they would be in a list or a paragraph?

Activities:

1. Conduct some research about food and nutrition trends in your school. First, make observations about the habits and behaviours of people in your school and community. Be curious and open-minded, focussing on new ideas, topics of conversation, or activities that you observe. To help focus your research, you can use one of the areas of emerging trends discussed in this chapter: health, sustainability, technology, authenticity, or convenience. Agriculture and Agri-Food Canada (2011) has also identified the following as upcoming food trends: healthy snacking; halal, kosher, and Mediterranean foods; and tea beverages.
2. From your observations, identify any trends that seem to be emerging. Use social media to see how much your trend or topic is being mentioned or discussed. Has it been identified as a future trend by others?
3. Create a survey or focus group to ask the public what their beliefs or attitudes are about the trend that you have identified. Ask questions that will help you determine if others are seeing the trend or believe that it is a trend, if consumers will adopt the trend, and whether it will be a short-lived fad, or a longer-lasting trend.
4. Analyze your observations and research to determine how this trend could be applied to food products or services. For example, trend predictor Faith Popcorn determined that consumers were increasingly concerned with how to make good food choices and forecast that a new career would emerge to help people make healthy decisions—a food coach (Day, 2012).
5. Write a report about your research and conclusions that could be given to media sources. Communicate your results in a clear, detailed, user-friendly way. Describe and explain the trend. Explain why you predict it will be a trend, and the effects the trend may have in the marketplace. Provide evidence for your conclusions.

Trends for Health

Food trends begin for many reasons. One of the most popular is people's desire to be healthy. More and more Canadians state they are interested in making healthier food choices (Canadian Council of Food and Nutrition, 2008). Increasingly, shoppers are purchasing food based on its nutrition profile and choosing products such as whole-grain breads and lower sodium products. In addition, increasing numbers of people reported having prepared a healthy recipe in the past year (Food Marketing Institute, 2012). As people make healthy choices, food companies, food-service operators, and retail establishments will make even more healthy options available.

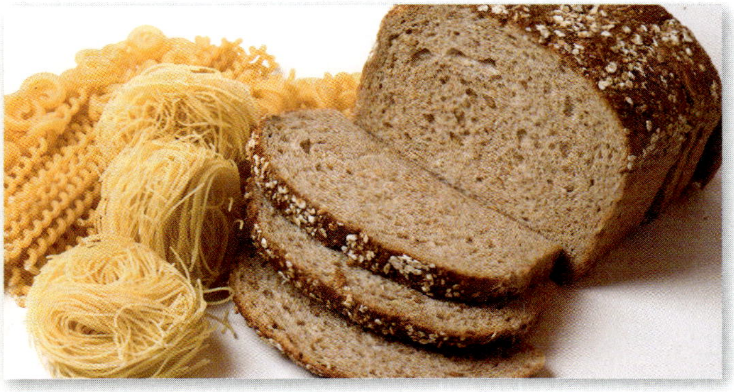

FIGURE 6.5 Increasingly, shoppers are choosing healthy options, such as whole-grain bread and pasta.

By researching consumers' attitudes and behaviours, companies can help to ensure that they are creating products that represent the needs of Canadians. As an example, people surveyed who buy "better-for-you" food products often buy them for their children (Agriculture and Agri-Food Canada, 2011). This knowledge may lead to the products being marketed differently than if those foods were used primarily by the purchaser.

Health Claims on Labels

Unfortunately, while consumers want to make healthier food choices, they find it difficult to do so. Research has shown that people worldwide have difficulty reading nutrition labels in order to make healthy choices (Nielsen Global Survey, 2012). In fact, when surveyed, more people said they find it easier to do their own taxes than to figure out how to make healthier choices (International Food Information Council, 2012). In response, food companies and other organizations have developed a range of tools to identify and promote healthy food options. Unfortunately, these are not always clear. In some systems, a symbol is used to identify healthy foods. The fairness of this system is not guaranteed, however. Even though only foods that satisfy certain specific criteria have the right to display the symbol, the results could be misleading. For example, if a hefty fee is charged to submit a food for evaluation, only large companies or companies with strong motivations to use the symbol will apply. Products produced by smaller companies may be just as healthy—or even more healthy—but may not display the symbol. If the use of the symbol is owned by one company, it may appear only on that company's products, and not on equally healthy competing products. It is always best to analyze the Nutrition Facts label yourself and make an informed decision about the healthfulness of a food.

NUTRITION LITERACY

Foods must meet specified criteria in order to make nutrient claims on their labels. For example, a food labelled "fat-free" can have up to 0.5 g of fat in one serving. A food labelled "good source of vitamin A" must contain at least 25 percent of the recommended daily intake in one serving.

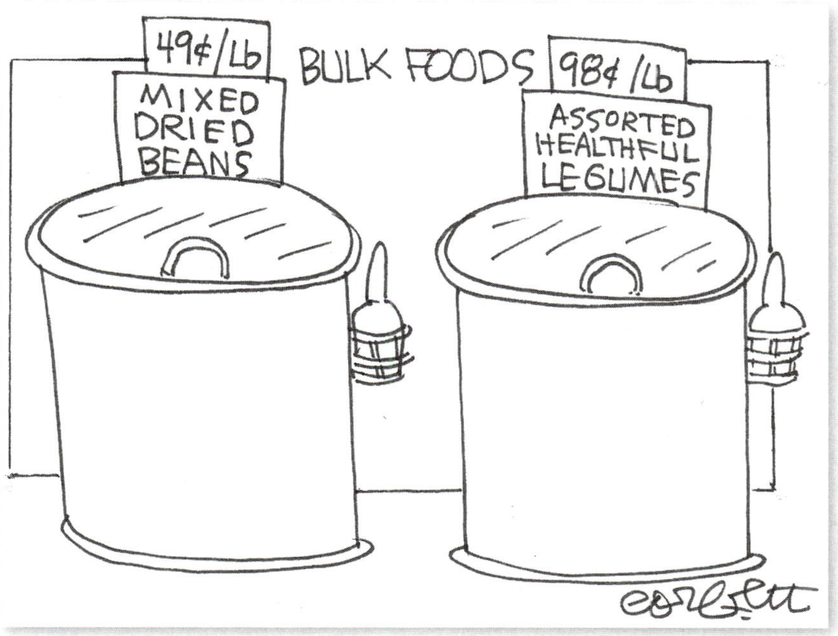

FIGURE 6.6 What message is this cartoon conveying about trends for healthy eating?

Food-Service Establishments

Food-service establishments have also focussed on consumers' desire to make healthy food choices. Some restaurant chains have created healthier menu options, with varied success. Unlike when cooking at home, or purchasing packaged food, it is not always possible for health-conscious consumers to learn the nutritional breakdown of food purchased in restaurants. Restaurant chains that use standardized recipes in each of their locations are able to post nutrition information on their Web sites. However, consumers may not have immediate access to such information when they are making dining decisions. In the United States, new legislation requires restaurant chains to post nutritional information on their menus or menu boards (Rosenbloom, 2010). Politicians and some members of the general public are pushing for similar legislation in Canada (Pynn, 2010).

TIP for Healthy Living

When eating in a restaurant, avoid rich dressings and creamy sauces. They often contain a lot of fat and extra Calories, and are nutrient-poor choices.

THINK CRITICALLY

1. What benefits would a food company likely receive if its labels included a logo showing the food was healthy? Would it receive similar benefits if the food was actually less healthy than a competing brand?
2. List reasons why consumers might have difficulty using nutrition labels to make healthy food choices.
3. Explain why restaurants' attempts to make and sell healthier choices are not always successful.

LIFE CONNECTION

Food Blogs

The term *weblog*, since shortened to *blog*, was coined in 1997 (BBC, 2007) as a way to log useful Web sites on an online journal. Blogs now run the gamut, from hobbyists writing personal musings, to corporations sharing expertise, as well as those who run their blog for profit. Blog search engine Technorati lists 25 000 blogs devoted to food as of June 2012, but that number increases daily.

The content of food blogs is varied. Some authors focus on a particular topic, such as food allergies, nutrition, reviews of restaurants, experiences working in food service, or current research. Other blogs offer detailed instructions for culinary techniques and recipes (complete with pictures). Many food corporations and organizations maintain their own blogs about their activities. Well-known chefs maintain blogs to promote upcoming projects.

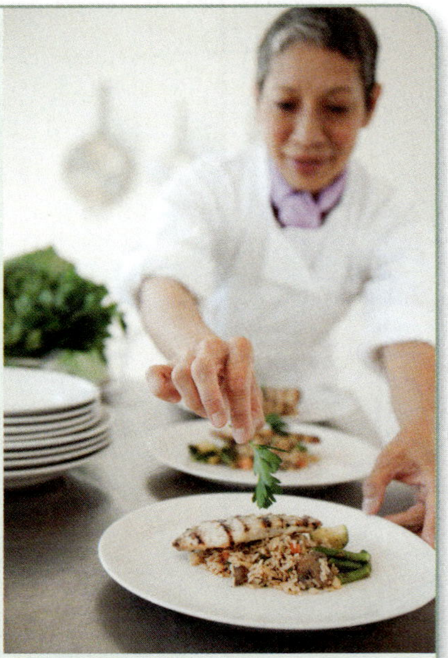

FIGURE 6.7 Some blogs include videos of specialized cooking techniques.

Blogging about research allows food scientists to increase communication with the public, as well as other scientists. As a blog can help to improve understanding of the scientific research process, social scientists may make postings throughout the research process, in addition to publishing the results of the inquiry. Blogging also can allow researchers to receive feedback about their topics of study, and analysis of their research. Postings allow information to be presented immediately, as well as allowing social scientists to receive instant feedback. Those giving feedback can be identified, allowing for a meaningful dialogue that may not occur if reviews are given anonymously.

As blogs can be read by social scientists and the public, they need to be written in a way that is accessible to all. Food scientists may have to rewrite content, reordering ideas and using more commonly used words, and giving some explanation of their research process. Visuals can be helpful, whether they are graphs of observations, or diagrams that help explain concepts.

Questions:

1. If you have looked at a food blog, describe what you learned from it.
2. What impact do you believe blogs have on food and nutrition trends?
3. How can a person determine the reliability of nutrition information presented on a blog?
4. If you were to create a food-related blog, what audience might you write for?
5. How would you write a post about the study that is presented on page 151?
6. Research blogs about food and nutrition. Choose one that you find particularly informative and interesting. Describe it to your classmates, including a summary of its most useful features.

Nutraceuticals

A combination of the words *nutrition* and *pharmaceutical*, **nutraceuticals** are considered beneficial or healthy beyond basic nutritional needs. For example, the Omega-3 fatty acids found in fish and flax products and the **phytochemicals** found in plants can be isolated as nutraceuticals. Nutraceuticals may be isolated, for example into pills, and sold as supplements, or may be added to other foods.

nutraceuticals: substances isolated from food that are considered beneficial beyond meeting basic nutritional needs

phytochemicals: chemical compounds in plants that are responsible for colour and odour; they are believed to aid in disease prevention

carotenoids: red and yellow pigments found in plants

Other examples of nutraceuticals:

- **Carotenoids** (including lycopene, lutein, and alpha- and beta-carotene) are found in foods such as carrots, tomato products, and green vegetables. These are believed to reduce the risk of prostate cancer and macular degeneration, and to neutralize free radicals.
- Soluble and insoluble fibre is found in wheat bran, oats, barley, and psyllium. In addition to reducing the risk of cardiovascular disease, these are also believed to reduce the risk of some types of cancers, and to lower LDL cholesterol.
- Conjugated linoleic acid (CLA) is found in cheese and meats. This fatty acid is also believed to reduce the risk of certain cancers.

The term *superfood* is a well-marketed term referring to nutraceuticals (Crowe, 2011). While no standard definition of superfoods exists, most who use the term refer to foods that are extremely high in nutrients or phytochemicals. The top superfoods will depend on who has coined the list. Blueberries, cranberries, watermelon, spinach and other dark leafy green vegetables, yams, pumpkin, seaweed, fatty fish such as salmon, various nuts and seeds, dark chocolate, and exotic fruits such as pomegranate, acai berries, and goji berries are commonly referred to as superfoods. However, other foods that contain similar beneficial components are not listed as often. For example, apples and pineapples are rarely included on superfood lists, but contain high levels of phytochemicals.

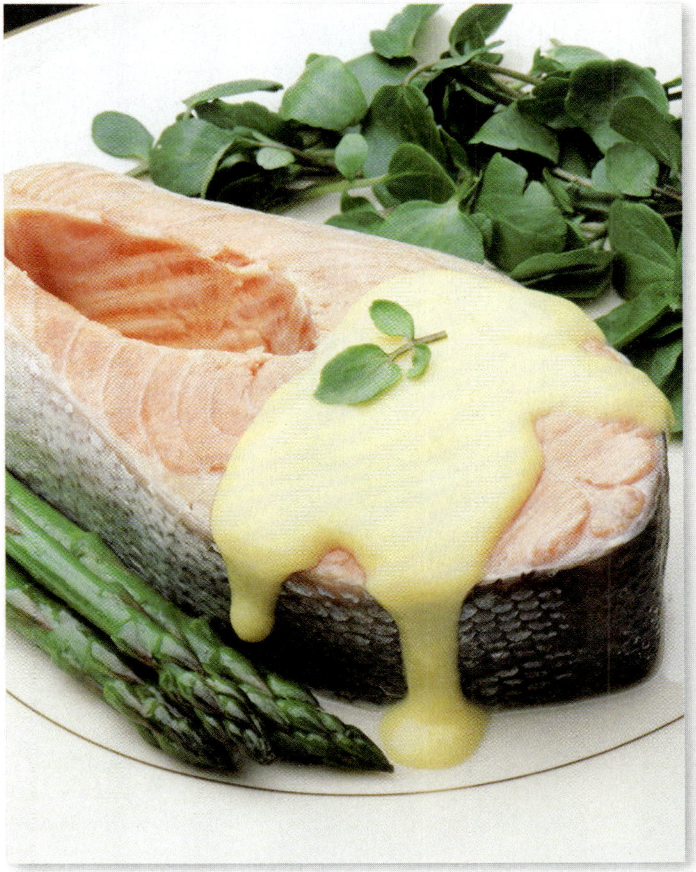

FIGURE 6.8 Omega-3 fatty acids are found in salmon and often added to other foods. What are the benefits of Omega-3 fatty acids?

Functional Foods

Despite the best intentions, many people have difficulty consistently eating healthy diets. For example, half of Canadian adults and 70 percent of children do not consume recommended daily servings of fruits and vegetables (Garriguet, 2004). Coupled with the increasing public concern about the rise in obesity rates, food and beverage companies as well as food-service operations have started making changes to the food that they produce, highlighting beneficial properties in certain foods.

functional foods:
foods that offer unique health benefits beyond meeting basic nutrient needs

bioactive compounds:
chemicals that occur naturally in foods and provide health benefits

probiotics:
beneficial bacteria

The term **functional foods** generally refers to foods that have had benefical ingredients added to them (Arvanitoyannis & van Houwelingen-Koukaliaroglou, 2005) to increase their healthfulness. Functional foods can also be described as foods with **bioactive compounds**. They can range from foods that naturally contain a nutraceutical, such as carrots (carotenoids) or some yogurts (**probiotics**), to foods that have had ingredients added during processing, such as orange juice with added calcium, and cereal with added fibre. Some foods have been enchanced through breeding, special feed, or genetic modification. For example, eggs can have increased Omega-3 levels from the flax fed to chickens, or tomatoes can be bred with higher levels of lycopene which may help prevent some types of cancer.

Are functional foods actually a healthier choice, or, as Nutrition Professor Marion Nestle states, are they more about marketing (Singer, 2011)? With increasing grocery-store shelf space devoted to these foods, consumers find the term *functional foods* confusing (Urala, Schultz, & Spinks, 2011).

proprietary:
owned; similar to a patent

The field of functional foods can indeed be confusing. In the case of probiotics, companies may develop a **proprietary** bacterial culture, and then advertise that they are the only brand with that particular type of bacteria. It is not necessarily true, however, that one bacterial strain is more healthful than another. Also, while a food may contain the bacteria, by the time that it reaches the consumer, many bacteria may have died, seriously reducing the number of live bacteria actually ingested. The amount of nutraceutical present in any food may not be enough to actually provide health benefits (Singer, 2011).

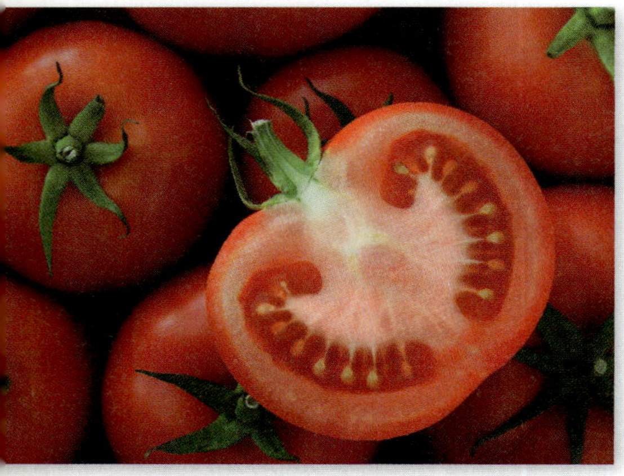

Some nutraceutical additions seem to be a natural fit, such as probiotic yogurt, since yogurt naturally contains bacteria. However, does adding vitamins and minerals to a cookie truly make the cookie a healthier choice? Singer (2011) reports that health professionals are concerned that consumers may focus only on the benefits that the functional food proclaims, while ignoring the entire ingredient list or full nutrition profile.

FIGURE 6.9 Do functional foods such as these tomatoes with higher levels of the antioxidant *lycopene* promote improved health, or just promote increased sales?

While researchers may determine the effects of a nutraceutical studied in isolation from food, it is often unclear whether those benefits can be applied when the nutraceutical is combined with other nutrients and with the components of our bodies. Food companies are required to follow strict guidelines for any health-related claims they make. For example, food companies may claim that nutraceuticals "reduce risk" of a particular disease, but cannot claim to cure or prevent a disease.

THINK CRITICALLY

1. What is the difference between a food fortified with vitamins and a functional food?
2. What effects does legislation have on the develoment and marketing of nutraceuticals and functional foods?

ACTIVE LEARNING

Incorporating Nutraceuticals/Functional Foods into Recipes

While some functional food products have had nutraceuticals added to them, there are functional foods that already contain the benefical substances. They can be incorporated into the diet by being consumed on their own, or added into recipes, helping to increase the nutritive value of the meal being consumed.

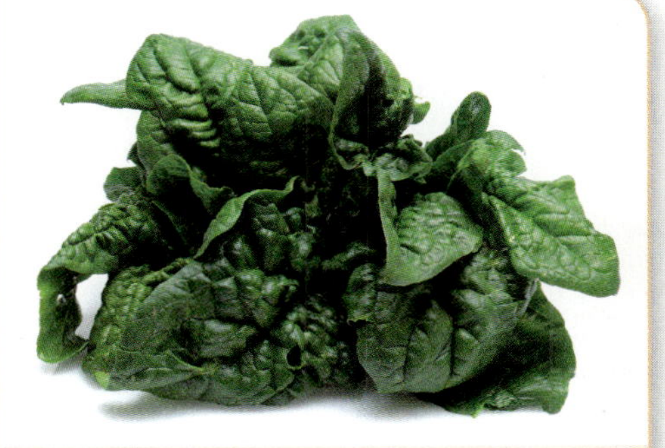

FIGURE 6.10 How could superfoods like spinach be incorporated into a person's diet?

Activities:

1. Describe how each food listed below could be incorporated into a person's diet.
2. Choose two of the foods below, and for each food, develop a healthy recipe.
3. Describe how the ingredients and cooking techniques were selected in order to make each recipe you developed healthy.
4. If possible, test one or both of the recipes and allow classmates to try the completed dishes.

Some Common Functional Foods:

Yogurt	Salmon	Avocados
Almonds	Flax seed	Tomatoes
Blueberries	Spinach	Grapes

NUTRITION LITERACY

The common allergens that must be identified on labels are peanuts, tree nuts (almonds, Brazil nuts, cashews, hazelnuts, macadamia nuts, pecans, pine nuts, pistachios, walnuts), milk, eggs, seafood, soy, wheat, sesame seeds, mustard, and sulphite (Health Canada, 2012a).

Other gluten sources, such as wheat, barley, oats, or rye must also be listed.

Allergies

There is an increased awareness in Canadian society about food allergies and intolerances (Agriculture and Agri-Food Canada, 2005). Current estimates are that five to six percent of children and three to four percent of adults in developed nations have a food allergy (Health Canada, 2011a). A food allergy is an immune response to a protein in a food. Food intolerances usually arise from the body's inability to digest a food or components of that food.

People with food allergies and intolerances rely on ingredient lists to determine whether they can safely eat a meal. As of 2012, Health Canada has strengthened allergy labelling requirements of packaged foods (2011a). In addition to listing all ingredients, any products containing the most common allergens must now identify them in the list of ingredients or in a special section at the end of the list of ingredients (Health Canada, 2011a).

People with allergies to other ingredients must read the entire Nutrition Facts label very closely to determine if foods are safe for them to eat.

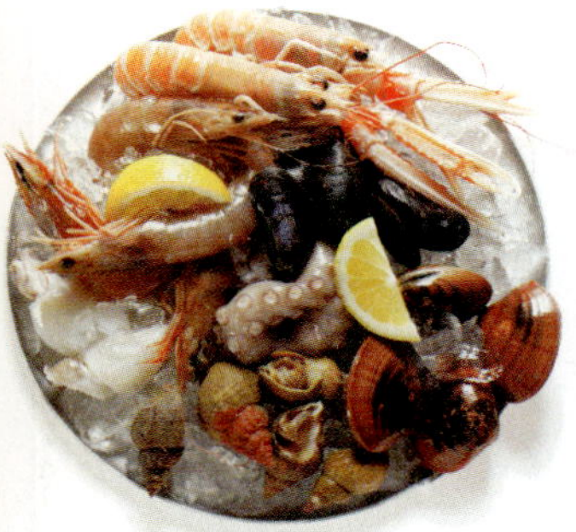

FIGURE 6.11 Shellfish are a common allergen. Why do you believe there is a heightened awareness of food allergies and intolerances?

Gluten-Free Foods

Approximately one in 133 Canadians suffers from celiac disease, an autoimmune condition in which the small intestine is damaged by the presence of gluten, a protein found in wheat, rye, triticale, and barley (Canadian Celiac Association, 2011). As a result, other nutrients cannot be absorbed by the body, leading to gastrointestinal problems, rashes, and in some cases, death. Gluten sensitivity or intolerance is a less serious condition also relieved by a gluten-free diet. Estimates are that there are 10 times more people who are gluten sensitive or intolerant than there are people with celiac disease (Katz, 2011).

Gluten-free products are one of the fastest growing segments of the food market (Nielsen, 2010). Because the gluten in wheat is responsible for the structure of some products, another ingredient that performs a similar role must be substituted. For those who have been unable to enjoy products such as bread, pasta, and cookies for years, these new gluten-free products can be a welcome addition to their diet. As with all other food choices, however, consumers need to be mindful of their selection. A gluten-free product may be high in sugar, salt, or fat. Simply eliminating gluten will not make a food any healthier than wheat-based versions of the same food.

THINK CRITICALLY

1. Explain how food products have been developed in response to people's increased attention to their health. Provide examples in your explanation.
2. Aside from gluten-free products, describe other food products or services that have been developed for people who have food allergies.

Active Learning

Wheat-Free Chocolate Chip Cookies

Yield: approximately 18 cookies

These cookies have been developed for those who can't have gluten in their diet. First make the flour mix. Store in an airtight container. There is enough to make three batches of cookies.

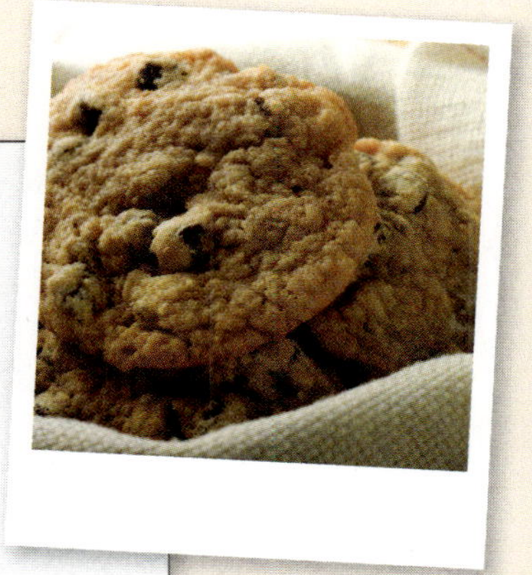

Figure 6.12 The ingredients for these cookies can be found in grocery stores, as well as health- and natural-food stores.

Brown Rice Flour Mix

500 mL (2 c) finely ground brown rice flour

150 mL (⅔ c) potato starch

80 mL (⅓ c) tapioca flour

1. Mix brown-rice flour, potato starch and tapioca flour together, mixing well.
2. Store in an airtight container.

Cookies

250 mL 1 cup brown-rice flour mix

5 mL (1 tsp) baking soda

2 mL (½ tsp) gluten-free baking powder

1 mL (¼ tsp) salt

2 mL (½ tsp) xanthan gum

125 mL (½ c) vegetable shortening

125 mL (½ c) granulated sugar

50 mL (¼ c) packed brown sugar

1 egg

5 mL (1 tsp) vanilla

125 mL (½ c) chocolate chips

Method

1. Preheat oven to 190 °C (375 °F). Lightly grease a large baking sheet, or cover with parchment paper.
2. In a medium bowl mix together flour mix, baking powder, baking soda, salt and xanthan gum. Set aside.
3. In a large bowl and using an electric mixer on medium speed, beat shortening, granulated sugar and brown sugar until creamed together. Add egg and vanilla and beat well.
4. Reduce electric mixer speed to low and mix flour mixture into shortening mixture, just until incorporated.
5. Stir in chocolate chips.
6. Drop rounded teaspoons of dough onto prepared baking sheet placing dough about 5 cm (2 inches) apart.
7. Bake for 9–11 min. Let stand for 1 min, then remove to a cooling rack.

Source: Adapted from Gourmet magazine (November, 2005).

Trends for Value

People generally agree that low-priced, nutritious, tasty food that doesn't spoil quickly has a high value. High-priced food that spoils easily has a low value. The food industry has developed many ingredients and processes to increase the value of foods. Some of these innovations affect the value of the food after it has been purchased. Others affect the value of the food as it is grown and transported. For example, breeding can produce crops that have a higher yield, thus decreasing the price of the end product and increasing its value.

Demographics also influence what qualities are perceived as valuable in foods. While large packages of food often cost less, increasing their value for a large family, people living in small households find that foods in smaller package sizes will not spoil. An increase in small households in Canada has prompted a trend to smaller package sizes (Sloan, 2011).

Pause and Think
How will a change (increase or decrease) in the number of teenagers in society affect the food products that a company may develop?

Food Additives

food additive:
any chemical substance that is added to food during preparation or storage and either becomes a part of the food or affects its characteristics for the purpose of achieving a particular chemical effect (Health Canada, 2012b)

Generally, the purpose of **food additives** is to

- maintain nutritive quality

  Vitamins and minerals enhance the nutrient profile of commonly consumed foods. For example, in Canada, vitamin D is commonly added to milk and iron is added to many breakfast cereals.

- enhance keeping quality (shelf life)

  Preservatives prevent bacteria from growing and inhibit oxidation. Vitamin C is added to some foods as an antioxidant, and high-maltose corn syrup is added to some baked goods to inhibit bacterial growth.

- make the food attractive

  Food dyes, both natural and artificial, as well as edible waxes, are used to add colour lost during the manufacturing process, as well as make foods more visually appealing.

- aid in processing, packaging, or storage

  Gum arabic is a thickening agent and gelatin helps marshmallows and other products gel. Calcium stearoyl lactylate is added to bread dough to produce a uniform grain and greater volume (Health Canada, 2012b).

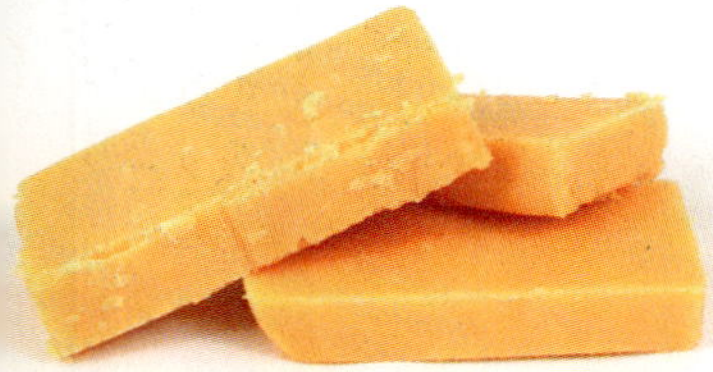

FIGURE 6.13 Added colour makes this cheddar cheese orange.

Health Canada, through the *Food and Drug Regulations*, is responsible for regulating the use of food additives, specifying not only which food additives can legally be used in Canada, but also how they can be used, on which foods they can be used, and in what quantities they can be used. Additives must be listed in a food product's ingredient list, though the specific chemical substance does not need to be named. For example, the generic ingredient *colour* can be listed.

Depending on its use, a substance may be classified as an additive or as a food processing aid. For example, an anti-foaming agent added to a fruit juice would be considered a food additive, but the same substance added to water when processing potatoes would be considered a food processing aid, as its purpose is to affect the water, not the potatoes. In addition, some nutrients may also be considered additives. Ascorbic acid (vitamin C) may be added to foods as a nutrient, and also may be used as an antioxidant. Flavour enhancers, such as salt, sugar, and monosodium glutamate (MSG), are not considered additives in Canada.

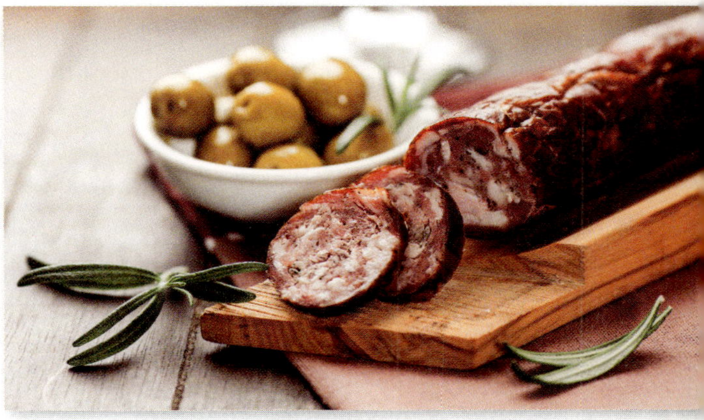

FIGURE 6.14 Ascorbic acid is often used as an antioxidant to prevent meats and sausages from turning brown.

Have you tried a packaged food in another country and noticed that it was different than the same food available here? The same product sold in different countries may have different compositions. This is due to a variety of factors, such as permissable additives in each country. For example, some additives allowable in the U.S. are not permitted in Canada, and vice versa. Other reasons for product variations include differences in flavour profiles (for example, one country preferring a sweeter or spicier version), and availability or price of ingredients. As a result, a product may look different, and, due to the ingredients used in making it, might also have a different flavour.

OPEN FOR DEBATE

Research the claims made about food additives. With your classmates, debate the following statement: "Food additives result in a safer food supply."

While food additives can increase the value of food by enhancing its nutritional profile and increasing its shelf life, additives have also been implicated by some in a wide variety of health issues, from allergies and learning disabilites to other, more serious health concerns. Others argue that each additive has been rigourously tested for safety in government laboratories and approved for use, so foods containing small amounts of additives are safe to consume. Both sides of the debate use evidence to support their claims. As with any research, however, not all evidence is credible. Anecdotal reports may sound convincing, but they represent a very small sample size. Even scientific research may use a small sample size, or may include bias. While studies initiated by manufacturers or lobby groups may follow acceptable research protocol, these groups do have a vested interest to ensure that their viewpoints are presented in the best possible light.

THINK CRITICALLY

1. A popular cereal has a different composition for its European version than the cereal available for purchase in Canada. Cereal A uses colouring from spinach, currant, carrot, and paprika extract. Cereal B uses artificial colouring. Cereal A has trans fats, while Cereal B does not. Cereal A has 12 g of sugar per serving, while Cereal B has 14 g. Which cereal would you choose to eat? Why?

2. Choose one of the following food additives approved for use in Canada. Research to determine its intended purpose(s) in food. Find credible evidence supporting its use in food and credible evidence opposing its use. Explain how you determined whether evidence was credible.

   Some Food Additives Approved for use in Canada:

Acesulfame Potassium (Acesulfame K)		Sodium Benzoate
Aspartame	Inulin	Sodium Nitrite
Caffeine	Rebiana (Stevia)	Transglutaminase

3. Based on your research in Question 2, state whether you believe that the food additive should continue to be used in Canada. Justify your position.

TRENDS AND CHANGE

Social Media

Social media, including blogs, microblogs, podcasts, social networks, crowd sourcing, and videos, has changed not only how food trends are shared with the public, but how quickly they get picked up by others.

- Before you go to a restaurant, you can check several reviews posted online by other diners. These may include ratings, photographs, and personal anecdotes. After dining, you can add your own impressions.
- Consumers can initiate online campaigns to persuade food retailers to change their product or service––for example, to stop using finely textured beef (Eng, 2012) or dyes made of insect carapaces (parts of the exoskeleton).
- Restaurants and food companies can use social media to interact with their customers, potentially increasing transparency about how their products are created and sold (Krashinsky, 2012).

FIGURE 6.15 QR codes that can be read with a mobile device can be used to obtain discounts and information about a food product. How does our increased use of technology impact our relationship with food?

Question:

What are the advantages and disadvantages of each use of social media described above?

Novel and GM/GE Foods

The CFIA defines *novel foods* as items that have not previously been used as foods, or foods produced using new manufacturing methods that cause a change to the food. Novel foods can be created to provide enhanced nutrition (such as the functional foods described earlier) or enhanced value (such as juice treated with ultraviolet light to reduce the numbers of micro-organisms and prevent spoilage).

"The only thing that is constant in life is change."
– François de la Rochefoucauld

Traditional agricultural practices result in modified foods and modified genetic profiles. Farmers breed livestock and crops to influence inherited characteristics and graft branches from one type of fruit tree onto another to create fruit that shares characteristics of both types. While these processes have been in use for centuries, GM (**genetically modified**) or GE (**genetically engineered**) foods have moved genetic change to a new level. Using modern biotechnology techniques, genetic modifications can now be carried out more rapidly and at increasingly detailed levels, including targeting individual genes. As a result, foods created using these technologies are commonly considered novel. Examples of GM/GE foods approved for use in Canada include corn that is tolerant to drought and pests; potatoes resistant to a common beetle; a tomato that ripens more slowly on the vine; and milk with an increased level of the fatty acid DHA (Health Canada, 2011b).

genetically modified/engineered: made from genetically modified organisms, in which the DNA of a plant or animal has been altered with biotechnology, often through the insertion of foreign or synthetic DNA

Any novel foods sold in Canada must first be approved by Health Canada, who determine if the food is safe for consumption. Current legislation does not require that products made with GM/GE ingredients be identified to consumers in Canada, though this labelling is mandatory in other jurisdictions, such as the European Union (Food Standards Agency, 2008). A voluntary labelling program does exist in Canada, in which manufacturers may identify if their product has been created through genetic engineering.

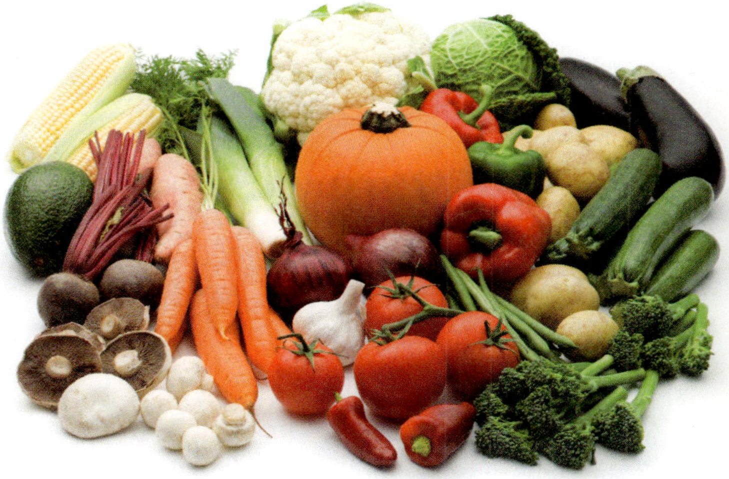

FIGURE 6.16 Most genetically modified foods look no different from unmodified varieties.

THINK CRITICALLY

1. What are the implications of labelling or not labelling foods as GM/GE?
2. Do you believe that GM/GE foods should be labelled as such in Canada? Justify your position.

POINT/COUNTERPOINT

Genetically Modified Foods

As with food additives, the use of GM/GE is controversial. Canadians state that while they are aware of GM/GE foods, they do not neccessarily understand them (Ipsos, 2000). Many also believe that the government has not provided them with enough information to make informed decisions about GM/GE foods (Leger, 2012). The largest concern raised is the safety of foods. Other fears point to potential environmental dangers and whether these foods are necessary. A quick search on the Internet will find thousands of Web pages attesting to the dangers of GM/GE foods. Are the concerns warranted?

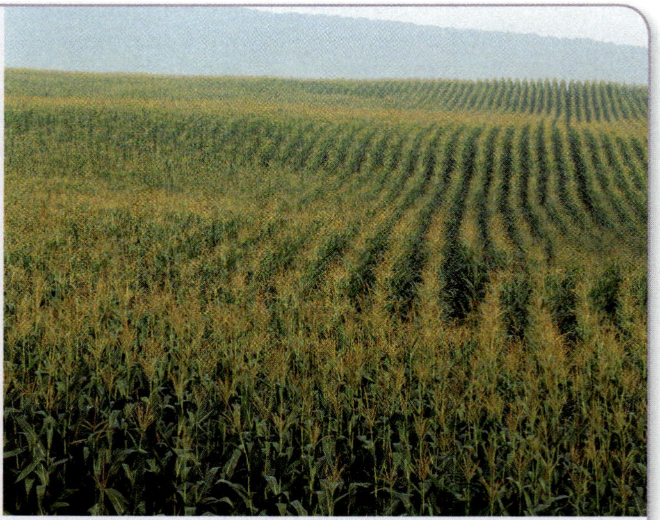

FIGURE 6.17 Does genetic modification result in more productive agriculture?

Activities:

1. Below are some of the arguments for and against the use of GM/GE foods. Classify each argument as For (that is, supporting genetic modification or engineering) or Against (that is, not supporting genetic modification or engineering).
   - GM/GE foods are widely available in our food supply.
   - GM/GE crops could adversely change the nutrient content of a food.
   - GM/GE foods may lead to an increase in allergic reactions, food intolerances, and antibiotic resistance.
   - GM/GE foods allow more efficient food production, and reduced prices for the consumer.
   - Non-GM/GE crops could become accidentally contaminated with the DNA of GM/GE crops.
   - Many GM/GE crops have improved resistance to pests and diseases.
   - The long-term effects of GM/GE foods are unknown.
   - Companies who create GM/GE seeds have an increased control over the food supply.
   - Food yields will increase using GM/GE crops, ensuring better access to food worldwide.
2. As a class, research each of the claims made. Determine the validity of each claim, and assess the degree of support each claim adds to the overall argument. How did you decide to what extent each claim supported the overall argument?

Trends for Convenience

Approximately 70 percent of meals are prepared at home, and only 20 percent are eaten in restaurants (Sloan, 2011). Sloan also notes that the number of meals prepared at home has increased over the past few years. However, the way meals are prepared has changed. Consumers are looking for meals that can be made quickly and easily, with little preparation and clean-up (Agriculture and Agri-Food Canada, 2010). Consumers are using more and more convenience products in their cooking, including meal kits, pre-washed salad greens, and frozen entrées.

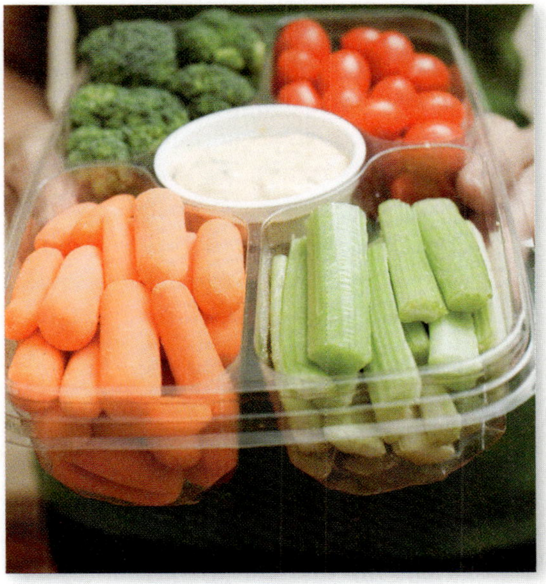

FIGURE 6.18 How might purchasing pre-cut produce affect the nutritional value of a meal or snack?

In addition to foods and food products that can be prepared quickly and easily, consumers are also looking for cooking methods that are fast and efficient. Appliances such as slow cookers, microwave ovens, and indoor grills have become increasingly popular (Agriculture and Agri-Food Canada, 2010). However, the same study notes that while consumers increasingly use convenience products, they are concerned about price, health, quality, and taste. In addition to being more expensive, convenience products are more likely to be higher in fat, sugar, and salt. But, if chosen and used carefully, convenience products may allow time-pressed consumers to still be able to prepare nutritious, tasty meals for themselves and their families.

THINK CRITICALLY

1. If 70 percent of meals are eaten at home, and 20 percent are eaten in restaurants, what might account for the other 10 percent of meals?
2. Explain how food companies have combined our renewed interest in preparing food at home with an increased demand for quick or convenience products.
3. Describe a convenience food and describe how you could use it in a meal to optimize taste and nutrition, while minimizing time spent preparing the meal.

NUTRITION LITERACY

An increasing body of research is showing that fat may be the sixth taste, besides sour, sweet, salty, bitter, and umami.

Career Connection

Mobile Food Service

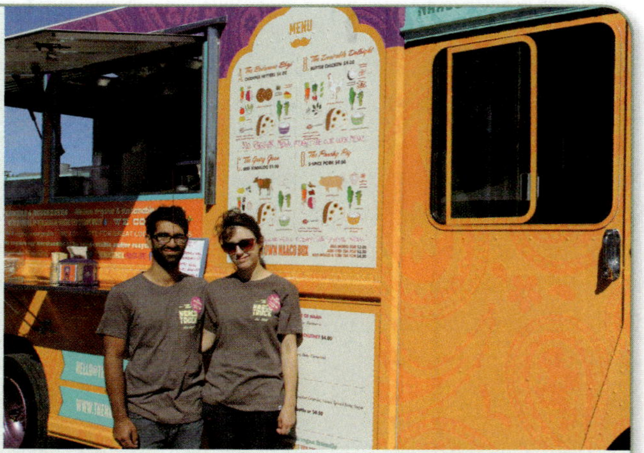

Figure 6.19 The Naaco Truck. What challenges might you encounter operating a food truck?

Food trucks have exploded in popularity in the past few years. They have also evolved to serve more upscale dishes, and are increasingly operated by classically trained chefs. With lower start-up costs than traditional brick-and-mortar restaurants, food trucks can allow those who might have difficulty opening a traditional restaurant to still become a part of the food-service industry.

Aman Adatia and Stephanie Shields both studied science in university. Aman went to culinary school and operated a catering company for many years. They decided to start a food truck just as Calgary changed its regulations allowing food trucks to operate. The Naaco Truck combines traditional flavours of India and East Africa with local ingredients. Aman believes that food trucks that have a unique, sustainable concept will succeed.

Aman and Stephanie believe in supporting local, organic, sustainable suppliers. Aman states, "If you don't support your neighbours, you can't survive as a small business". They compost as much as possible, and only use eco-friendly products. They have the first LEAF (Leaders in Environmentally Accountable Foodservice) certified food truck in Canada. In addition, each month, customers can donate money to a different charity that parallels the philosophy of The Naaco Truck.

Social media plays a major role in the success of almost any small business. Stephanie and Aman use social media to promote themselves and to communicate their changing location. For The Naaco Truck, choice of location is often based on feedback and emails from their customers. Reviews from customers, whether by word of mouth or on restaurant-review sites, help them build a following.

While many skills needed to successfully run a food-service establishment are the same no matter what type is operated, food-truck operators have unique challenges that may not be seen in other types of establishments. Operators need to forge strong connections with their customers, as they will need customers who will follow them wherever their truck goes, as well as acquire new customers with each location. They also need to be flexible, dealing not only with the food side of the business, but also with traffic and the mechanics of the truck, for example.

Questions:

1. What food and nutrition trends do small food-service businesses like Stephanie's and Aman's food truck support?
2. Do you believe that the food-truck industry is a fad or will it become a permanent option for food service?
3. What skills would be needed to run any small food-service establishment?
4. "Restaurants have customers, food trucks have followers." Explain the meaning of this quote.

Trends for Authenticity

Over the past hundred years, our society has undergone significant technological innovations in areas relating to foods, entertainment, transportation, and in other parts of our lives. While these innovations have presented us with many advantages—more nutritious and readily available foods, the ability to travel long distances in a day, and music downloads, for example—they have also presented us with some disadvantages. A trend toward authenticity in food is borne partly of a desire to do away with disadvantages that may come with the modern food production and delivery systems.

Natural Foods

Due to concerns about additives in food products and the use of technologies such as genetic engineering, an increasing number of consumers are looking for natural food products (Agriculture and Agri-Food Canada, 2011). Some people buy raw ingredients from health-food stores and farms and prepare foods from scratch at home. Others seek out prepared foods that claim to be natural in the supermarket.

Nutrition Literacy

As food companies do not have to list the source of their natural colourings or flavourings, vegetarians, vegans, and others wanting to avoid animal products need to be aware that they may be derived from animal sources.

Unfortunately, the word *natural* or *nature* on a label does not ensure superior nutritional content. While there is no legal definition for these terms, the Canadian Food Inspection Agency's *Guide to Food Labelling and Advertising* does state that foods labelled *natural* are expected to have had no vitamins, minerals, artificial flavourings, or food additives added or removed, and to have undergone minimal to no processing. While foods labelled *natural* will not have preservatives added to them, neither will they be fortified with vitamins.

Artificial and natural colours and flavourings appear commonly on lists of ingredients. These may have similar chemical compositions, but differ in their source. Natural colourings and flavourings come from natural sources, but that does not mean that the flavour or colour is naturally found in that particular food. Flavourists extract natural flavours from a wide variety of sources, incuding plants, animals, and fermented products. These are used to flavour an assortment of food products. For example, an extract from cochineal, an insect, is used as red colouring in many candies.

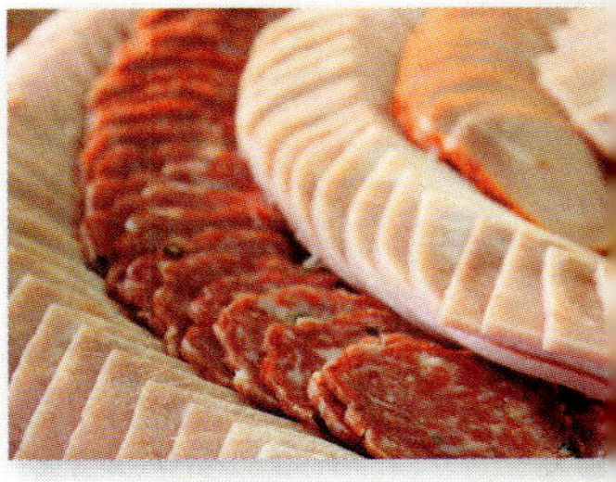

Figure 6.20 A food company advertises that their deli meats are cured with natural ingredients, such as celery-seed extract. Why can't the company state that the deli meats are a natural product?

Food manufacturers who use colours, flavours, or other additives from natural sources may claim that natural ingredients are used in their product. However, they may not claim that the food product itself is natural. In addition, if one of many common types of processing is used, the resulting food product cannot be labelled *natural*. For example, the CFIA considers that chopping, baking, drying, and canning constitute enough of a change that a food produced by one of these techniques cannot be called *natural*.

Global Foods

In Canada's multicultural environment, we are becoming more and more aware of cultures different from our own. Through personal interaction, the arts, and the media, we can learn about the traditions and foods of many of these cultures. As demand for them has grown, authentic ingredients, foods, and meals of many ethnic groups have become available across Canada. As part of the trend toward authenticity, many Canadians are trying foods from a variety of cultures. To date, the demographic group called *Generation Y* or *Millennials* are most likely to try eating and preparing a variety of foods from different ethnic groups (Sloan, 2011).

THINK CRITICALLY

1. How would you expect the cost of foods labelled *natural* to compare with other foods? Why?
2. Describe advantages and disadvantages of purchasing natural foods.
3. Describe how the trend to global foods has affected your eating habits.
4. Compare the foods you choose to eat with those your parents or grandparents ate. What has changed? What has stayed the same?

CAREER CONNECTION

Food Scientist

It takes teams of people with many different skills to develop a new food product. Food production companies rely on market researchers to analyze consumers' needs, and on food scientists to apply their knowledge of food chemistry to develop products with the desired characteristics. A food scientist combines a background in several areas including biology, chemistry, and nutrition. Some food scientists work in research laboratories, using chemical principles to predict the effects of modifying food products and testing the results. Others work in quality-assurance facilities to ensure that food products meet established criteria for safety and healthfulness. When you see that a food product has been modified to be tastier, lower in fat, or easier to prepare, you can be sure that at least one food scientist has been involved.

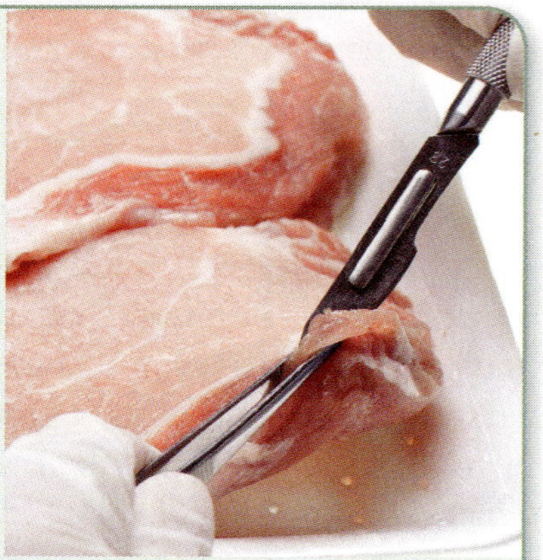

FIGURE 6.21 Why is it important for food scientists to follow established scientific procedures in their work?

Questions:

1. In what situations might market researchers and food scientists work together?
2. What universities in your region offer programs in food chemistry? What are the prerequisites for these programs?

Trends for Sustainability

As Canadians become more concerned about the environment and the conditions under which food is grown and produced, there is increasing demand for local and organic food products (Canadian Council of Food and Nutrition, 2008). Many consumers believe that sustainable foods—that is, foods grown locally, without using manufactured fertilizers and pesticides—and providing a fair wage to growers and producers results in less negative impact on the ecosystem and can help to improve the lives and communities of those who produce the food. However, food products grown and produced sustainably are usually more expensive than conventionally grown or raised foods, creating a barrier to purchase for some consumers.

"Let's finally embrace the truth that food is not something to be taken for granted."
– Chef David Chang

Local Foods

Many Canadians see benefits in purchasing locally produced foods. These include helping the local economy, enjoying better taste, and reducing the greenhouse gases required to transport food long distances (Ipsos, 2006). **Locavores** seek out food produced locally. One result of the locavore movement is *The 100-Mile Diet* (MacKinnon & Smith, 2007), a book written by a Canadian couple that detailed their year of consuming foods that were produced within a 100 mile (160 km) radius of where they lived.

locavore: a person focussed on consuming locally grown or produced foods

The trend towards local foods is reflected in a number of ways. Farmers' markets are increasingly popular across the country—sales are over $1 billion per year (Farmers' Markets Canada, 2009). Many restaurants highlight the growers or producers of their ingredients. Some cities have made urban agriculture a possibility by creating plots for residents to grow produce, allowing chickens in backyards for egg production, and promoting beekeeping.

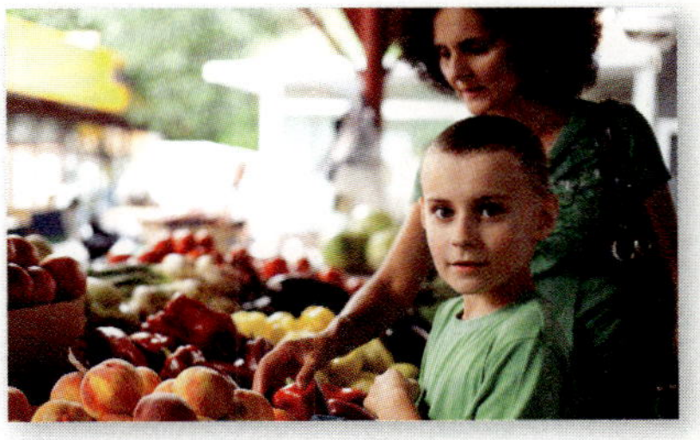

FIGURE 6.22 Canada-wide, sales at farmers' markets are over $1 billion per year (Farmers' Markets Canada, 2009).

Proponents of local food point to the fact that produce loses nutrients once it is harvested, therefore local produce would retain more nutrients than food that is produced elsewhere and shipped. In fact, a variety of factors work together to determine the nutrient content of produce (Frith, 2007). Researchers have found that the average nutrient content of produce has declined over the past few decades (Davis, Epp, & Riordan, 2004). Production methods, the degree of ripeness when the produce is harvested, as well as how the produce is handled and stored after harvesting all play a role in determining nutrient content at the time of purchase. Locally grown and harvested produce spends less time in shipping, and growers focussing on a local market can offer varieties that emphasize nutrient content and taste as opposed to durability. On the other hand, local produce may be grown using unsustainable or unfair practices, while produce shipped from other countries may provide much-needed employment to the population.

Organic Foods

Sales of organic foods have increased about 20 percent per year for the past decade (CBC, 2009). While natural-food stores and farmers' markets were the traditional source for organic foods and food products, almost half of current sales occur in major grocery stores.

SAFETY AND SANITATION

Whether it is grown conventionally or organically, all produce should be washed thoroughly prior to consumption.

Some people choose organic foods because they believe foods grown organically are more sustainable—that is, they do not deplete the soil and other resources as conventionally grown foods do. For example, instead of manufactured pesticides and fertilizers, crops may be alternated in a field from one year to the next. Compost and natural predators may also be used.

The term *organic* and the Canada Organic logo are regulated by the Canadian Food Inspection Agency and its Canada Organic Regime. The CFIA's *Guide to Food Labelling and Advertising* stipulates that in order for a food to be considered organic, 95 percent of the ingredients in the food must be organic. Food products that contain less than this percent may identify which specific ingredients are organic but cannot state that the food product itself is organic.

While many farmers use organic methods to produce their crops, in order to be marketed as organic, the growers must be certified to the Canadian Organic Standards. This regulation also applies to foods imported into Canada. In addition to the national organic system, both British Columbia and Québec have provincial certification systems, and there are a number of other certification systems worldwide. In Canada, growers or operators pay yearly fees and undergo certification every year. Certification can take some time, so growers often incur the expenses of organic certification long before they are able to label their foods as organic.

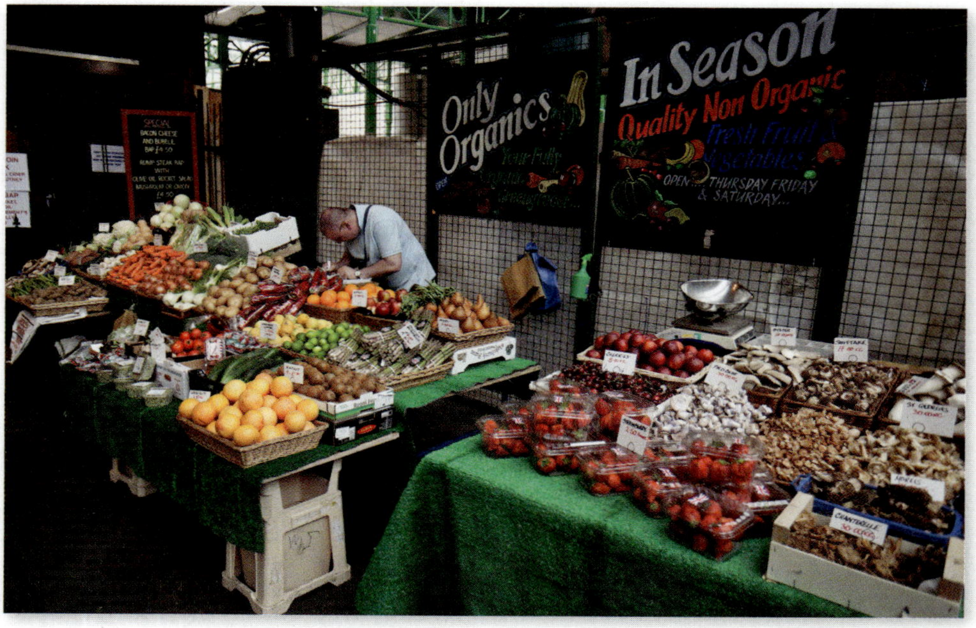

FIGURE 6.23 Organic produce. What foods are most likely to be grown organically in Canada?

While many consumers believe that organic food is healthier, research results have been inconclusive. A review of the literature finds that there is little difference in the amount of nutrients in organically grown food compared to conventionally grown food (Rosen, 2010). Rosen states that some earlier research concluding that organic food was healthier did not take into account differences in geography and soil, both of which can influence the nutrient content of a food.

FIGURE 6.24 The Canada Organic logo. What benefits other than nutrient value could be attained by choosing organic foods?

Sustainable Fisheries

An increased consumption of fish worldwide has led to an increase in harvesting. While some fish are grown in fish farms, others are harvested from the wild. Unfortunately, as technology has improved, humans have used it to deplete several important global fish stocks. Also, some fishing technology results in damage to the ecosystem, including harming other species of wildlife. For example, some practices used to catch tuna also result in killing dolphins (Perrin, Wursig, & Thewissen , 2002).

To allow fish stocks to recover, many experts recommend that we not consume certain types of fish. Other types of fish are harvested in a sustainable way. Their populations are stable and there is little concern about eating them. To help consumers choose fish from sustainable environments, several groups publish lists of fish categorized by the sustainability of their harvest. These lists are available online, and as apps that can be used as restaurant patrons scan a restaurant menu.

THINK CRITICALLY

1. What are benefits and disadvantages of having provincial organic certification systems in addition to a national system?
2. Describe ways to handle and store produce in order to retain its nutrients.
3. After reading about local and organic food, which would you choose: a locally grown apple or an organic one that is grown in another country? Fully explain your answer.
4. How might your answer to Question 3 change depending on the time of year when you were buying the apple? Explain.

SKILLS FOCUS

Think of what you have learned about communicating information effectively. How would you communicate your answer to Question 2 to shoppers in a supermarket?

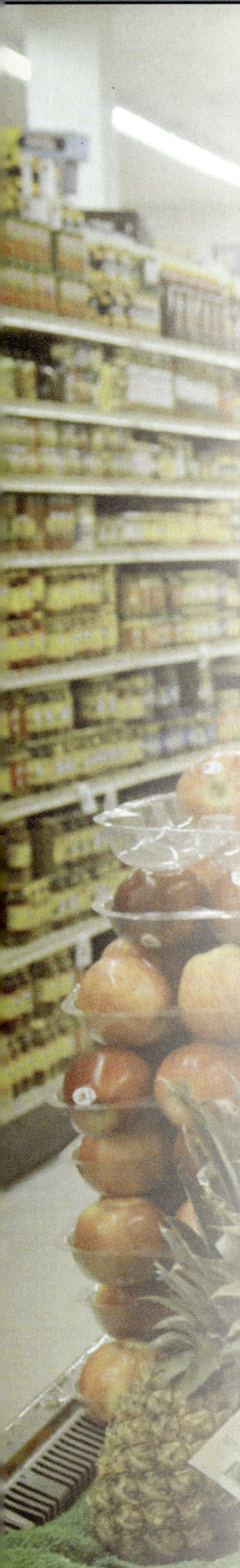

Chapter Review

Knowledge and Understanding/Thinking

1. Describe some cautions that a consumer should take into account when reading a list of superfoods.
2. Some companies and organizations have their own programs that they use to rate the relative healthfulness of their products. Describe and explain issues that could arise with these programs.
3. Summarize the arguments for and against the use of functional foods in the diet.
4. Often, the terms *organic* and *local* are used interchangeably, when they are quite different terms. Explain what each means.
5. Describe some behaviours that a locavore may exhibit when making food purchasing decisions.
6. List and explain nutritional and economic advantages and disadvantages of choosing to support local growers and producers.
7. Describe how legislation has allowed those with allergies and intolerances to make informed food choices.
8. Explain some advantages and disadvantages to consumers receiving much of their food, nutrition, and recipe information online as opposed to more traditional print sources.

Thinking/Communication

9. Compare the positive and negative impacts of food additives on food consumption and health.
10. Investigate to find other certified-organic logos used in Canada, aside from the one pictured in the textbook. Create a display for the school showing the logos and the foods on which they might be found.
11. Explain how current food trends have influenced the foods available in your home or in the school cafeteria.
12. Rank the five food-related trends discussed in this chapter (health, value, convenience, authenticity, and sustainability) in order of their importance to you. Explain why you ranked each trend as you did.
13. Find one article supporting the use of GM/GE products and one against. Summarize the findings of each article.
14. "If a product is not certified as organic, it could still be considered organic." Explain the meaning of this statement.

Communication/Application

15. Choose a functional food. Research to determine how much of the nutraceutical is in one serving of the product. How many servings would need to be consumed to receive a benefit from the nutraceutical?
16. Research to determine what kinds of urban agriculture are allowed in your community. What are the requirements for use?
17. Choose an additive that is approved for use in Canada but not in the United States. Research to find credible information about the additive. Based on your research, would you recommend that Health Canada continue to allow its use?
18. Describe ways in which technology can be used to help people make more informed food choices.

Putting It All Together

In this chapter, you have

- identified various trends in food products and services
- investigated the advantages and disadvantages of food trends
- prepared food products that incorporated a nutraceutical
- used research to predict future trends in food products and services

Create a concept map to show various trends in food and how those trends are represented in food products and services. Part of a sample concept map is shown below:

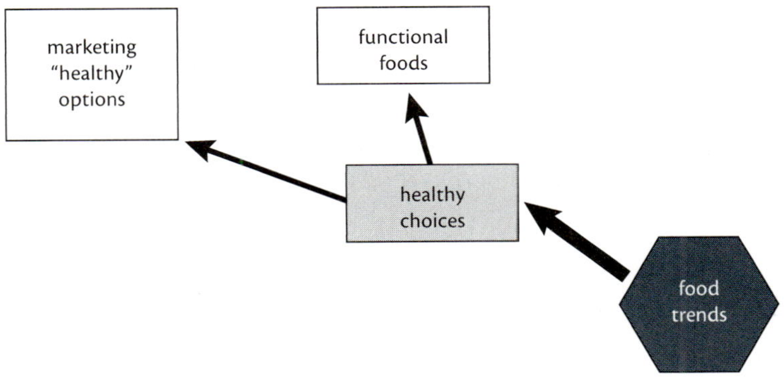

Glossary

A

absorption: the movement of nutrients through the walls of the intestine into the bloodstream

adipose tissue: body tissue that contains stored fat cells

allergen: a substance that causes allergic reactions

anaphylaxis: the most serious type of allergic reaction, often including throat swelling and low blood-pressure; it can progress very quickly and can cause death without proper medical attention

anemia: a lack of healthy red blood cells; symptoms can include weakness, fatigue, trouble concentrating, and shortness of breath

B

basal metabolic rate (BMR): the amount of energy used *per kilogram of body mass* to carry out basal metabolic functions

basal metabolism: the chemical processes by which the body uses energy to carry out functions necessary to sustain life; does not include energy used for daily activities

bioactive compounds: chemicals that occur naturally in foods and provide health benefits

bioavailability: the degree to which the amount of an ingested nutrient is absorbed and available to the body

C

caries: cavities in teeth, caused by decay of tooth enamel

carotenoids: red and yellow pigments found in plants

coenzyme: a vitamin that combines with another molecule to form an organic compound

colostrum: the thick, yellow breastmilk that is produced immediately after birth, continuing through the early days of breastfeeding

D

digestion: the process by which the body breaks food down to its component nutrients

E

empty Calorie: describes foods that are high in Calories and low in other nutrients, also known as nutrient-poor foods

energy dense: describes the relationship between the caloric value of a food and its size, weight, or volume. A food that is energy dense will have a larger Calorie content, while a food that is not energy dense will have fewer Calories relative to the amount of food

F

food additive: any chemical substance that is added to food during preparation or storage and either becomes a part of the food or affects its characteristics for the purpose of achieving a particular chemical effect (Health Canada, 2012b)

food neophobia: fear of and unwillingness to try new foods

foremilk: the watery milk produced early in a breastfeeding session

free radical: a highly reactive substance, produced by oxidation, that can cause cell damage

functional foods: foods that offer unique health benefits beyond meeting basic nutrient needs

G

gastrointestinal (GI) tract: a tubular passage of specialized mucous membrane and muscle from mouth to anus that carries out the processes of digestion and excretion

genetically modified/engineered: made from genetically modified organisms, in which the DNA of a plant or animal has been altered with biotechnology, often through the insertion of foreign or synthetic DNA

H

hemorrhoids: a condition in which the veins in the rectum become enlarged and may be painful

hindmilk: the thicker, almost cream-like milk produced later in breastfeeding that is high in fat

histamine: a powerful chemical produced by the body that can cause an inflammatory reaction in the respiratory system, gastrointestinal tract, skin, or cardiovascular system

hyperglycemia: abnormally high levels of glucose in the blood

I

insulin: a hormone produced by the pancreas that regulates blood sugar (glucose)

insulin resistance: the body's inability to use insulin efficiently to absorb glucose into cells, which leads to a rise in blood-glucose levels

intrinsic factor: a substance that binds with vitamin B12 in food so that the nutrient can be absorbed

K

kilocalorie: A kilocalorie is the amount of heat energy required to raise one kilogram of water one degree Celsius

L

lipid: a nutrient in foods; fats, oils, and cholesterol are lipids

locavore: a person focussed on consuming locally grown or produced foods

M

malnutrition: a condition in which a person's diet is inadequate to meet minimum daily requirements for nutrients

N

neural tube: in a developing fetus, the neural tube eventually becomes the central nervous system, including the brain and spinal cord

neuropathy: an abnormal and usually degenerative state of the nervous system or nerves

nutraceuticals: substances isolated from food that are considered beneficial beyond meeting basic nutritional needs

nutrient deficiency: inadequate amounts in the diet of nutrients necessary for good health and the prevention of disease

nutrient dense: describes foods that are relatively low in Calories, while high in a variety of nutrients

O

obesogenic: describes environmental factors and influences that encourage or promote obesity

oxidation: the chemical combination of a substance with oxygen; in cells, oxidation causes damage and can lead to cancer, heart disease, and premature aging

P

percentage daily value (% daily value): listed on nutrient fact labels, it provides the percent of an average daily healthy diet that a particular nutrient provides

peristalsis: a wave-like movement in the esophagus created by muscle contraction and relaxation

phytochemicals: chemical compounds in plants that are responsible for colour and odour; they are believed to aid in disease prevention

portion distortion: large serving sizes that are more than one portion of food, but seem normal due to the size and type of packaging, dinnerware, and serving utensils

probiotics: beneficial bacteria

proprietary: owned; similar to a patent

pulses: dried seeds from certain pod-bearing plants, such as lentils, kidney beans, and chickpeas

R

RDA (Recommended Dietary Allowance): the minimum levels of nutrients needed daily by different groups to satisfy health requirements

S

starvation mode: a state in which the body perceives a threat of starvation, and conserves Calories and slows metabolism in order to survive

stress: excessive pressure that causes a physical or emotional response

T

teratogenic: describing a genetic or environmental factor that can cause abnormal fetal development and lead to birth defects

References

Chapter 1

Beck, L. (2011, January 11). Test your nutrition IQ. *The Globe and Mail*. Retrieved on March 16, 2012, from http://www.theglobeandmail.com/life/health/new-health/health-nutrition/leslie-beck/article1866041.ece

Daniel, L. J. (2012). *Vitamin*. Encyclopedia Americana. Retrieved on May 1, 2012, from Grolier Online http://ea.grolier.com/article?id=0405670-00

Health Canada. (2005). *Dietary Reference Intakes Table, Reference Values for Elements*. Retrieved on March 18, 2012, from http://www.hc-sc.gc.ca/fn-an/nutrition/reference/table/ref_elements_tbl-eng.php

Health Canada. (2007). *Reference Values for Macronutrients*. Retrieved from: http://www.hc-sc.gc.ca/fn-an/nutrition/reference/table/ref_macronutr_tbl-eng.php

Health Canada. (2012). *Allergen labelling*. Retrieved from: http://www.healthycanadians.gc.ca/kids-enfants/food-aliment/allergen-allergenes-eng.php

King, H. (2003). *Carbohydrates for a healthy body*. Chicago, IL: Heinemann Library.

Royston, A. (2011). *Why we need proteins*. St. Catharines, ON: Crabtree Publishing Co.

Royston, A. (2011). *Why we need water and fiber*. New York, NY: Crabtree Publishing Co.

Chapter 2

Abdoler, E., Emanuel, E., & Stunkel, L. (n.d.). *Research ethics: How to Treat People who Participate in Research*. Retrieved on May 3, 2012, from http://www.bioethics.nih.gov/education/FNIH_BioethicsBrochure_WEB.PDF

Alaimo, K., Olson, C. M., & Frongillo, E. A. (2001). Food Insufficiency and American School-Aged Children's Cognitive, Academic, and Psychosocial Development. *Pediatrics, 108(1), 44*. Retrieved on April 24, 2012, from EBSCO Database.

Alpert, P. T. (2012). Portion Size: A Disconnect Among Americans? *Home Health Care Management & Practice; 24(1) 59-61*. Retrieved on February 29, 2012, from EBSCO Database.

Downs, A. & Ashton, J. (2011). Vigorous Physical Activity, Sports Participation, and Athletic Identity: Implications for Mental and Physical Health in College Students. *Journal of Sport Behavior 34(3) 228-249*. Retrieved on February 29, 2012, from EBSCO database.

Fröding, K., Elander, I., & Eriksson, C. (2012). Neighbourhood development and public health initiatives: Who participates?. *Health Promotion International, 27(1), 102-116*. Retrieved on May 3, 2012, from Ebsco Database.

Health Canada. (2011). *Canadians' Awareness, Knowledge and Behaviours Related to Dietary Fats (2010): Research Synthesis*. Retrieved on April 24, 2012, from http://www.hc-sc.gc.ca/fn-an/label-etiquet/nutrition/res-rech/fats-lipides-2010-synth-eng.php

Malik, V.S., Schulze, M.B., & Hu, F.B. (2006) Intake of sugar-sweetened beverages and weight gain: A systematic review. *American Journal of Clinical Nutrition, 84*, 274-288.

Nestle, M. (2006). *What to eat*. New York, NY: North Point Press.

Popkin, B.M., Armstrong, L.E., Bray, G.M,. Caballero, B., Frei, B., & Willett, W.C. (2006). A new proposed guidance system for beverage consumption in the United States. *American Journal of Clinical Nutrition, 83*, 529-542.

Seifert, S. M., Schaechter, J. L., Hershorin, E. R., & Lipschultz, S. E. (2011). Health Effects of Energy Drinks on Children, Adolescents, and Young Adults. *Pediatrics, 127(3), 511-528*. doi:10.1542/Deds.2009-3592

Statistics Canada. (2004a). *Percentage of daily calories derived from beverages, by gender and age group, household population aged 1 to 18, Canada excluding territories, 2004*. Retrieved on January 17, 2012 from http://www.statcan.gc.ca/pub/82-003-x/2008004/article/10715/t/6500235-eng.htm

Statistics Canada (2004b). *Percentage of daily calories derived from beverages, by gender and age group, household population aged 19 or older, Canada excluding territories, 2004* Retrieved on January 17, 2012 http://www.statcan.gc.ca/pub/82-003-x/2008004/article/10716/t/6500249-eng.htm

Wansink, B. & Park, S. (2001), At the Movies: How External Cues and Perceived Taste Impact Consumption Volume. *Food Quality and Preference, 12:1 (January)*, 69-74. Retrieved on April 25, 2012, from http://dx.doi.org/10.1016/j.bbr.2011.03.031

Chapter 3

Beck, L. (2012). Healthy ways to gain weight. In *www.lesliebeck.com*. Retrieved from http://www.lesliebeck.com/page.php?id=10&type=sec

CSEP. (2012). Canadian physical activity guidelines and Canadian sedentary behaviour guidelines. Retrieved from http://www.csep.ca/english/view.asp?x=949

Dietitians of Canada. (2010). Guidelines for choosing a weight loss program. Retrieved from http://www.dietitians.ca/getattachment/ed3f9bba-1bb9-47cd-b23c-da256467eb94/FactSheet-Guidelines-for-choosing-Weight-Loss-Program.pdf.aspx

Dietitians of Canada. (2011, November 2). 5 steps to a healthy body weight for teens. Retrieved from http://www.dietitians.ca/Nutrition-Resources-A-Z/Factsheets/Teens/5-Steps-to-a-Healthy-Body-Weight-for-Teens.aspx

Fessler, T. A. (2010, June). Gastric residuals: Understand their significance to optimize care. *Today's Dietitian* 12,5,8. Retrieved from http://www.todaysdietitian.com/newarchives/060210p8.shtml

Health Canada. (2012). *Do Canadian adults meet their nutrient requirements through food intake alone?* Retrieved from http://www.hc-sc.gc.ca/fn-an/surveill/nutrition/commun/art-nutr-adult-eng.php#a1

Leeder, J. (2011). Teaching food literacy, one school lunch at a time. *The Globe and Mail*. October 7, 2011. Retrieved from: www.theglobeandmail.com/news/national/time-to-lead/teaching-food-literacy-one-school-lunch-at-a-time/article556784/

McCabe, R. E. (1999). Exposing the diet myth: Diets make you eat less. Retrieved from http://www.nedic.ca/knowthefacts/documents/Exposingthedietmyth.pdf

Chapter 4

Anderson, S.E. (2005). Interpreting the Continued Decline in the Average Age at Menarche: Results from Two Nationally Representative Surveys of U.S. Girls Studied 10 Years Apart. *Journal of Pediatrics, 147(6)*, 753-760 http://dx.doi.org/10.1016/j.jpeds.2005.07.016. Retrieved on May 4, 2012

Arim. R., Shapka, J.D., Dahinten, V., & Willms, J. D. (2007). Patterns and Correlates of Pubertal Development in *Canadian Youth: Effects of Family Context Canadian Journal of Public Health 98(2)*, 91-96

Attaman, J. A., Toth, T. L., Furtado, J., Campos, H., Hauser, R., & Chavarro, J. E. (2012). Dietary fat and semen quality among men attending a fertility clinic. *Human Reproduction, 27(5)*, 1466-1474. Retrieved on July 11, 2012, from EBSCO Host.

Baylor College of Medicine. (2004). *How do the Daily Values found on food labels compare to the nutritional recommendations for children*. Retrieved on July 5, 2012, from http://www.bcm.edu/cnrc/consumer/archives/percentDV.htm

Benton, D. (2004) Role of parents in the determination of the food preferences of children and the development of obesity. *International Journal of Obesity & Related Metabolic Disorders, 28(7)*, 858-869.

Bischoff-Ferrari, H. A., Dawson-Hughes, B. B., Staehelin, H. B., Orav, J. E., Stuck, A. E., Theiler, R. R., Wong, J.B., Egli, A., Kiel, D.P., & Henschkowski, J. J. (2009). Fall prevention with supplemental and active forms of vitamin D: a meta-analysis of randomised controlled trials. *BMJ: British Medical Journal (Overseas & Retired Doctors Edition)*, 339(7724), 843-846. doi:10.1136/bmj.b3692

Canadian Council on Food and Nutrition (2008). *Tracking Nutrition Trends VII*. Retrieved on April 24, 2012, from http://www.ccfn.ca/in_action/trends.asp

Canadian Dental Association. (2012). *Early Childhood Tooth Decay*. Retrieved on July 4, 2012, from http://www.cda-adc.ca/en/oral_health/cfyt/dental_care_children/tooth_decay.asp

Canadian Society for Exercise Physiology. (2012). *Canadian Physical Activity Guidelines*. Retrieved on April 4, 2012, from http://www.csep.ca/english/view.asp?x=804

Chalmers, B., Levitt, C., Heaman, M., O'Brien, B., Sauve, & R., Kaczorowski, J., for the Maternity Experiences Study Group of the Canadian Perinatal Surveillance System, Public Health Agency of Canada. (2009). Breastfeeding Rates and Hospital Breastfeeding Practices in Canada: A National Survey of Women. *Birth*, 36, 122–132. doi: 10.1111/j.1523-536X.2009.00309.x

Cheng, G., Buyken, A., Shi, L., Karaolis-Danckert, N., Kroke, A., Wudy, S., Degen, G. & Remer, T. (2012). Beyond overweight: nutrition as an important lifestyle factor influencing timing of puberty. *Nutrition Reviews, 70(3)*, 133-152. doi:10.1111/j.1753-4887.2011.00461.x. Retrieved on April 6, 2012, from Ebsco Database

Cheng, G., Gerlach, S., Libuda, L., Kranz, S., Günther, A. B., Karaolis-Danckert, N., ... & Buyken, A. E. (2010). Diet Quality in Childhood Is Prospectively Associated with the Timing of Puberty but Not with Body Composition at Puberty Onset 1,2. *Journal Of Nutrition, 140(1)*, 95-102. doi:10.3945/jn.109.113365

Derbyshire, E. (2012). Strategies to improve iron status in women at risk of developing anaemia. *Nursing Standard, 26(20)*, 51-57.

Exline, J. J., Zell, A. L., Bratslavsky, E., Hamilton, M., & Swenson, A. (2012). People-Pleasing Through Eating: Sociotropy Predicts Greater Eating in Response to Perceived Social Pressure. *Journal Of Social & Clinical Psychology, 31(2)*, 169-193. doi:10.1521/jscp.2012.31.2.169. Retrieved on May 6, 2012

Galloway, A. T., Fiorito, L. M., Francis, L. A., & Birch, L. L. (2006). 'Finish your soup': Counterproductive effects of pressuring children to eat on intake and affect. *Appetite, 46(3)*, 318-323. doi:10.1016/j.appet.2006.01.019 Retrieved on July 6, 2012, from EBSCO Database

Greene-Finestone, L. S., Campbell, M., Gutmanis, I. A., & Evers, S. E. (2005). Dietary intake among young adolescents in Ontario: Associations with vegetarian status and attitude toward health. *Preventive Medicine, 40(1)*, 105-111. doi:10.1016/j.ypmed.2004.05.009. Retrieved on April 17, 2012, from Ebsco Database

Greer, F., Sicherer, S., Burks, W., & the Committee on Nutrition and Section on Allergy and Immunology. (2008). Effects of Early Nutritional Interventions on the Development of Atopic Disease in Infants and Children: The Role of Maternal Dietary Restriction, Breastfeeding, Timing of Introduction of Complementary Foods, and Hydrolyzed Formulas *Pediatrics. 121(1)* 183–191 (doi: 10.1542/peds.2007-3022)

Guadalupe-Grau, A., Fuentes, T., Guerra, B., & Calbet, J. L. (2009). Exercise and Bone Mass in Adults. *Sports Medicine, 39(6)*, 439-468. Retrieved on July 16, 2012, from EBSCO Database

Halford, J. G., Boyland, E. J., Hughes, G., Oliveira, L. P., & Dovey, T. M. (2007). Beyond-brand effect of television (TV) food advertisements/commercials on caloric intake and food choice of 5–7-year-old children. *Appetite, 49(1)*, 263-267. doi:10.1016/j.appet.2006.12.003

Health Canada. (2007). *Nutrition for Healthy Term Infants—Statement of the Joint Working Group: Canadian Paediatric Society, Dietitians of Canada and Health Canada.* Retrieved on April 2, 2012, from http://www.hc-sc.gc.ca/fn-an/pubs/infant-nourrisson/nut_infant_nourrisson_term-eng.php#a3

Health Canada. (2009). *Do Canadian Adolescents Meet Their Nutrient Requirements Through Food Intake Alone?* Retrieved on July 8, 2012, from http://www.hc-sc.gc.ca/fn-an/surveill/nutrition/commun/art-nutr-adol-eng.php

Health Canada. (2010). Safe Food Handling for Pregnant Women. Retrieved on March 31, 2012, from http://www.hc-sc.gc.ca/fn-an/securit/kitchen-cuisine/pregnant-women-femmes-enceintes-eng.php

Jacobs Starkey, L., Johnson-Down, L., & Gray-Donald, K. (2001). Food habits of Canadians: Comparison of intakes in adults and adolescents to Canada's food guide to healthy eating. *Canadian Journal of Dietetic Practice and Research, 62(2)*, 61-9. Retrieved on July 8, 2012, from http://ezproxy.library.ubc.ca/login?url=http://search.proquest.com/docview/220777033?accountid=14656

Kaiser Family Foundation (2004). *The Role of Media in Childhood Obesity.* Retrieved on July 6, 2012, from http://www.kff.org/entmedia/upload/the-role-of-media-in-childhood-obesity.pdf

Kaufman, L., Deenadayalan, S., & Karpati, A. (2009). *Breastfeeding or formula? Women's infant feeding experiences in North and Central Brooklyn.* New York, NY: New York City Department of Health and Mental Hygiene.

Kirk, S. L., Penney, T. L., & McHugh, T. F. (2010). Characterizing the obesogenic environment: The state of the evidence with directions for future research. *Obesity Reviews*, 11(2), 109-117. doi:10.1111/j.1467-789X.2009.00611.x

Kniskern, M. A., & Johnston, C. S. (2011). Protein dietary reference intakes may be inadequate for vegetarians if low amounts of animal protein are consumed. *Nutrition*, 27(6), 727-730. doi:10.1016/j.nut.2010.08.024

Lindemann, B., Ogiwara, Y., & Ninomiya, Y. (2002). The Discovery of Umami. *Chemical Senses, 27(9)*, 843-844. doi: 10.1093/chemse/27.9.843

Lorson, B. A., Melgar-Quinonez, H. R., & Taylor C. A. (2009). Correlates of Fruit and Vegetable Intakes in US Children. *Journal Of The American Dietetic Association, 109(3)*, 474-478. doi:10.1016/j.jada.2008.11.022

Mennella, J., Jagnow, C., & Beauchamp, G. (2001). Prenatal and Postnatal Flavor Learning by Human Infants. *Pediatrics, 107(6)*, e88 doi: 10.1542/peds.107.6.e88

Mumby, H.S., Elks, C.E., Li, S., Sharp, S.J., Khaw, K,T., Luben, R.N., Wareham, N.J., Loos, R.J., et al. (2011). Mendelian Randomisation Study of Childhood BMI and Early Menarche. *Journal of Obesity* doi: 180729. Retrieved on April 17, 2012, from http://www.ncbi.nlm.nih.gov/pmc/articles/PMC3136158/?tool=pmcentrez

Nguyen-Rodriguez, S. T., Unger, J. B., & Spruijt-Metz, D. (2009). Psychological Determinants of Emotional Eating in Adolescence. *Eating Disorders, 17(3)*, 211-224. doi:10.1080/10640260902848543. Retrieved on May 6, 2012

Nichols, J. A., Curtis, E. P., Rayman, M. P., & Taylor, A. (2008). A survey to estimate total nutrient intake at conception—Dietary and supplementary. *Journal Of Nutritional & Environmental Medicine, 17(1)*, 12-43. doi:10.1080/13590840801934355

Nied, R.J , & Franklin, B. (2002). Promoting and Prescribing Exercise for the Elderly. *American Family Physician, 65(3)*,419-427. Retrieved on May 6, 2012, from http://www.aafp.org/afp/2002/0201/p419.html

Olesen, A. W., Jeune, B., & Boldsen, J. L. (2000). A continuous decline in menarcheal age in Denmark. *Annals Of Human Biology, 27(4)*, 377-386. doi:10.1080/03014460050044856

Physicians Committee for Responsible Medicine. (2008). *Nutritional Requirements Throughout the Lifecyle.* Retrieved on July 11, 2012, from http://www.tcolincampbell.org/courses-resources/article/nutritional-requirements-throughout-the-life-cycle/category/general-nutrition/?tx_ttnews%5BbackPid%5D=76&cHash=63267af816af0791e4e83985c4ddb77d

Saad, G. (October 31, 2010). Food Preferences Develop In Utero and During Breastfeeding. *Psychology Today.* Retrieved on July 3, 2012, from http://www.psychologytoday.com/blog/homo-consumericus/201010/food-preferences-develop-in-utero-and-during-breastfeeding

Scully, M., Wakefield, M., Niven, P., Chapman, K., Crawford, D., Pratt, I. S., Baurr, L., Flood, V., & Morley, B. (2012). Association between food marketing exposure and adolescents' food choices and eating behaviors. *Appetite,* 58(1), 1-5. doi:10.1016/j.appet.2011.09.020. Retrieved on July 6, 2012, from EBSCO Database

Statistics Canada. (2010). *Canadian Health Measures Survey.* Retrieved on April 6, 2012, from http://www.statcan.gc.ca/daily-quotidien/100113/dq100113a-eng.htm

Troisi, J. D., & Gabriel, S. (2011). Chicken Soup Really Is Good for the Soul: "Comfort Food" Fulfills the Need to Belong. *Psychological Science,* 22(6), 747-753. doi:10.1177/0956797611407931

University of Copenhagen. (2008, December 16). *Girls Have Superior Sense Of Taste To Boys.* ScienceDaily. Retrieved on July 5, 2012, from http://www.sciencedaily.com/releases/2008/12/081216104035.htm

Wansink, B. & Park, S. (2001), At the Movies: How External Cues and Perceived Taste Impact Consumption Volume, *Food Quality and Preference,* 12:1 (January), 69-74. Retrieved on April 25, 2012, from http://dx.doi.org/10.1016/j.bbr.2011.03.031

Wardle, J., Carnell, S., & Cooke, L. (2005). Parental control over feeding and children's fruit and vegetable intake: How are they related? *Journal Of The American Dietetic Association,* 105(2), 227-232. doi:10.1016/j.jada.2004.11.006

Wells, T. T., & Cruess, D. G. (2006). Effects of partial sleep deprivation on food consumption and food choice. *Psychology & Health,* 21(1), 79-86. doi:10.1080/14768320500102301

WHO. (2012). *Breastfeeding.* Retrieved on July 3, 2012, from http://www.who.int/topics/breastfeeding/en/

Chapter 5

Beiser, M. (2005, March-April). The Health of Immigrants and Refugees in Canada. *Journal of Public Health,* 96, Sup. 2. Retrieved from journal.cpha.ca/index.php/cjph/article/download/1494/1683

Blackwell, T. (2012, October 23). MDs accused of demonizing fatty, sugary snacks after call for graphic junk food warnings. *The National Post.* Retrieved from http://news.nationalpost.com/2012/10/23/mds-accused-of-demonizing-fatty-surgery-foods-after-call-for-graphic-junk-food-warnings/

Canadian Cancer Society. (2011). *Potential years of life lost due to cancer: 2008.* Retrieved form http://www.cancer.ca/Canada-wide/About%20cancer/Cancer%20statistics/Past%20statistics/Potential%20Years%20of%20Life%20Lost%20Due%20to%20Cancer%20-%202008.aspx?sc_lang=en

Canadian Cancer Society. (2012) *Meat intake.* Retrieved from http://info.cancer.ca/cce-ecc/default.aspx?cceid=29&toc=1&Lang=E

Canadian Celiac Association. (2008). *Nutrition complications for Celiac disease.* Retrieved from http://www.celiacguide.org/articles/Nutrition_Complications_CCA.pdf

Canadian Diabetes Association. (2012). *Research progress: Diabetes in special populations.* Retrieved from http://www.diabetes.ca/research/researchprogress/

Canadian Liver Foundation. (2012) *Fatty Liver Disease.* Retrieved from http://www.liver.ca/liver-disease/types/fatty-liver.aspx?gclid=CNHi1tnH_rMCFeJ9OgodlS0AKg

CBC. (2012, October 23). Ontario doctors urge junk food warning labels and taxes. Retrieved from http://www.cbc.ca/news/health/story/2012/10/23/obesity-tax-oma.html

Chapel, H., Haeney, M., Misbah, S., & Snowden, N. (2006, June). *Essentials of Clinical Immunology.* Case 4.8 Nut allergy. Retrieved from http://www.immunologyclinic.com/case.asp?chap=04&case=8

Dietitians of Canada. (2012). *nutritionDay in Canada.* Retrieved from http://www.dietitians.ca/Dietitians-Views/Health-Care-System/nutritionDay-in-Canada.aspx

Haddy, F.J., Vanhoutte, P. M., and Feletou, M. (2005, September 16). Role of potassium in regulating blood flow and blood pressure. *American Physiological Society.* Retrieved from http://ajpregu.physiology.org/content/290/3/R546.full

Health Canada. (2004). *Canadian community health survey, Cycle 2.2, Nutrition (2004) A guide to accessing and interpreting the data.* Retrieved from http://www.hc-sc.gc.ca/fn-an/surveill/nutrition/commun/cchs_guide_escc-eng.php

Health Canada. (2009) Food allergies. Retrieved from http://www.hc-sc.gc.ca/hl-vs/iyh-vsv/food-aliment/allerg-eng.php

Healthhype.com. (2012). Gastroenteritis Diet. Retrieved from http://www.healthhype.com/gastroenteritis-diet.html

Kline. D. A. (2008, September). Stressed out: Health and nutritional implications of modern lifestyles. *Today's Dietitian,* 10, 9, 10.

Koc, M. & Welsh, J. (2001, November). *Food, Foodways and Immigrant Experience.* Paper written for the Multiculturalism Program, Department of Canadian Heritage at the Canadian Ethnic Studies Association Conference, November 2001, Halifax. Retrieved from http://canada.metropolis.net/events/ethnocultural/publications/aliments_e.pdf

References

Kromhout, D. (2001). Diet and cardiovascular diseases. *Journal of Nutrition, Health, and Aging.5(3)*,144-9. Retrieved from http://www.ncbi.nlm.nih.gov/pubmed/11458283

Livestrong Foundation. (2009). *Tips on preparing food for cancer patients.* Retrieved from http://www.livestrong.com/article/23651-tips-preparing-cancer-patients/

Mayi TH, Daoudi M, Derudas B, Gross B, Bories G, Wouters K, Brozek J, Caiazzo R, Raverdi V, Pigeyre M, Allavena P, Mantovani A, Pattou F, Staels B, and Chinetti-Gbaguidi G. (2012, April 17). Human adipose tissue macrophages display activation of cancer-related pathways. *The Journal of Biological Chamistry.* doi: 10.1074/jbc.M111.315200. Retrieved from http://www.ncbi.nlm.nih.gov/pubmed/22511784

National Institutes of Health. (2009). *Dietary Supplement Fact Sheet: Magnesium.* Retrieved from http://ods.od.nih.gov/factsheets/Magnesium-HealthProfessional/

National Kidney Foundation. (2006). *Nutrition and chronic kidney disease.* Retrieved from http://www.kidney.org/atoz/pdf/nutri_chronic.pdf

Public Health Agency of Canada. (2012). What makes people healthy? Retrieved from http://www.phac-aspc.gc.ca/ph-sp/approach-approche/qa-qr6-eng.php

Svoboda, E. (2012, September 3). Lessons For Living: Five surprising principles for living, loving, and playing well with others. *Psychology Today Magazine.* Retrieved from http://www.psychologytoday.com/articles/201208/lessons-living?

Therien, E. (2012, October 31). Graphic warning labels for junk food won't work. *The Toronto Star.* Retrieved from http://www.thestar.com/opinion/editorialopinion/article/1280679--graphic-warning-labels-for-junk-food-won-t-work

Thomas, R, (2006, April 5). *The impacts of neighbourhood food choices and acculturation on immigrant diets. University of British Columbia, School of Community and Regional Planning.* Retrieved from renthomas.ca/wp-content/.../Acculturation%20food%20choices.pdf

Web.M.D. (2012). Eating to Prevent Colorectal Cancer. Retrieved from http://www.webmd.com/colorectal-cancer/guide/eating-prevent-cancer

WHO. (2012). Preventing chronic diseases: A vital investment. Retrieved from http://www.who.int/chp/chronic_disease_report/part1/en/index4.html

Zhao, J., Xue. L. & Gilkinson, T. (2010). *Health Status and Social Capital of Recent Immigrants in Canada: Evidence from the Longitudinal Survey of Immigrants to Canada.* Citizenship and Immigration Canada. This paper was originally published as a chapter in: McDonald, T., E. Ruddick, A. Sweetman, and C. Worswick, eds. 2010. *Canadian Immigration: Economic Evidence for a Dynamic Policy Environment.* Montreal and Kingston: Queen's Policy Studies Series, McGill-Queen's University Press. Retrieved from http://www.cic.gc.ca/english/resources/research/immigrant-survey/index.asp

Chapter 6

Agriculture and Agri-Food Canada. (2005). *Canadian Food Trends to 2020 - A Long Range Consumer Outlook.* Retrieved on July 30, 2012, from http://www4.agr.gc.ca/AAFC-AAC/display-afficher.do?id=1288812085312&lang=eng#chp25

Agriculture and Agri-Food Canada, (2010). *The Canadian Consumer: Behaviour, Attitudes and Perceptions Toward Food Products.* Retrieved on August 14, 2012, from http://www.gov.mb.ca/agriculture/statistics/food/canada_consumer_report_en.pdf

Agriculture and Agri-Food Canada. (2011). *Agri-Food Trade Service: Health and Wellness Trends for Canada and the World.* Retrieved on August 0, 2012, from http://www.ats-sea.agr.gc.ca/inter/4367-eng.htm#f

Arvanitoyannis, I. S., & Van Houwelingen-Koukaliaroglou, M. (2005). Functional Foods: A Survey of Health Claims, Pros and Cons, and Current Legislation. *Critical Reviews In Food Science & Nutrition, 45(5)*, 385-404. Retrieved on March 12, 2012, from EBSCOHost Database

BBC. (2007). *Weblogs rack up a decade of posts.* Retrieved on June 24, 2012, from http://news.bbc.co.uk/2/hi/7147728.stm

Canadian Celiac Association. (2011). *About Celiac Disease.* Retrieved on January 25, 2012, from http://www.celiac.ca/index.php/about-celiac-disease-2/symptoms-treatment-cd/

Canadian Council of Food and Nutrition. (2008). *Tracking Nutrition Trends VII.* Retrieved on April 24, 2012, from http://www.ccfn.ca/in_action/trends.asp

Crowe, T. (2011). Superfoods or Supermyths? *Nutridate, 22(4)*, 2-5. Retrieved on July 20, 2012, from EBSCO Database.

Davis, D.R., Epp, M.D., & Riordan, H.D. (2004). Changes in USDA food composition data for 43 garden crops, 1950 to 1999. *Journal of American College of Nutrition.* 23(6),669-82. Retrieved on July 19, 2012, from http://www.ncbi.nlm.nih.gov/pubmed/15637215.

Day, P.K. (2012). *Faith Popcorn's predictions five years later.* Retrieved on July 25, 2012, from http://www.latimes.com/entertainment/la-et-popcorn-predicts01-2008oct01,0,4915463,full.story

Eng, M. (March 28, 2012). *Social media turn up heat on food industry.* Retrieved on August 21, 2012, from http://articles.chicagotribune.com/2012-03-28/business/ct-met-pink-slime-safety-20120328_1_beef-products-ammonia-treated-beef-social-media

Farmers Markets Canada. (2009). *The National Farmers' Market Impact Study 2009 Report.* Retrieved on August 28, 2012, from http://www.farmersmarketscanada.ca/Documents/FMC%20FINAL%20Brochure%202009-ENG.pdf

Food Marketing Institute. (July 17, 2012). *Prevention Magazine and Food Marketing Institute Reveal 20th Annual "Shopping For Health" Survey Results.* Retrieved on July 20, 2012, from http://www.fmi.org/news-room/latest-news/view/2012/07/17/prevention-magazine-and-food-marketing-institute-reveal-20th-annual-shopping-for-health-survey-results

Food Standards Agency. (April 8, 2008). *GM Labelling.* Retrieved on July 2, 2012, from http://www.food.gov.uk/safereating/gm/gm_labelling

Frith, K. (2007). *Is Local More Nutritious?* Retrieved on July 19, 2012, from http://chge.med.harvard.edu/resource/local-more-nutritious

Garriguet, D. (2004). *Nutrition: Findings from the Canadian Community Health Survey. Overview of Canadians' Eating Habits.* Statistics Canada. Retrieved on August 15, 2012, from http://publications.gc.ca

Health Canada. (2011a). *Food Allergies and Intolerances.* Retrieved on January 25, 2012, from http://www.hc-sc.gc.ca/fn-an/securit/allerg/index-eng.php

Health Canada. (2011b). *Novel Food Decisions.* Retrieved on July 2, 2012, from http://www.hc-sc.gc.ca/fn-an/gmf-agm/appro/index-eng.php/Collection/Statcan/82-620-M/82-620-MIE2006002.pdf

Health Canada. (2012a). *What to Look for on Food Labels—Allergy Awareness.* Retrieved September 5, 2012, from http://www.hc-sc.gc.ca/ahc-asc/media/nr-cp/_2012/2012-130fs-eng.php

Health Canada. (2012b). *Food Additives.* Retrieved on June 16, 2012, from http://www.hc-sc.gc.ca/fn-an/securit/addit/index-eng.php

International Food Information Council. (May 2012). *2012 Food and Health Survey: Consumer Attitudes towards Food Safety, Nutrition and Health.* Retrieved on June 14, 2012, from http://www.foodinsight.org/Content/3840/FINAL%202012%20Food%20and%20Health%20Exec%20Summary.pdf

Ipsos. (June 8, 2000). *Awareness of Genetically Modified Foods Wide But Knowledge Inch Deep.* Retrieved on August 23, 2012, from http://www.ipsos-na.com/news-polls/pressrelease.aspx?id=1040

Katz, D. (7 August 2011). *Is Gluten Free Just a Fad?* Retrieved on January 25, 2012, from http://blog.fooducate.com/2011/08/07/is-gluten-free-just-a-fad/

Krashinsky, S. (June 21, 2012). McDonald's marketing tries a transparent approach. *The Globe and Mail.* Retrieved on August 20, 2012, from http://m.theglobeandmail.com/report-on-business/industry-news/marketing/mcdonalds-marketing-tries-a-transparent-approach/article4357943/?service=mobile

MacKinnon, J.B. & Smith, A. (2007). *The 100 Mile Diet: A Year of Local Eating.* Random House Canada.

Nielsen. (January 26, 2010). *Healthy Eating Trends and Myths.* Retrieved on July 2, 2012, from http://blog.nielsen.com/nielsenwire/consumer/healthy-eating-trends-pt-1-commitment-trumps-the-economic-pinch/

Nielsen Global Survey. (2012). *Healthy Eating Trends Around the World.* Retrieved on January 29, 2012, from http://www.nielsen.com/us/en/insights/reports-downloads/2012/healthy-eating-trends-around-the-world.html?status=successHealthy

Perrin, W.F, Wursig, B. & Thewissen, J.G.M. (2002). *The Tuna-Dolphin Issue.* Updated on Southwest Fisheries Science Center, NOAA Fisheries Service. Retrieved September 5, 2012, from http://swfsc.noaa.gov/textblock.aspx?Division=PRD&ParentMenuId=228&id=1408

Pynn, L. (January 2, 2010). *Lack of BC food labelling laws leaves restaurant diners in peril.* Vancouver Sun. Retrieved on July 26, 2012, from www.vancouversun.com

Rosen, J.D. (2010). A Review of the Nutrition Claims Made by Proponents of Organic Food. *Comprehensive Reviews in Food Science and Food Safety*, 9(3) 270-277. DOI: 10.1111/j.1541-4337.2010.00108.x . Retrieved on July 20, 2012.

Rosenbloom, S. (March 23, 2010). *Calorie Data to Be Posted at Most Chains.* New York Times. Retrieved on January 29, 2012, from http://www.nytimes.com

Singer, N. (May 14, 2011). *Foods With Benefits, or So They Say.* New York Times. Retrieved on July 1, 2012, from http://www.nytimes.com

Sloan, E. (April 2011). Top 10 Food Trends. *Food Technology*, 65(4). Retrieved on January 29, 2012, from http://www.ift.org/food-technology/past-issues/2011/april/features/food-trends.aspx?page=viewall

Urala, N., Schutz, H., & Spinks, J. (2011). Consumer Perceptions of 'Functional Food' in the United States. *Journal Of Food Products Marketing*, 17(4), 407-419. doi:10.1080/10454446.2011.583181. Retrieved on July 1, 2012.

Index

Text Credits

Chapter 1
5 Courtesy of Leslie Beck

Chapter 4
115 Source: Canadian Consumers: Spending on Food and Beverages, 2005, http://www4.agr.gc.ca/AAFC-AAC/display-afficher.do?id=1170942402619&lang=eng, Agriculture and Agri-Food Canada, 2005, reproduced with the permission of the Minister of Public Works and Government Services Canada, 2012.

Chapter 6
163 Annalise Roberts, www.foodphilosopher.com

Photo Credits

Chapter 1
2-3 Digital Vision/Getty Images; **4-5** © Ersler Dmitry/Shutterstock, **5 (insert)** UpperCut Images/Alamy; **6** Richard G. Bingham II/Alamy; **7** Jupiterimages/ThinkStock; **8** Dustin Dennis/Shutterstock; **9** Goodluz/Shutterstock; **11** svry/Shutterstock; **13** Jkwchui/Wikipedia; **14t** Evgeny Karandaev/Shutterstock, **14c** Alexander Kalina/Shutterstock, **14b** Cathy Britcliffe/iStockphoto; **15** © Truembie/Dreamstime.com; **16** Gareth Morgans/Getty Images; **17** Getty Images; **18** iStockphoto/ThinkStock; **19t** © Food-micro/Dreamstime.com, **19b** Pixtal/AGE Fotostock; **21** Thinkstock/Getty Images; **22** Robyn Mackenzie/Shutterstock; **23** bokan/Shutterstock; **24** Digital Vision/ThinkStock; **25** Nancy R. Cohen/Getty Images; **26** © Tamsindove/Dreamstime.com; **27t** Robyn Mackenzie/Shutterstock, **27b** Copyright © Foodcollection; **28** Reproduced with kind permission of Unilever PLC and group companies.; **29** © Gvictoria/Dreamstime.com; **31** Monkey Business Images/Shutterstock

Chapter 2
32-33 oznuroz/Shutterstock, **33 (insert)** Liz Whitaker/Photodisc/Getty Images; **35** © Nikolay Okhitin/Dreamstime.com; **36** Buccina Studios/ThinkStock; **37 (left and right)** Ingram Publishing/SuperStock; **38** Courtesy of Melodie Yong; **39** © Her Majesty the Queen in Right of Canada, represented by the Minister of Health Canada, 2011. This publication may be reproduced without permission. No changes permitted. HC Pub.: 4651 Cat.: H164-38/1-2011E-PDF ISBN: 978-1-100-19255-0; **40** © Her Majesty the Queen in Right of Canada, represented by the Minister of Health Canada, 2007. This publication may be reproduced without permission. No changes permitted. HC Pub.: 3426 Cat.: H34-159/2007E ISBN: 0662-44562-7; **41** Peter Carroll/Alamy; **42** © 2010 Government of Nunavut; **44l** www.choosemyplate.gov, **44r** Nutrition Austrailia; **45t** © 2011 Oldways Preservation & Exchange Trust, www.oldwayspt.org, **45b** VeganFoodPyramid.com; **46** © kate_sept2004/iStockphoto; **48** Shelby Allison/Shutterstock; **50** Paul Binet/Shutterstock; **51 (left to right)** © Monika Adamczyk/Dreamstime.com, Copyright © Foodcollection, © Dynamic Graphics/PunchStock, © Prapann stock photo/Shutterstock, Copyright © Foodcollection; **53** Copyright © Foodcollection; **55** ARLO AND JANIS © 2011 Jimmy Johnson. Reprinted by permission of Universal Uclick for UFS. All rights reserved.; **56** © Elena Moiseeva/Dreamstime.com; **58** Chris Jobs/Alamy; **59** Copyright © Foodcollection; **60** Bernard Weil/GetStock.com; **61** Mary Kate Denny/PhotoEdit Inc.

Chapter 3
64-65 Abel Tumik/Shutterstock.com, **65 (insert)** John A Rizzo/Pixtal/SuperStock; **66** Paul Schlemmer/Shutterstock; **67** desire/Shutterstock; **68** Simone van den Berg/Shutterstock; **70** Courtesy of May Hughes; **73** © Stockbyte/PunchStock; **74 (left to right)** Stockbyte/Thinkstock, Ryan McVay/Thinkstock, iStockphoto/Thinkstock; **76** Monkey Business Images/Shutterstock; **77** Thinkstock Images/Jupiterimages; **78** CLS Design/Shutterstock; **79** Mike Flippo/Shutterstock; **80** Zurijeta/Shutterstock; **81** Grant Cravens; **82** Ryan McVay/Photodisc/Getty Images; **85** © Cato-Symonds, Shaun/Maxx Images; **86** Rubberball/Erik Isakson/Getty Images; **87** AP Photo/Ed Ou/CP Images; **89** Bon Appetit/Alamy; **90** gresei/Shutterstock; **91** Jen Voo Photography/Flickr/Getty Images

Chapter 4

94-95 © Jacqueline Veissid/Blend Images/Corbis; **96-97** Robert Kneschke/Shutterstock, **97 (insert)** © Brand X Pictures/Jupiterimages; **98** © Digital Vision/PunchStock; **99** iStockphoto/ThinkStock; **100** Bubbles Photolibrary/Alamy; **101** Alexander Raths/Shutterstock; **102** Copyright © 2012 breastfeedingsymbol.org; **104** Hemera/ThinkStock; **105** © IT Stock/PunchStock; **106** Rita Maas/FoodPix/Getty Images; **107** Stockbyte/ThinkStock; **108** Michael Newman/PhotoEdit Inc.; **110** AdamEdwards/Shutterstock; **111** Noe Montes/FoodPix/Getty Images; **113** Kuzma/Shutterstock; **114** Purestock/SuperStock; **115** © Jiri Miklo/Dreamstime.com; **116** Images-USA/Alamy; **117** ZUMA Wire Service/Alamy; **118** © Ted Horowitz/Corbis; **119** Dirk Ott/Shutterstock

Chapter 5

122-123 Markus Mainka/Shutterstock, **123 (insert)** l i g h t p o e t/Shutterstock; **124** iStockphoto/ThinkStock; **126** Dahlgren G, Whitehead M (1993). Tackling inequalities in health: what can we learn from what has been tried? Working paper prepared for the King's Fund International Seminar on Tackling Inequalities in Health, September 1993, Ditchley Park, Oxfordshire. London, King's Fund, accessible in: Dahlgren G, Whitehead M. (2007) European strategies for tackling social inequities in health: Levelling up Part 2. Copenhagen: WHO Regional office for Europe: http://www.euro.who.int/__data/assets/pdf_file/0018/103824/E89384.pdf; **128** oliveromg/Shutterstock; **129** Rubberball/Getty Images; **130** ray Laskowitz/Alamy; **131** © Mehmet Dilsiz/Dreamstime.com; **132** iStockphoto/ThinkStock; **133** wong sze yuen/Shutterstock; **134** PhotoLink/Getty Images; **135** Kevin Van Paassen/The Globe and Mail/CP Images; **136** marco mayer/Shutterstock; **138t (cigarette box)** Givaga/Shutterstock, **(french fries)** sashas/Shutterstock; **138** Monkey Business Images/Shutterstock; **140** Kzenon/Shutterstock; **141** iStockphoto/ThinkStock; **142** Kasia Bialasiewicz/Shutterstock; **143** Liv friis-larsen/Shutterstock; **144** Copyright © FoodCollection; **145** Peter Dazeley/Photographer's Choice/Getty Images; **146** © Envision/Corbis; **147** The Image Works

Chapter 6

152-153 Jonathan Feinstein/Shutterstock, **153 (insert)** John Kasawa/Shutterstock; **154** Frances Roberts/Alamy; **156** iStockphoto/ThinkStock; **157** www.CartoonStock.com; **158** © JGI/Tom Grill/Blend Images/Corbis; **159** Jackson Vereen/Cole Group/Getty Images; **160** Gytis Mikulicius/Shutterstock; **161** Alessio Cola/Shutterstock; **162** Copyright © Foodcollection; **163** iStockphoto/ThinkStock; **164** BW Folsom/Shutterstock; **165** barbaradudzinska/Shutterstock; **166** Colin Underhill/Alamy; **167** Hemera/ThinkStock; **168** Ingram Publishing/SuperStock; **169** Foodcollection.com/Alamy; **170** Photo by: JOLAYNE REHM; **171** val lawless/Shutterstock; **172** Shawn Hempel/Shutterstock; **173** Catalin Petolea/Shutterstock; **174** Fotomaton/Alamy; **175** Canada Organic Office

Brief Workbook for Writers

Lennet J. Daigle
and
Allen D. Towery

Georgia Southwestern College

Prentice-Hall, Englewood Cliffs, New Jersey 07632

© 1986 by Prentice-Hall
A Division of Simon & Schuster, Inc.
Englewood Cliffs, New Jersey 07632

All rights reserved. No part of this book may be reproduced, in any form or by any means, without permission in writing from the publisher.

Printed in the United States of America

10 9 8 7 6 5 4 3 2 1

ISBN 0-13-082066-0 01

Prentice-Hall International (UK) Limited, London
Prentice-Hall of Australia Pty. Limited, Sydney
Prentice-Hall of Canada Inc., Toronto
Prentice-Hall Hispanoamericana, S.A., Mexico
Prentice-Hall of India Private Limited, New Delhi
Prentice-Hall of Japan, Inc., Tokyo
Prentice-Hall of Southeast Asia Pte. Ltd., Singapore
Editora Prentice-Hall do Brasil, Ltda., Rio de Janeiro
Whitehall Books Limited,, Wellington, New Zealand